Manual of Canine and Feline Cardiology

Second Edition

MICHAEL S. MILLER, M.S., V.M.D.

Diplomate, American Board of Veterinary Practitioners;
Director, Cardiology Ultrasound Referral Service
Thornton, Pennsylvania

LARRY PATRICK TILLEY, D.V.M.

Diplomate, American College of Veterinary Internal Medicine
(Internal Medicine);
Adjunct Professor, Department of Clinical Studies
Ontario Veterinary College, University of Guelph and
Vice President, Corporate Development, Lifelearn V Inc.
Guelph, Ontario, Canada;
President, Vet Med Fax Consultation Service, Santa Fe, New Mexico;
Consultant, Veterinary Research Associates, Diagnostic Laboratory
Farmingdale, New York

W.B. SAUNDERS COMPANY

A Division of Harcourt Brace & Company

PHILADELPHIA, LONDON, TORONTO, MONTREAL, SYDNEY, TOKYO

W.B. SAUNDERS COMPANY

A Division of Harcourt Brace & Company

The Curtis Center
Independence Square West
Philadelphia, Pennsylvania 19106

Library of Congress Cataloging-in-Publication Data

Manual of canine and feline cardiology   /   [edited by] Michael S. Miller, Larry Patrick Tilley. —2nd. ed.
    p.   cm.
    Rev. ed. of: Manual of small animal cardiology. 1985. Includes bibliographical references and index.
    ISBN 0–7216–5940–3
    1. Dogs—Diseases.   2. Cats—Diseases.   3. Veterinary cardiology.
I. Miller, Michael S. (Michael Steven),   II. Tilley, Lawrence P.   III. Manual of small animal cardiology.
    SF992.C37M36   1995
    636.7'089612—dc20

94-30552

Manual of Canine and Feline Cardiology   ISBN   0–7216–5940–3

Last digit is the print number: 9   8   7   6   5   4   3   2   1

Contributors

DANA G. ALLEN, D.V.M., MSc.

Diplomate, American College of Veterinary Internal Medicine (Internal Medicine); Professor and Head, Small Animal Clinic, Department of Clinical Studies, Ontario Veterinary College, University of Guelph, Guelph, Ontario, Canada

Cor Pulmonale

CLARKE E. ATKINS, D.V.M.

Diplomate, American College of Veterinary Internal Medicine (Internal Medicine); Professor, Department of Companion Animal and Special Species Medicine, North Carolina State University, College of Veterinary Medicine, Raleigh, North Carolina

Acquired Valvular Insufficiency

ANDREW W. BEARDOW, B.V.M.&S., M.R.C.V.S.

Diplomate, American College of Veterinary Internal Medicine (Cardiology); Vice President, Cardiopet, Inc., Floral Park, New York

Cardiopulmonary Arrest and Resuscitation; Emergency Management and Critical Care

JOHN V. CALI, Jr., D.V.M.

Diplomate, American Board of Veterinary Practitioners; Vice President and Staff Consultant, Brookside Veterinary Clinic; Director, Holter Monitoring Services, Bloomfield, New Jersey

Cardiovascular Disorders in Systemic Diseases

CLAY A. CALVERT, D.V.M.

Diplomate, American College of Veterinary Internal Medicine (Internal Medicine); Associate Professor, Department of Small Animal Medicine, University of Georgia, College of Veterinary Medicine, Athens, Georgia

Canine Cardiomyopathy; Heartworm Disease

NISHI DHUPA, B.V.M., M.R.C.V.S.

Diplomate, American College of Veterinary Emergency and Critical Care; Diplomate, American College of Veterinary Internal Medicine (Internal Medicine); Staff Veterinarin, Emergency and Critical Care, Tufts University, School of Veterinary Medicine, Foster Hospital for Small Animals, North Grafton, Massachusetts

Cardiopulmonary Arrest and Resuscitation

PHILIP R. FOX, D.V.M., M.Sc.

Diplomate, American College of Veterinary Internal Medicine (Cardiology); Staff Cardiologist and Chairman, Department of Clinic Services, The Animal Medical Center, New York, New York
Cardiovascular Disorders in Systemic Diseases

REBECCA E. GOMPF, D.V.M., M.S.

Diplomate, American College of Veterinary Internal Medicine (Cardiology); Associate Professor, Department of Urban Practice, University of Tennessee, College of Veterinary Medicine, Knoxville, Tennessee
History Taking and Physical Examination of the Cardiovascular System

JOHN-KARL GOODWIN, D.V.M.

Diplomate, American College of Veterinary Internal Medicine (Cardiology); Assistant Professor, Mississippi State University, College of Veterinary Medicine, Mississippi State, Mississippi
Congenital Heart Disease

DEBORAH J. HADLOCK, V.M.D.

Staff Consultant, Cardiopet, Inc., Floral Park, New York
Electrocardiography

ROSEMARY A. HENIK, D.V.M., M.S.

Diplomate, American College of Veterinary Internal Medicine (Internal Medicine); Clinical Assistant Professor, Department of Medical Sciences, The University of Wisconsin-Madison, School of Veterinary Medicine, Madison, Wisconsin
Echocardiography and Doppler Ultrasound

RICHARD D. KIENLE, D.V.M.

University of California, School of Veterinary Medicine; Veterinary Medicine Teaching Hospital, Davis, California
Feline Cardiomyopathy

MARK D. KITTLESON, D.V.M., Ph.D.

Diplomate, American College of Veterinary Internal Medicine (Cardiology); Professor, Department of Medicine, University of California, School of Veterinary Medicine, Davis, California
Pathophysiology and Treatment of Heart Failure

ANDREW MACKIN, B.Sc., B.V.M.S., M.V.S., D.V.Sc.

Fellow, Australian College of Veterinary Scientists; Waltham Lecturer, Internal Medicine and Clinical Nutrition, Department of Veterinary Clinical Studies, Royal (Dick) School of Veterinary Studies, University of Edinburgh, Edinburgh, Scotland
Cor Pulmonale

MATTHEW W. MILLER, D.V.M., M.S.

Diplomate, American College of Veterinary Internal Medicine (Cardiology); Associate Professor, Department of Small Animal Medicine and Surgery, Texas A&M University, College of Veterinary Medicine; Staff Cardiologist, Texas Veterinary Medical Center, College Station, Texas
Pericardial Disease

MICHAEL S. MILLER, M.S., V.M.D.

Diplomate, American Board of Veterinary Practitioners; Director, Cardiology Ultrasound Referral Service, Thornton, Pennsylvania

Treatment of Cardiac Arrhythmias and Conduction Disturbances

PHILIP A. PADRID, D.V.M.

Assistant Professor, Section of Pulmonary and Critical Care, Department of Medicine, and Committee on Comparative Medicine and Pathology, University of Chicago Division of the Biological Sciences Pritzker School of Medicine; Chief, Clinical Services, Animal Resources Center, Chicago, Illinois

Key Treatment Principles for Cor Pulmonale

PAUL D. PION, D.V.M.

Diplomate, American College of Veterinary Internal Medicine (Cardiology); University of California, School of Veterinary Medicine; Veterinary Medicine Teaching Hospital, Davis, California

Feline Cardiomyopathy

JOHN E. RUSH, D.V.M., M.S.

Diplomate, American College of Veterinary Internal Medicine (Cardiology); American College of Veterinary Emergency and Critical Care; Assistant Professor, Department of Medicine, Tufts University, School of Veterinary Medicine, North Grafton, Massachusetts

Special Diagnostic Techniques for Evaluation of Cardiac Disease

CURTIS G. SCHELLING, V.M.D.

Diplomate, American College of Veterinary Radiology; President, Veterinary Diagnostic Imaging Associates, Wynnewood, Pennsylvania

Radiology of the Heart

FRANCIS W.K. SMITH, Jr., D.V.M.

Diplomate, American College of Veterinary Internal Medicine (Internal Medicine); Clinical Instructor, Department of Medicine, Tufts University, School of Veterinary Medicine, North Grafton, Massachusetts; Chief of Medicine, Cardiopet, Inc., Floral Park, New York

Electrocardiography; Cardiovascular Disorders in Systemic Diseases; Common Cardiovascular Drugs

LARRY PATRICK TILLEY, D.V.M.

Diplomate, American College of Veterinary Internal Medicine (Internal Medicine); Adjunct Professor, Department of Clinical Studies, Ontario Veterinary College, University of Guelph; Vice President, Corporate Development, Lifelearn V Inc., Guelph, Ontario, Canada; President, Vet Med Fax Consultation Service, Santa Fe, New Mexico; Consultant, Veterinary Research Associates, Diagnostic Laboratory, Farmingdale, New York

Treatment of Cardiac Arrhythmias and Conduction Disturbances

Acknowledgments

The completion of this manual provides a welcome opportunity to recognize in writing the many individuals who have helped along the way. The majority of the authors have Board Certification or are uniquely qualified to give an update or review of their respective disciplines.

In addition to thanking veterinarians who have referred cases to us, we would like to express our gratitude to each of the veterinary students, interns, and residents whom we have had the pleasure of teaching. Their curiosity and intellectual stimulation has enabled us to grow and prompted us to undertake the task of writing this manual.

We gratefully acknowledge the assistance of the numerous secretaries involved in this project.

NOTICE

Preface

In the last decade there have been a number of excellent textbook chapters and journal articles describing new findings in the field of canine and feline cardiology. However, for the practicing veterinarian and veterinary student who are new in the field, the amount of information is overwhelming. Many veterinarians and students have stated, in past surveys, the need to keep up with cardiovascular advances in the most time-effective way. The *Manual of Canine and Feline Cardiology* has been written to meet that need for a textbook that can provide useful and practical information on cardiac disease in the dog and cat. We have worked hard to make this book a most reliable source for practicing cardiovascular medicine in the dog and cat today. We have also worked to conserve reading time by using an outline format.

This practical approach to the diagnosis and therapy of cardiac disease will be useful to a wide audience, from the veterinary student to the fully trained cardiologist. The approach is largely clinical and includes the practical as well as the most sophisticated methods for diagnosis and therapy.

Cardiovascular disorders in the dog and cat represent a substantial portion of diseases seen in the average veterinary practice. It is important for veterinary students and practitioners to understand the principles of diagnosis and treatment of the numerous cardiovascular disorders.

The basic examination of a dog or cat with a suspected cardiovascular disorder still consists of obtaining a history and performing a physical examination, routine electrocardiography, and thoracic radiography. More advanced procedures may be indicated in certain situations. For example, in radiography, we can not utilize fluoroscopy, cardiac catherterization, and angiocardiography. In electrocardiography, continuous (Holter) electrocardiographic monitoring and His bundle recordings are now available. Echocardiography is now an important noninvasive diagnostic method in veterinary medicine.

The methods of diagnosis of heart diseases in the dog and cat are described in Section I. The first five chapters follow the sequence that the veterinarian uses in his approach to the patient. Chapter 1 covers the history and physical examination; Chapter 2, the radiologic examination of the heart; Chapter 3, electrocardiography; Chapter 4, echocardiography and Doppler ultrasound; and Chapter 5, special diagnostic techniques for evaluation of cardiac disease, including Holter ECG monitoring, blood pressure measurement, endomyocardial biopsy, computed tomography, and radionuclide imaging.

Section II presents in a step-by-step fashion a description of the various cardiac disorders that occur in the dog and cat, starting in each chapter with general considerations (e.g., definitions, incidence, pathophysiology, etiology), history, physical examination, electrocardiography, thoracic radiography, special diagnostic techniques, differential diagnosis, and finally, the therapeutic approach.

Section III includes chapters describing the treatment of cardiac failure, disturbances of cardiac rhythm, conduction disturbances, and two separate chapters on cardiopulmonary arrest and resuscitation and critical care in cardiology.

Appendix 1—Recommendations for the Diagnosis of Heart Disease and the Treatment of Heart Failure in Small Animals—was created by the recently established International Small Animal Cardiac Health Council, a group comprised of eminent veterinary clinical cardiologists from around the world. This document provides guidelines for diagnosing common cardiac diseases in small animals and for treating the heart failure that occurs secondary to these diseases.

Appendix 2 represents a cardiopulmonary drug formulary that contains extensive cardiopulmonary drug tables with indications, dosages, side effects, contraindications, and drug interactions. An extraordinary array of new cardiovascular drugs had become available, and both students and veterinarians have difficulty deciding which drugs from various drug classes should be prescribed. Dr. Smith's uniquely designed tables provide a practical, rational approach.

Although this manual includes discussions of the majority of cardiac disorders, many of these conditions can only be evaluated and treated satisfactorily by a specialist situated in a veterinary school or private practice. Necessary facilities and skills must be available for the evaluation of many cardiac disorders.

The *Manual of Canine and Feline Cardiology* will help to eliminate the aura of mystery that surrounds the diagnostic and therapeutic principles of veterinary cardiology. The teaching principles that are presented will allow even the novice to make an intelligent assessment of a cardiac case. This manual will be useful to a wide audience, but comprehensive enough to serve as reference for the advanced student and the veterinarian with expertise in cardiology.

MICHAEL S. MILLER, M.S., V.M.D.
LARRY PATRICK TILLEY, D.V.M.

Contents

1

History Taking and Physical Examination of the Cardiovascular System

Rebecca E. Gompf

INTRODUCTION

A patient suspected of having a cardiac problem needs to have a complete history taken and physical examination performed; these procedures will establish the correct diagnosis and permit appropriate therapy. The cardiac examination is an extension of the complete physical examination. It includes the signalment (age, breed, sex of the animal), current and previous complaints, clinical history of the complaint, physical examination, radiography, electrocardiography, laboratory examination, and other special procedures (phonocardiography, angiocardiogram, echocardiogram, Doppler) as indicated. The purposes of performing these examinations are as follows:

1. To determine whether a cardiac problem exists
2. To identify the disease process
3. To determine the severity and prognosis of the disease
4. To determine the best treatment of the disease
5. To determine the expected cost of the therapy

MEDICAL HISTORY

SIGNALMENT

Age

  I. Young animals usually present with a congenital (e.g., patent ductus arteriosus) or infectious cardiac disease (e.g., parvovirus).
  II. Older animals usually present with acquired disease, such as degenerative (e.g., mitral and tricuspid insufficiencies) or neoplastic diseases (e.g., heart base tumor).
  III. Exceptions
    A. Cardiomyopathy can occur in young dogs and cats (i.e., aged 6 months or younger).

    B. Older dogs can have congenital heart defects that were not diagnosed when they were young (e.g., patent ductus arteriosus, atrial septal defect).
IV. Cardiac disease in older animals can be modified or affected by other concurrent disease processes (e.g., collapsing trachea, renal or liver disease).

Breed

    I. Certain congenital heart defects are more common in specific breeds of dogs.
        A. Patent ductus arteriosus (PDA): poodles, collies, Pomeranians, Maltese, Shetland sheepdogs, English springer spaniels, keeshonds, bichons frises
        B. Subaortic stenosis (SAS): Newfoundlands, golden retrievers, rottweilers, boxers, samoyeds, bulldogs, Great Danes, German shepherds
        C. Pulmonic stenosis (PS): English bulldogs, mastiffs, samoyeds, miniature schnauzers, West Highland white terriers, cocker spaniels
        D. Tetralogy of Fallot: keeshonds
  II. Large breeds of dogs (e.g., German shepherds, Great Danes, Doberman pinschers) are more susceptible to the development of dilated cardiomyopathy.
III. Boxers are susceptible to neoplasms and myocarditis.
IV. Siamese cats are more susceptible to the development of cardiomyopathy.

Sex of the Animal

    I. Males are more susceptible to cardiac disease (e.g., male cocker spaniels to fibrosis of the mitral valve, and large-breed males to dilated cardiomyopathy).
  II. Sick sinus syndrome occurs in the female miniature schnauzer.
III. PDAs are more common in the female than the male.

Weight

    I. The animal's weight influences several aspects of treatment.
        A. Dosing cardiac medication
        B. Evaluating the response to diuretic medication
        C. Monitoring cardiac cachexia
  II. A "Pickwickian" syndrome (characterized by severe obesity, somnolence, and hypoventilation) can occur in an animal that is so obese that its ability to breathe is restricted.

Utilization of the Animal

    I. A hunting dog with severe heartworm disease may not be able to hunt again after treatment.
  II. Some animals with congenital heart defects may have normal lifespans and

make good pets. However, they should not be used for breeding purposes, as the defect could be perpetuated.

HISTORY

I. Obtain a complete history
   A. Establishes the presence of a cardiac problem
   B. Helps differentiate between cardiac and respiratory problems
   C. Determines the course of the disease and the response to therapy
   D. Must be carefully done to prevent an owner from giving a misleading history
   E. Includes several key questions
      1. Reason the animal is being presented
      2. Onset and duration of the problem(s)
      3. Progression of the disease
      4. Problems noted by the owner
      5. Any known exposure to infectious diseases, as well as vaccination history
      6. Animal's response to any medications that have been given
      7. Any current medications the animal is receiving
      8. The owner's ability to give the medication
   F. Defines the animal's attitude and behavior
      1. Is the animal listless and depressed or alert and playful?
      2. Does the animal tire easily on exercise?
   G. Covers other relevant information to identify the problem
      1. Appetite (what and how much is being fed)
      2. Water consumption
      3. Urinary habits
      4. Bowel movements
      5. Vomiting or regurgitation
      6. Pruritus, biting, or licking
      7. Seizures or snycopal episodes
      8. Reproductive status
      9. Lameness or paresis
      10. Previous diseases or trauma
      11. Coughing, sneezing, difficult breathing
      12. Environment
   H. Includes more specific, follow-up questions
      1. Character of the cough
      2. When the cough occurs
      3. Stimuli evoking the cough
II. Symptoms most commonly associated with cardiac disease
   A. Coughing
   B. Swelling (edema or ascites)
   C. Tiring on exercise
   D. Fainting or syncopal episodes
   E. Dyspnea, orthopnea, or difficult breathing

  F. Cyanosis
  G. Poor growth or performance
 III. Other symptoms associated with cardiovascular disease
  A. Changes in urinary habits
   1. Polydipsia and polyuria are common in animals on diuretics or having a concurrent disease (e.g., renal disease).
   2. Oliguria occurs with severe left-heart failure.
   3. Hemoglobinuria is found with the postcaval syndrome of heartworm disease.
  B. Vomiting and/or diarrhea
   1. Cardiac drugs such as digitalis, quinidine, and procainamide can be responsible.
   2. Supplemental drugs such as aminophylline can be causative.
   3. Regurgitation occurs with congenital vascular ring anomalies.
   4. Right-heart failure can cause intestinal edema and a protein-losing enteropathy, which results in diarrhea.
   5. Cats with cardiomyopathy can develop a hemorrhagic enteritis secondary to thromboemboli of the gastric or mesenteric arteries.
   6. Concurrent diseases can be causative.
  C. Sneezing
   1. It is a sign of a nasal disease.
   2. It is not a cardiac problem.
 IV. Specific Symptoms
  A. Coughing
   1. The most common complaint
   2. A sudden, forced expiration; a normal defense mechanism to clear debris from the tracheobronchial tree
   3. Can be initiated in the following structures
    a) Pharynx
    b) Trachea
    c) Bronchi
    d) Bronchioli
    e) Pleura
    f) Pericardium
    g) Diaphragm
   4. Causes
    a) Acute coughs: tonsillitis—pharyngitis, tracheobronchitis, acute bronchitis, pleuritis, or pneumonia
    b) Chronic coughs: right- or left-sided heart disease, heartworm disease, asthma
   5. Characteristics that often help determine its cause
    a) Loud, harsh, dry cough of sudden onset followed by a nonproductive gag: common in tracheobronchitis
    b) Cardiac coughs: usually harsher and lower pitched
    c) Chronic nonproductive cough: may indicate a neoplasm or extrinsic pressure on the trachea, such as that due to an enlarged left atrium with bronchial collapse
    d) Honking, high-pitched cough: often found with a collapsing trachea and/or collapsed bronchi

        e) Coughing after drinking: found with cardiac disease, collapsing trachea, chronic tracheitis, tracheobronchitis, laryngeal incompetence, or other causes of dysphagia

        f) Coughing without an inciting factor: may indicate cardiac, pulmonary, or extrapulmonary disease

        g) Coughing after eating: found with pharyngeal dysphagia, megaesophagus, vascular ring anomalies, esophageal diverticula, esophageal foreign bodies, and esophageal tumors

    6. Harmful effects of chronic coughing

        a) Dissemination of infection to new areas of the lung

        b) Ruptured lung abscesses

        c) Localized emphysema

        d) Pneumomediastinum

        e) Pneumothorax

        f) Increased weakness and exhaustion of animal

B. Dyspnea

    1. Difficult, labored, or painful breathing

    2. Can be accompanied in cardiac patients by

        a) Stridor (harsh, high-pitched respiratory sounds)

        b) Rhonchus (dry, course rale)

        c) Wheezing

    3. Characteristics

        a) Paroxysmal: comes and goes

        b) Exertional: occurs after or during activity

        c) Orthopneic: occurs in recumbency

    4. Occurs whenever anything increases the amount of air that must be breathed

        a) Decrease in environmental oxygen (high altitudes)

        b) Strenuous exercise

        c) Cardiac disease, primary and secondary

        d) Pulmonary disease, primary and secondary

        e) Central nervous system disorders

    5. Most common cardiac cause of dyspnea: left-heart failure causing pulmonary edema

    6. Types of dyspnea

        a) Inspiratory dyspnea: prolonged and labored on inspiration; due to upper airway obstruction

        b) Expiratory dyspnea: prolonged and labored on expiration; due to lower respiratory tract obstruction

        c) Mixed dyspnea: due to severe pulmonary edema caused by left-heart failure or to severe pneumonia

        d) Simple dyspnea or polypnea: increased rate of respiration due to fever, fear, pain, or excitement

C. Hemoptysis

    1. Coughing up of blood

    2. Uncommon in animals, as they usually swallow their sputum

    3. A sign of very severe pulmonary disease

    4. Causes

    a) Trauma that causes severe pulmonary contusions
    b) Severe heartworm disease
    c) Neoplasms
    d) Foreign bodies
    e) Lung abscesses
    f) Fungal infections
    g) Lung lobe torsions
    h) Acute and chronic bronchitis
    i) Severe pneumonia
    j) Chronic granulomas
    k) Pulmonary embolism (e.g., in heartworm disease)
    l) Clotting disorders including disseminated intravascular coagulopathy (DIC)
    m) Severe pulmonary edema (e.g., ruptured chordae tendineae)

PHYSICAL EXAMINATION

OBSERVATION

I. Attitude and behavior
  A. Depressed or alert?
  B. Listless or active?
II. Posture
  A. Refusal to lie down may indicate pulmonary edema or pleural effusion.
  B. Standing with elbows abducted and head extended as well as open-mouth breathing with flared nostrils indicates severe respiratory distress.
III. Rate and rhythm of respiration
  A. Tachypnea and panting are usually due to excitement.
  B. Expiratory dyspnea usually indicates lower airway disease, and inspiratory dyspnea usually indicates upper airway disease.
  C. Coughing
IV. Dependent ventral edema
  A. If edema is present in the neck, head, and forelimbs only, it usually indicates an obstruction of the cranial vena cava or a mediastinal mass.
  B. If edema is present in the entire body, pleural effusion with or without ascites is usually present. Other causes of edema (e.g., hypoproteinemia) should be considered.
V. Elevated temperature may be seen with an infectious disease or subacute bacterial endocarditis.

CARDIAC EXAMINATION

Head

I. Check for any asymmetry and swellings.
II. The eyes should be examined for changes that could indicate systemic diseases.
III. The ears have no significant changes associated with the cardiovascular sys-

tem. Cyanosis can sometimes be recognized by evaluating the color of the pinna.

IV. Examine the nose for signs of disease and patency.

V. In the mouth, mucous membrane color and perfusion should be noted.
  A. A perfusion time of greater than 2 seconds suggests decreased cardiac output.
  B. Cyanosis is due to hypoventilation or to poor diffusion across the alveoli produced by
    1. Large airway obstruction (e.g., tracheal collapse)
    2. Small airway obstruction (e.g., bronchitis)
    3. Fluid-filled small airways (e.g., edema)
    4. Right-to-left vascular shunts (e.g., tetralogy of Fallot)
    5. Peripheral extraction of more oxygen from a slow systemic circulation (e.g., severe heart failure)
  C. Hyperemic mucous membranes may indicate an increased packed cell volume, which can be secondary to a chronic right-to-left vascular shunt.
  D. Pale mucous membranes indicate anemia or poor perfusion.
  E. The mucous membranes of the mouth should be compared with the posterior membranes (e.g., vagina, prepuce), as differential cyanosis can occur in a right-to-left shunting PDA.
  F. Check the oral cavity for severe dental tartar, gingivitis, or pyorrhea, which can serve as sources of sepsis, leading to bacteremia and possibly endocarditis.

Neck

I. The jugular pulse should be evaluated while the animal is standing, with its head in a normal position. Any pulse going over one-third of the way up to the neck is abnormal and can be due to any of several factors.
  A. Right-heart failure with tricuspid insufficiency
  B. Heart block or premature beat
  C. Pulmonic stenosis
  D. Pulmonary hypertension
  E. Heartworm disease
  F. Right heart failure with cardiomyopathy

II. The entire jugular vein can be distended due to congestive heart failure, pericardial disease, or obstruction of cranial vena cava (e.g., heart base tumor).

III. Arterial pulses can mimic a jugular pulse; however, when light pressure is applied to the area of the jugular pulse, the arterial pulse will continue, while the jugular pulse will stop.

PALPATION

Trachea

I. The trachea should be palpated for abnormalities such as collapsing, masses, or increased sensitivity.

II. This step is best postponed until after auscultation of the thorax, as a cough may be elicited that makes auscultation difficult.

Thorax

  I. The point of maximum intensity (PMI) should be on the left side between the fourth to sixth intercostal spaces. Shifting of the PMI is due to
  A. Cardiac enlargement
  B. Masses displacing the heart
  C. Collapsed lung lobes allowing the heart to shift
  D. Lying down in right lateral recumbency such that the heart falls to the right
  II. A decreased intensity of heartbeat may be due to
  A. Obesity
  B. Pleural effusion
  C. Pericardial effusion
  D. Thoracic masses
  E. Pneumothorax
 III. Loud cardiac murmurs can be palpated as "thrills," which are due to vibrations caused by blood flow.

Abdomen

  I. Check for ascites.
 II. Check for signs of hepatomegaly and splenomegaly due to right-sided heart failure.
III. Palpate for other concurrent related or unrelated masses.

Skin

Palpate for evidence of edema due to right-heart failure or venous obstruction.

Femoral Pulses

  I. Both pulses should be compared, as one could be obstructed.
 II. It is difficult to palpate the femoral pulse in a normal cat; therefore, the absence of palpable femoral pulses in a cat should not be interpreted as definite arterial obstruction.
III. The rate should be taken.
  A. Normal rates in dogs are 70 to 180 beats/min (bpm), with smaller dogs having faster rates. Puppies can have a normal rate of 220 bpm.
  B. Normal rate in cats is 160 to 240 bpm.
IV. The rhythm of the pulses should be noted.
  A. There should be a pulse for every heartbeat.
  B. Pulse deficits usually indicate incomplete ventricular filling, as seen in arrhythmias.
  V. The intensity of the pulse should be palpated.
  A. Normal pulses are strong and have a rapid rate of rise and fall.
  B. Hypokinetic (weak) pulses are due to decreased cardiac output or slower rate of rise due to delayed emptying of the left ventricle.

   C. Hyperkinetic (strong) pulses rise and fall quickly and are due to large left-ventricular stroke volumes with rapid diastolic runoffs (e.g., PDA and aortic insufficiency). They are called "B-B shot" or "water-hammer" pulses. Fear and fevers can also produce this type of pulse.
   D. Pulsus alternans occurs when the pulse is alternately weak and then strong. It is frequently associated with myocardial failure.
   E. Pulsus paradoxus is an alteration of the pulse strength during respiration due to changes in ventricular filling. This is sometimes a sign of cardiac tamponade.

PERCUSSION

   I. Determines the presence of masses or fluid lines, especially in the thorax
  II. Elicits a hollow sound over the lungs
 III. Elicits a dull sound over solid structures

AUSCULTATION

   I. The Stethoscope
   A. The main components of the stethoscope are the bell, diaphragm, tubing, and ear pieces. The bell transmits both low-frequency (20 to 10 cps) and high-frequency (100 to 1000 cps) sounds.
   B. The diaphragm attenuates low frequencies (200 to 100 cps) and selectively transmits the high frequencies.
   C. Most stethoscopes combine the bell and diaphragm into a dual-sided, combination-style chest piece.
   D. A new stethoscope (Littman "Master") design by 3M Health Care, St. Paul, MN, combines the bell and diaphragm into a single-sided chest piece.
   E. With the Master Classic, simple fingertip pressure allows one to switch from low-frequency to high-frequency sounds. There is no interruption in sound as there is in a traditional two-sided stethoscope, resulting in added convenience and efficiency in auscultation.
   F. A practical tubing length is approximately 14 to 18 inches.
   G. Ear tubes should angle forward to conform to the anatomy of the ear canal.
   H. For dog and cats under 15 lbs., a pediatric stethoscope (3M Health Care) that has a smaller head-piece should only be used.
  II. This is the most helpful part of the cardiac examination; it should be done carefully and systematically. The animal should be standing, so that the heart is in its normal position.
   A. Common artifacts heard
      1. Respiratory clicks and murmurs
      2. Rumbles due to shivering and twitching
      3. Movement sounds
      4. Crackling sounds due to the rubbing of hair
      5. Extraneous sounds if auscultation is not performed in a quiet area
   B. Auscultate the heart and lungs separately.

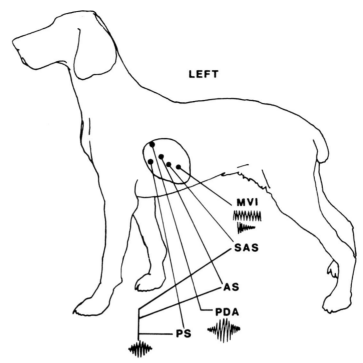

Fig. 1-1. Phonocardiographic configurations of various cardiac murmurs as recorded at the usual points of maximal murmur intensity. View of left hemithorax of the dog. MVI, mitral valve insufficiency; SAS, subaortic stenosis; AS, valvular aortic stenosis; PDA, patent ductus arteriosus; PS, pulmonic stenosis. (From Bonagura JD, Berkwitt L: Cardiovascular and pulmonary disorders. p. 119. In: Quick Reference to Veterinary Medicine. JB Lippincott, Philadelphia, 1982, with permission.)

III. The areas of auscultation (Figs. 1-1 and 1-2) are as follows
    A. Pulmonic area—left side
        1. In the dog, it is between the second and fourth intercostal spaces just above the sternum.
        2. In the cat, it is located at the second to third intercostal space one-third to one-half of the way up the thorax from the sternum.
    B. Aortic area—left side
        1. In the dog, it is at the fourth intercostal space just above the costrochondral junction.
        2. In the cat, it is at the second to third intercostal space just dorsal to the pulmonic area.
    C. Mitral area—left side
        1. In the dog, it is at the fifth intercostal space at the costochondral junction.
        2. In the cat, it is at the fifth to sixth intercostal space one-fourth of the way up the thorax from the sternum.
    D. Tricuspid area—right side
        1. In the dog, it is at the third to fifth intercostal space near the costochondral junction.

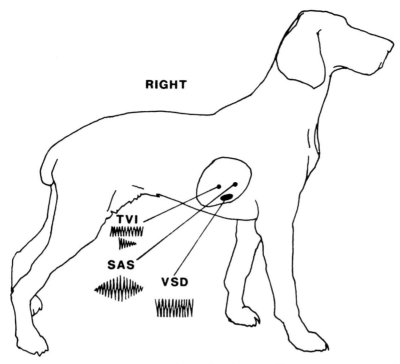

Fig. 1-2. Phonocardiographic configurations of various cardiac murmurs as recorded at the usual points of maximal intensity. View of the right hemithorax of the dog. TVI, tricuspid valve insufficiency; VSD, ventricular septal defect; SAS, subaortic stenosis. (From Bonagura JD, Berkwitt L: Cardiovascular and pulmonary disorders. p. 119. In: Quick Reference to Veterinary Medicine. JB Lippincott, Philadelphia, 1982, with permission.)

2. In the cat, it is at the fourth or fifth intercostal space, at a level opposite the mitral area.
IV. The area in which murmurs are loudest and in which they radiate should be noted. This can help identify the heart problem.
V. Heart rate and rhythm should be identified.
   A. The effects of inspiration and expiration on heart rate, rhythm, and heart sounds should be noted.
   B. The presence or absence of heart sounds should be noted.

NORMAL HEART SOUNDS

I. Heart sounds are due to the abrupt acceleration or deceleration of blood and the vibrations of the heart and vessels.
II. The first heart sound (S_1) (Fig. 1-3) is due to passive closure of the mitral and tricuspid valves.
   A. S_1 is longer, louder, duller, and lower pitched than the second heart sound.
   B. It is loudest over the mitral area.
   C. Its intensity increases due to fever, fear, or tachycardia.

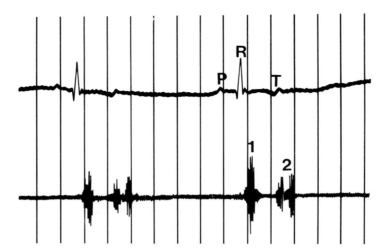

Fig. 1-3. Lead II electrocardiogram recorded simultaneously with medium-frequency band phonocardiogram from a dog. The second heart sound (S_2) is split. First heart sound (S_1). Paper speed, 100 mm/sec. (From Gompf RE: Physical examination of the cardiopulmonary system. Vet Clin North Am 131:201, 1983, with permission.)

  D. Its intensity decreases due to obesity, pleural or pericardial effusion, thoracic masses, diaphragmatic hernias, bradycardias, and insufficient filling of the ventricles.

  E. It varies in intensity with arrhythmias.

  F. It has four parts that can be seen on a phonocardiogram.

  G. It can be split in large breeds of dogs, right bundle branch block, or ventricular premature beats.

III. The second heart sound (S_2) is produced by passive closure of the aortic and pulmonic valves.

  A. It is short, high pitched, and sharp.

  B. It is loudest over the aortic area.

  C. A split S_2 (Fig. 1-3) is due to closure of the pulmonic valve after the aortic valve. This occurs in

   1. Pulmonary hypertension (e.g., heartworm disease)

   2. Right bundle branch block

   3. Ventricular premature beats originating in the left ventricle

   4. Atrial septal defect

   5. Pulmonic stenosis

  D. Paradoxical splitting is due to delayed closure of the aortic valve. This results from

   1. Left bundle branch block

   2. Premature beats originating from the right ventricle

   3. Subaortic stenosis

   4. Severe systemic hypertension

   5. Left ventricular failure

  E. S_2 may be absent in arrhythmias where there is incomplete filling of the ventricles and insufficient pressure to open the semilunar valves.

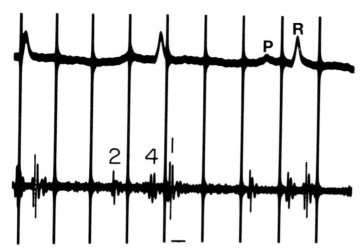

Fig. 1-4. Lead II electrocardiogram recorded simultaneously with a low-frequency band phonocardiogram from a cat with hypertrophic cardiomyopathy. A gallop rhythm or fourth heart sound (S_4) is present. First heart sound (S_1); second heart sound (S_2). Paper speed, 100 mm/sec. (From Gompf RE: Physical examination of the cardiopulmonary system. Vet Clin North Am 131:201, 1983, with permission.)

Abnormal Heart Sounds

I. The third heart sound (S_3) is due to rapid ventricular filling.
    A. It is lower pitched than the second heart sound.
    B. It is heard best in the mitral area.
    C. In dogs and cats, its presence indicates dilated ventricles, which most commonly occur with dilated cardiomyopathy, or decompensated mitral or tricuspid insufficiency.

II. The fourth heart sound (S_4) is due to atrial contraction.
    A. It is heard best over the aortic or pulmonic areas but sometimes can be heard over the mitral area as well.
    B. It is present in dogs or cats when the atria dilate in response to ventricular diastolic dysfunction, such as hypertrophic cardiomyopathy.

III. A gallop rhythm is an S_3, S_4, (Fig. 1-4) or combination of the two.
    A. Gallops are of a low frequency and can be difficult to hear.
    B. A gallop can be a very early sign of heart failure, preceding clinical signs.

IV. Systolic clicks are clicking noises that occur in systole between S_1 and S_2.
    A. It may come and go and may change its position in systole (gets closer to or further away from S_2).
    B. The precise cause of the click is unknown, but many animals develop a mitral insufficiency murmur later in life.
    C. This is a benign finding and not usually associated with heart failure.

Arrhythmias Heard on Auscultation

I. Arrhythmias that increase the heart rate

   A. Atrial fibrillation
      1. A rapid, irregular rhythm with heart sounds that vary in intensity.
      2. Pulse deficits are present.
      3. It has been described as being irregularly irregular and rarely is mistaken for other tachycardias.
   B. Ventricular tachycardias are usually intermittent and tend to be more regular than atrial fibrillation. Pulse deficits are frequently present.
   C. Sinus and atrial tachycardias are rapid and regular. All the heart sounds are of a uniform intensity, but an atrial tachycardia tends to be intermittent.
   D. An electrocardiogram is necessary to distinguish among sinus, atrial, and ventricular tachycardia.
 II. Arrhythmias that decrease the heart rate
   A. Sinus arrhythmia has a cyclic pattern.
      1. The heart rate will increase during inspiration and decrease during expiration due to changes in vagal tone.
      2. The intensity of the pulse and heart sounds may vary.
      3. It is normal in dogs, but in cats is usually associated with heart disease.
   B. Sinus bradycardia has a very slow rhythm.
      1. The heart sounds may vary.
      2. The heart rate in dogs is 50 to 100 beats/min, depending on size.
      3. The heart rate in cats is less than 120 bpm.
   C. Second- and third-degree heart blocks have slow heart rates.
      1. The heart sounds will vary in intensity.
      2. A fourth heart sound may be present in third-degree block.
      3. The pulses will be slow and hyperkinetic, but there are no pulse deficits.
      4. A jugular pulse is usually present.
      5. Extra sounds may be generated by escape beats.
III. Atrial and ventricular premature beats: generation of extra sounds that mimic S_3 and S_4
   A. It is hard to differentiate between the two types of premature beats as well as S_3 and S_4 on physical examination. An electrocardiogram (ECG) and phonocardiogram may be necessary.
   B. Both premature beats interrupt the normal rhythm and are usually followed by a pause.
   C. Usually only an S_1 is heard with a premature beat, although sometimes S_1-S_2 is heard very close together. S_2 is usually absent.
   D. Ventricular premature beats can also cause a split S_1 or S_2.
 IV. Unexpected pauses
   A. Sinoatrial (SA) arrest occurs when an impulse does not leave the SA node. The pause continues until the next normal beat or an escape beat occurs.
   B. The heart sound following a pause may be louder than usual as the ventricles have had longer to fill and eject a larger amount of blood.

MURMURS

Murmurs are due to turbulent blood flow through the heart and vessels.

 I. Classification

    A. Functional murmurs are divided into two types.
       1. Physiologic murmurs have a known cause such as anemia, hypoproteinemia, hyperkinetic circulation (e.g., fever), and an athletic heart.
       2. Innocent murmurs have no known cause and are not associated with any cardiac problem.
    B. Pathologic murmurs are caused by underlying heart or vessel disease.
       1. Stenosis of valves, outflow tract, or great vessels
       2. Valvular insufficiency
       3. Abnormal intra- or extracardiac shunts
II. Description
    A. Site at which the murmur is loudest (e.g., valve area)
    B. Timing in the cardiac style (e.g., systole or diastole)
    C. Duration of the murmur (e.g., early systolic, holosystolic, pansystolic, continuous)
    D. Intensity of the murmur
       1. Grade 1/6 can only be heard after listening for several minutes and sounds like a prolonged first heart sound.
       2. Grade 2/6 is very soft and can be heard immediately.
       3. Grade 3/6 is low to moderate in intensity.
       4. Grade 4/6 is very loud but a "thrill" cannot be palpated on the thorax.
       5. Grade 5/6 is very loud and a "thrill" can be palpated on the thorax.
       6. Grade 6/6 can be heard without the use of a stethoscope or with the stethoscope slightly off the thoracic wall.
    E. Quality of the murmur: subjective, but can be evaluated according to graphic appearance on phonocardiogram (Figs. 1-1 and 1-2)
       1. Regurgitant murmurs: plateau shaped
       2. Ejection murmurs: decrescendo, crescendo, or diamond shaped
       3. Machinery murmur: diamond shaped and peaking at S_2, continuing through all of systole and most of diastole
       4. Blowing murmur: decrescendo murmur
    F. Radiation of the murmur
       1. Can help identify the problem
       2. Many cardiac problems have murmurs that are loud over one valve area and that radiate to another

OTHER SOUNDS AUSCULTATED IN THE THORAX

  I. Normal respiratory sounds
    A. Referred sounds from the trachea are commonly heard over the lungs and bronchi.
    B. Vesicular sounds are due to air moving through the small bronchi and are louder on inspiration.
    C. Bronchial sounds are due to air moving through the large bronchi and trachea and are heard best on expiration.
    D. Bronchovesicular sounds are the combination of the above two and are heard best over the hilar area.
  II. Abnormal respiratory sounds

    A. Attenuated bronchovesicular sounds are due to
        1. Thoracic masses
        2. Pleural effusion
        3. Pneumothorax
        4. Obesity
        5. Pneumonia
        6. Shallow breathing
        7. Early consolidation of the pulmonary parenchyma
    B. Rhonchi are due to air passing through partially obstructed airways in the bronchial tubes or smallest airways.
        1. Rhonchi from the large bronchi are low pitched, sonorous, and almost continuous. They are heard best on inspiration.
        2. Rhonchi from the small bronchi are high pitched, sibilant, or squeaky and are heard best on expiration.
    C. Rales are interrupted, crepitant, inspiratory sounds heard in many disease conditions and are not pathognomonic for pulmonary edema.
        1. Opening of alveoli or airways that are collapsed or partially filled with fluid
        2. Bubbles bursting in the airways
III. Other sounds auscultated
    A. Pleural friction rubs: grading, rubbing sounds heard during inspiration and expiration due to the moving of two relatively dry, roughened pleural surfaces against each other
    B. Pericardial friction rubs: short, scratchy noises produced by pericarditis and heart movement
    C. Pericardial knocks: diastolic sounds that occur in animals with constrictive pericarditis

SUGGESTED READINGS

Bonagura JD, Berkwitt L: Cardiovascular and pulmonary disorders. p. 119. In: Quick Reference to Veterinary Medicine. JB Lippincott, Philadelphia, 1982

Buchanan JW: Causes and prevalence of cardiovascular disease. p. 647. In Kirk RW (ed): Current Veterinary Therapy XI. WB Saunders, Philadelphia, 1992

Ettinger SJ, Suter PF: Canine Cardiology. WB Saunders, Philadelphia, 1970

Gompf RE: Physical examination of the cardiopulmonary system. Vet Clin North Am Small Anim Pract 13:201, 1983

Gompf RE: Heart murmur. p. 151. In Ford RB (ed): Clinical Signs and Diagnosis in Small Animal Practice. Churchill Livingstone, New York, 1988

Harpster NK: Clinical examination of the feline cardiovascular system. Vet Clin North Am Small Anim Pract 7:241, 1977

Roudebush P: Lung sounds. J Am Vet Med Assoc 181:122, 1982

Tilley LP: Essentials of Canine and Feline Electrocardiography, Interpretation and Treatment. 3rd Ed. Lea & Febiger, Philadelphia, 1992

2

Radiology of the Heart
Curtis G. Schelling

INTRODUCTION

Thoracic radiography is a key component of the cardiovascular evaluation. Careful attention to proper positioning is of primary importance to the use of radiographic guidelines for interpretation. Radiographic interpretation relies heavily on possible disease considerations (i.e., differential diagnosis) derived from signalment, physical examination, and clinical pathology. Radiographic findings are not consistently specific enough to lead to the derivation of a definitive diagnosis without supportive clinical evidence. The radiographic study isolated from clinical information will not provide a diagnosis. The clinician must be aware of certain parameters and guidelines for interpretation in order to derive information from the radiographic image.

RADIOGRAPHIC TECHNIQUE

EXPOSURE TECHNIQUE AND FILM QUALITY

Exposure technique will vary depending on equipment and film-screen combinations. The current standard for veterinary radiographic equipment is a 300 mA/125-175 kVp machine. The current standard for economic film-screen combination imaging systems is the rare earth systems. Because of the motion created by respiration, relatively high speed (400) film-screen combinations that allow shorter exposure times are best suited for thoracic radiography. Use of a grid is imperative for adequate image quality when chest thickness exceeds 10 cms. Table 2-1 is a representative thoracic technique chart using a 400 speed imaging system and 300 mA/125 kVp X-ray equipment.

RADIOGRAPHIC PROJECTIONS

Lateral Projection

There are subtle differences in cardiac conformation and position when comparing the right versus the left lateral radiographic projection. These differences are not significant enough to warrant further discussion except to note that the same

TABLE 2-1. SMALL ANIMAL THORACIC RADIOGRAPHIC TECHNIQUE CHART USING A 400 SPEED FILM-SCREEN SYSTEM AND STANDARD RADIOGRAPHIC EQUIPMENT[a]

	mA	TIME	mAs	Thickness (cm)												
				kVp												
				Table Top												
				3	4	5	6	7	8	9	10 cm					
Thorax	100	1/60	1.7	48	50	52	54	56	58	60	62					
				In the Table (using Grid)												
				4	5	6	7	8	9	10	11	12	13	14	15	16 cm
Thorax	200	1/60	3.3	52	54	56	58	60	62	64	66	68	70	72	74	76
				17	18	19	20	21	22	23	24	25	26	27	28 cm	
	300	1/60	5	76	78	80	82	84	86	88	90	92	95	98	101	

Technique rules of thumb: Change exposure: (1) ± 10% kVp. (2) ± 2/3 rds of mAs
[a] Single-phase fully rectified 300 mA, 125 kVp generator focal-film distance = 38"

projection should be used on all serial radiographic examinations when repeated evaluation is required.

Patient positioning and adequate radiographic exposure are critical to an accurate radiographic interpretation in the lateral projection. A normal heart can appear diseased and vice versa when positioning is not adequate. Guidelines for proper exposure and positioning include (Fig. 2-1)

I. Radiographic exposure should be adequate to define the dorsal spinous process of the cranial thoracic vertebrae superimposed on the scapula.
II. To ensure a lateral projection, the dorsal heads of the ribs should be superimposed.
III. The forelimbs should be pulled forward so they are not superimposed over the cranial thorax or cranial margin of the heart.
IV. The radiographic exposure is taken during full inspiration, identified as an adequate lung field spacing between the caudal margin of the heart and cupula of the diagram. Two primary disease considerations for consistent expiratory phase radiographs are
    A. Obesity and Pickwickian Syndrome where the overabundance of abdominal fat prevents adequate inspiratory distraction of the diaphragm
    B. Upper airway disease, which most commonly causes obstruction during the inspiratory phase of respiration

Dorsoventral/Ventrodorsal Projection

The dorsoventral (DV) radiographic projection is preferred over the ventrodorsal (VD) for cardiac evaluation for two reasons: (1) The anatomic positioning of the heart in the DV projection is less dependent on thoracic cavity conformation (deep-chested v. barrel-chested breeds). (2) The dorsal lung fields are hyperinflated and the vessels to the caudal lung fields are magnified due to increased object-film distance. This produces an improved radiographic definition of the large pulmonary arteries and veins of the caudal lung fields. The DV projection also allows increased detection of early pulmonary infiltrates (most commonly with cardiac

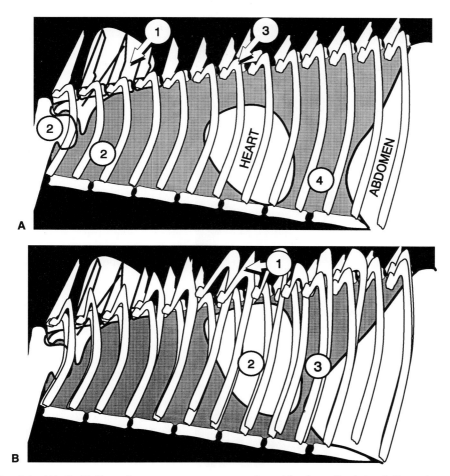

Fig. 2-1. (A) Guidelines for proper exposure and positioning of a lateral thoracic radiographic projection. *(1)* Exposure should allow delineation of the thoracic vertebral dorsal spinous process superimposed over the scapula. *(2)* The forelimbs should be pulled forward to provide an unsuperimposed view of the cranial thorax. *(3)* The dorsal rib heads should be superimposed (compare to Fig. B). *(4)* The exposure should be performed during inspiration, which provides maximum separation between caudal cardiac margin and diaphragmatic cupula. **(B)** Improperly positioned lateral thoracic radiographic projection (compare to Fig. A): *(1)* Non-superimposed left and right rib heads. *(2)* The oblique projection markedly distorts cardiac silhouette conformation and intrathoracic position. *(3)* Expiratory phase radiographic exposure with poor lung volume between caudal cardiac margin and cupula of the diaphragm.

disease in the hilar and caudodorsal lung fields). However, an improperly positioned DV/VD projection is worthless for cardiac radiographic interpretation. Although the DV projection is preferred, a straight (symmetrical) projection is the ultimate goal, with patient compliance determining which projection (DV v. VD) is attainable. Guidelines for proper exposure and positioning for the DV/VD projections include (Fig. 2-2):

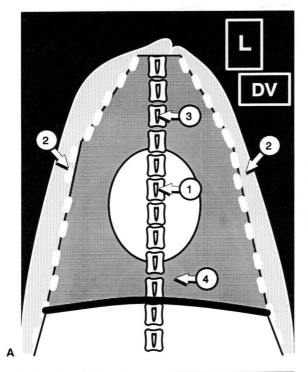

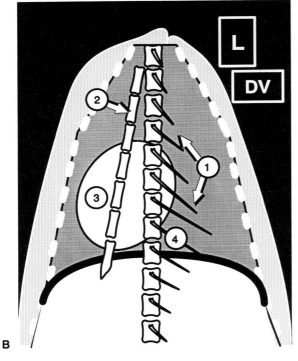

Fig. 2-2. (A) Guidelines for proper exposure and positioning of a dorso-ventral/ventrodorsal thoracic radiographic projection. *(1)* The radiographic exposure should provide outline definition of thoracic vertebra superimposed over the cardiac silhouette. *(2)* Exposure should be increased (usually a 10% kVp increase with obesity as suggested by an increase in thoracic body wall thickness). *(3)* The thoracic vertebral dorsal spinous processes should be superimposed over the body portions for the entire length of the thoracic spine. *(4)* Adequate lung volume between caudal cardiac margin and cupula indicates an inspiratory phase radiographic exposure. **(B)** Improperly positioned dorsoventral radiographic projection. Thoracic vertebral dorsal spinous processes projected over the left hemithorax *(1)* and the sternal vertebra projected over right hemithorax *(2)*, indicating an oblique thoracic dorsoventral radiographic projection. A lack of lung volume between caudal cardiac margin *(3)* and cupula *(4)* indicates an expiratory phase radiographic exposure.

   I. Radiographic exposure should be sufficient to define the outline of the thoracic vertebrae superimposed over the cardiac silhouette.

  II. The kVp should be increased 10% from technique-chart values for obese patients. Examination of the thoracic body-wall thickness on the VD view should assist in evaluation of obesity.

 III. The dorsal spinous processes of the thoracic vertebrae should be centered over the vertebral bodies along the full length of the thoracic spine. The thoracic sternebrae also should be superimposed over the thoracic spine and be essentially indistinguishable radiographically.

 IV. The radiograph is taken during full inspiration, identified as an adequate lung field spacing between caudal cardiac margin and cupula of the diaphragm.

PROJECTION SELECTION IN CARDIAC-RELATED PATHOLOGY

PULMONARY EDEMA

The dorsoventral is preferred over the ventrodorsal projection for radiographic detection of pulmonary edema. The dorsoventral view accentuates pathology in the dorsal lung field, which is the most common location for the formation of early cardiogenic pulmonary edema. Adequate exposure is critical to ensure definition of caudal pulmonary vasculature superimposed over the cupula of the diaphragm.

The radiographic detection of caudodorsal pulmonary vasculature is the best objective parameter for the detection of pulmonary edema. Vessels in the normal lung are detected by their soft tissue opacity contrasting with the normal radiolucent gas-filled lung parenchyma surrounding them. As pulmonary parenchyma (interstitial spaces as well as alveoli) become filled with edema fluid, the normal radiographic soft tissue-gas contrast is lost and delineation of the vessels diminishes. In other words, the vessels start to "disappear" from radiographic detection with the increased opacity of the surrounding edematous lung parenchyma (Fig. 2-3).

Phase of inspiration is critical when using this method for interpretation both in the DV/VD and lateral projections. Pulmonary pathology can be mimicked when underinflation decreases the parenchymal gas content per unit volume, thus decreasing the radiographic contrast between lung parenchyma and associated vasculature. This is especially true in older patients, which already have slightly increased pulmonary parenchymal radiographic opacity due to age-related pulmonary degenerative changes (interstitial fibrosis, bronchial mineralization, heterotopic pulmonary bone formation).

PLEURAL EFFUSION

Pleural effusion is radiographically evident as focal areas of increased soft tissue opacity located within the thoracic cavity. It causes separation of lung lobes from both the thoracic wall and adjacent lobes. This is seen on the lateral projection as an increase in the soft tissue thickness of the caudodorsal thoracophrenic angle

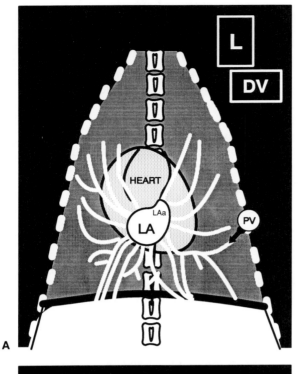

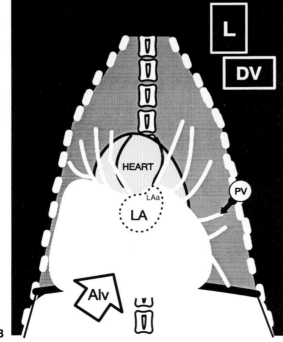

Fig. 2-3. (A) Normal radiographic definition and contrast of pulmonary venous vasculature (PV) with surrounding normal radiolucent lung parenchyma. LA, left atrium; LAa, left atrial auricular appendage. **(B)** Radiographic obliteration of pulmonary venous vasculature (PV) by alveolar consolidation (Alv) of hilar and caudal lung lobes, a characteristic distribution for cardiogenic pulmonary edema.

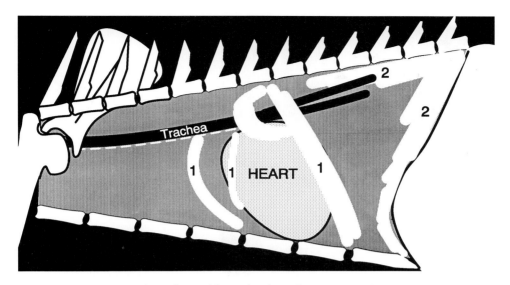

Fig. 2-4. Lateral thoracic radiographic projection of pleural effusion. Intrathoracic fluid accumulation causes separation of adjacent lung lobes by *(1)* linear interlobar opacities, radiographically defined as pleural fissures, and *(2)* separation of lung lobes from the thoracic wall.

and diaphragm as well as linear soft tissue opacities (pleural fissures) at anatomic locations comparable with interlobar fissures (Fig. 2-4). Pleural effusion also contributes to loss of definition of the cranial and caudal margins of the heart, producing a radiographic positive silhouette sign.

In cases of pleural effusion, the VD projection is much preferred over the DV view for detection and delineation of cardiac size and shape. If intrathoracic fluid volumes are severe enough, the heart can effectively disappear on the DV view because of the relative distribution of the fluid and heart in the thoracic cavity. The positive-silhouette phenomenon is accentuated in the DV compared to the VD view (Fig. 2-5). However, patient positioning for the DV projection puts less physiologic demand on the patient compromised by pleural effusion and thus is favored over the VD projection. The patient's physiologic stability and degree of respiratory compromise should always be assessed prior to thoracic imaging. If significant amounts of pleural effusion are suspected, increasing radiographic exposure to abdominal technique-chart levels results in better intrathoracic radiographic contrast. When possible, thoracocentesis and fluid drainage prior to radiography is always preferred.

RADIOGRAPHIC ANATOMY

LATERAL THORACIC RADIOGRAPHIC PROJECTION

Cardiac Parameters

Even though the lateral radiographic projection defines the cranial-caudal and dorsal-ventral dimensions of the thorax, the anatomy of the heart of the dog and cat as it resides in the thorax also allows this projection to detail the left and right

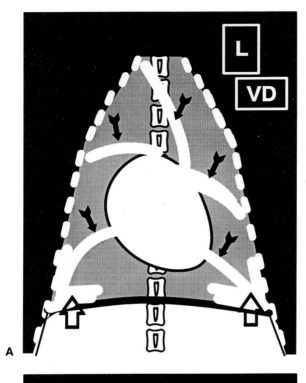

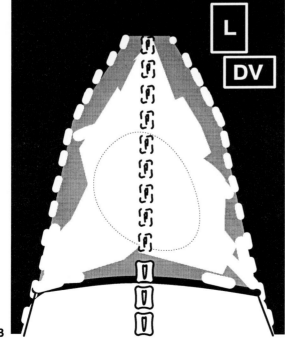

Fig. 2-5. (A) Ventrodorsal thoracic radiographic projection of pleural effusion consisting of pleural fissure lines *(closed arrows)* with blunting of the thoracophrenic angles *(open arrows)*. Note that the cardiac silhouette is still well outlined. **(B)** Dorsoventral thoracic radiographic projection of pleural effusion. The intrathoracic fluid distribution creates a "positive silhouette sign" where a complete loss of the cardiac silhouette has occurred. Thus, the VD projection **(A)** is preferred for cardiac silhouette definition in the presence of pleural effusion.

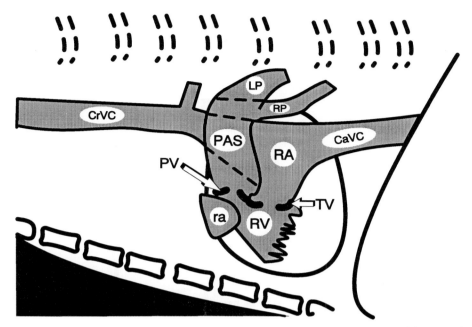

Fig. 2-6. Schematic lateral thoracic radiographic projection of the relative position and size of the right-side structures of the heart. Note the more cranial position of the right chambers of the heart. CrVC, cranial vena cava; PAS, main pulmonary artery; PV, pulmonic valve; ra, right atrial auricular appendage; RV, right ventricle; RA, right atrium; LP, left pulmonary artery; RP, right pulmonary artery; TV, tricuspid valve; CaVC, caudal vena cava.

aspects of the heart. This is because in the dog and the cat the heart is slightly rotated along its base-apex axis, such that the right cardiac chambers are positioned more cranially and the left chambers positioned more caudally. Thus, the cardiac silhouette as it appears on the lateral projection defines the right side of the heart along the cranial margin and the left side is defined by its caudal margin (Figs. 2-6 to 2-8).

The canine and feline heart shape or radiographic silhouette is ovoid, with the apex more pointed in conformation than the broader base. This base/apex difference in conformation is accentuated in the cat. The heart axis is defined by drawing a line from the tracheal bifurcation (carina) to the apex at an angle approximately 45 degrees to the sternal vertebrae. This angle can decrease in the cat with age and is often called a "lazy" heart. It has been postulated that this may be related to a loss of aortic connective tissue elasticity. This is most often seen in cats older than 7 years of age. Shallow, barrel-chested dog breeds (dachshund, Lhasa apso, bulldogs) tend to have more globular-shaped hearts, with increased sternal contact of the cranial margin of the heart. The heart chambers can be roughly defined by a line connecting the apex to the tracheal bifurcation and a second line perpendicular to the base-apex axis and positioned at the level of the ventral aspect of the caudal vena cava (Fig. 2-8).

The dorsal cardiac margin includes both atria, pulmonary arteries and veins, the cranial and caudal vena cavae and the aortic arch (Figs. 2-6 to 2-8). The cranial

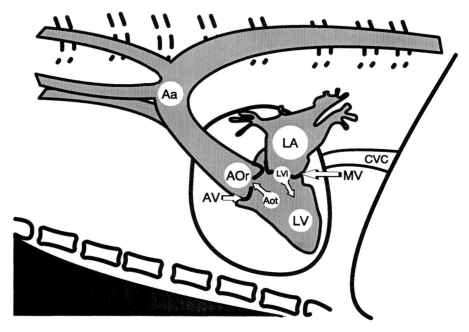

Fig. 2-7. Schematic lateral thoracic radiographic projection of the relative position and size of the left-side structures of the heart. Note the more caudal position of the left chambers of the heart. Aa, aortic arch; AOr, aorta; AV, aortic valve; Aot, aortic outflow tract; LV, left ventricle; LVi, left ventricular inflow tract; LA, left atrium; MV, mitral valve; CVC, caudal vena cava.

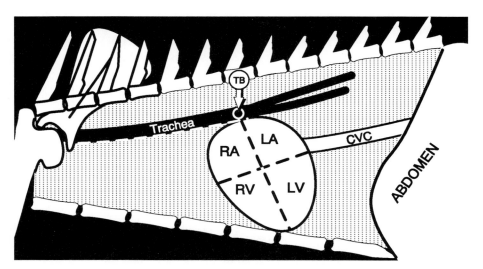

Fig. 2-8. Schematic lateral thoracic radiographic projection outlining the approximate location of the four heart chambers. TB, tracheal bifurcation; CVC, caudal vena cava; RA, right atrium; LA, left atrium; RV, right ventricle; LV, left ventricle.

border is formed both by the right ventricle and the right atrial appendage, resulting in the radiographically defined "cranial waist" (Figs. 2-6 and 2-8). The caudal margin is formed by the left atrium and left ventricle with the atrioventricular junction defined as the radiographic "caudal waist."

The base-to-apex cardiac dimension or length occupies approximately 70 percent of the dorsoventral distance of the thoracic cavity at its position within the thorax. For objective measurements it is important to measure thoracic cavity distance between the thoracic spine and sternum *at an axis perpendicular to the thoracic spine.*

The cranial-caudal dimension or width as it appears on the lateral projection is measured at its maximum width (which is usually at the level of the ventral aspect of the insertion of the caudal vena cava) and perpendicular to the base-apex axis. This classically has been defined as between 2.5 (deep-chested conformation breeds, setters, Afghans, collies) and 3.5 (barrel-chested conformation breeds, dachshunds, bulldogs) intercostal spaces (ICS) in the dog and 2.5 to 3.0 ICS in the cat. The ICS measurement is made at an axis *perpendicular to the long axis of the ribs.* Thus, the cardiac width distance determination may have to be shifted in axis angle before comparison to ICS length.

A more objective determination of cardiac size has been formulated for the dog and uses a vertebral scale system in which cardiac dimensions are scaled against the length of specific thoracic vertebrae (Fig. 2-9). In lateral radiographs, the long axis of the heart (L) is measured with a caliper extending from the ventral aspect of the left main stem bronchus (tracheal bifurcation hilus, carina) to the left ventricular apex. The caliper is repositioned along the vertebral column beginning at the cranial edge of the 4th thoracic vertebra. The length of the heart is recorded as the number of vertebrae caudal to that point and estimated to the nearest $\frac{1}{10}$ of a

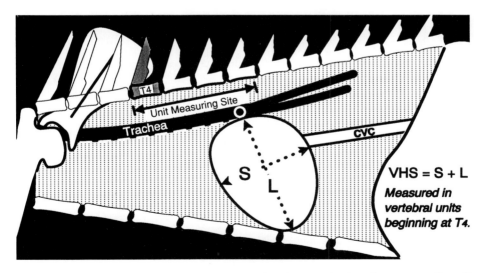

Fig. 2-9. Schematic representation parameters for the vertebral scale system of cardiac size. The vertebral heart sum (VHS) is the sum of the long axis cardiac dimension (L) and the maximal perpendicular short axis dimension (S). S and L are measured in vertebral units beginning at T4.

vertebra. The maximum perpendicular short axis (S) is measured in the same manner beginning at the 4th thoracic vertebra. If obvious left atrial enlargement is present, the short axis measurement is made at the ventral juncture of left atrial and caudal vena caval silhouettes.

The lengths in vertebrae (v) of the long and short axes are then added to obtain a vertebral heart sum (VHS) which provides a single number representing heart size proportionate to the size of the dog. The average VHS in the dog is 9.7 v (range 8.5–10.5 v). Caution must be exercised in some breeds that have excessively disproportionate skeletal-body weight conformations. An example is the English bulldogs, which have relatively small thoracic vertebrae and commonly have hemivertebrae as well; thus, a normal heart may be interpreted as large with the VHS method. Although the VHS concept is more precise, clinical judgment is still necessary to avoid over or under diagnosing heart disease.

Vessel Parameters

The main pulmonary artery (pulmonary trunk) cannot be seen on the lateral projection due to a positive silhouette sign with the craniodorsal base of the heart. The left pulmonary artery can sometimes be seen extending dorsal and caudal to the tracheal bifurcation (carina). The right pulmonary artery is frequently seen end-on as it leaves the main pulmonary artery immediately ventral to the carina (Fig. 2-10). This end-on appearance may be confused with a mass lesion on normal

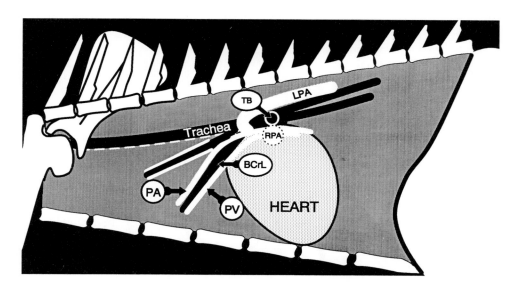

Fig. 2-10. Pulmonary vascular anatomy in the lateral thoracic projection: cranial lung lobe branch of the pulmonary artery (PA), cranial lung lobe branch of the pulmonary vein (PV), end-on view of the right main pulmonary artery as it traverses the thorax from left to right (RPA), and left main pulmonary artery (LPA). TB, tracheal bifurcation (carina); BCrL, bronchus to a cranial lung lobe.

radiographs and is accentuated in cases of pulmonary hypertension such as heart-worm disease. The pulmonary veins are best identified as they enter the left atrium caudal to the heart base.

Using the larger, more proximal segments of the mainstem bronchi as a reference, the pulmonary arteries are dorsal to the bronchus and the pulmonary veins are ventral to the bronchus (Fig. 2-10).

The vessels to the cranial lung lobes are usually seen as two pairs of vessels, each with their respective bronchi. The more cranial pair of vessels generally corresponds to the side on which the lateral projection was made. Thus, in the right lateral projection, the right cranial lobar vessels are more cranial than vessels of the left cranial lung lobe. The pulmonary arteries and veins should be equal in size. The width of the vessels where they cross the 4th rib should not exceed the width of the narrowest portion of that rib at its juncture with the rib head (the dorsal aspect of the rib near the thoracic spine). The dorsal section of the rib is used as a reference to adjust for radiographic magnification due to thoracic conformation.

DORSOVENTRAL AND VENTRODORSAL PROJECTIONS

Cardiac Parameters

The heart is rotated on its long axis such that the right chambers are oriented both right and cranially, and the left chambers reside both left and caudal. The degree of rotation is less in the cat. The cranial-caudal rotation is most significant when defining the location of the left and right atria respectively.

The canine heart appears radiographically as an elliptical opacity with its base-apex axis orientation approximately 30 degrees to the left of the midline. The width of the heart across its widest point is usually 60 to 65 percent of the thoracic width at its location within the thorax. In the cat, the cardiac axis is most commonly on or close to midline, and its width does not usually exceed 50 percent of the width of the thoracic cavity during full inspiration. The cardiac silhouette may be artificially increased in the obese patient due to an excessive amount of pericardial fat. In these cases, the cardiac silhouette margin appears to be less well defined or blurred because the margin of contrast between soft tissue (heart), fat (pericardial), and air is not as distinct as between soft tissue and air.

Evaluating the obesity of the patient by evaluating the thickness of the abaxial thoracic wall and width of the mediastinum (as well as examining the patient) will assist in the determination of pericardial fat contribution to cardiac size. In deep, narrow-chested breeds the heart stands more vertical in the thorax and thus produces a smaller and more circular cardiac silhouette conformation. The broad, barrel-chested breeds produce a radiographic silhouette that appears wider than standard breeds.

The margins of the heart that create the cardiac silhouette contain a number of structures that often overlap. A clockface analogy can be used to simplify the location of these structures. The aortic arch extends from the 11 to 1 o'clock

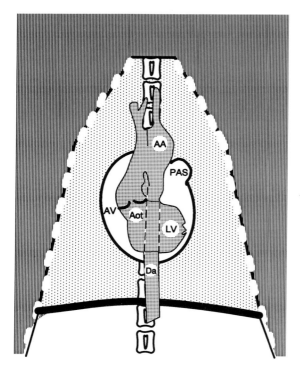

Fig. 2-11. Schematic anatomy of the chambers and vasculature of the left ventricular outflow tract of the heart in the dorsoventral radiographic projection. LV, left ventricle; Aot, aortic outflow tract; AV, aortic valve; AA, aortic arch; PAS, pulmonary artery segment; Da, descending aorta.

position (Fig. 2-11). The main pulmonary artery is located from the 1 to 2 o'clock position, with its radiographic designation as the "pulmonary artery segment" (PAS) (Figs. 2-12 and 2-13). In the cat, the body of the left atrium proper forms the 2 to 3 o'clock position of the cardiac silhouette. In the dog, the left atrium is superimposed over the caudal portion of the cardiac silhouette in the DV projection (Fig. 2-12). With severe cases of left atrial enlargement in the dog, the left atrial appendage contributes to the definition and enlargement of the cardiac silhouette at the 2 to 3 o'clock position (Fig. 2-13). The left ventricle forms the left heart margin from the 2 to 6 o'clock position (Fig. 2-11). The right ventricle is located from the 7 to 11 o'clock position (the right ventricle does not extend to the apex of the heart) (Fig. 2-14). The right atrium is located at the 9 to 11 o'clock position (Fig. 2-14). Pericardial fat in the dog can asymmetrically contribute to cardiac silhouette enlargement at the 4 to 5 and 8 to 11 o'clock positions.

Vessel Parameters

The pulmonary arteries originate from the main pulmonary artery or the pulmonary artery segment (PAS) with the right branch coursing transversely, superimposed over the cranial portion of the heart silhouette, extending beyond the right heart margin at approximately the 8 o'clock position (Fig. 2-12). The left pulmonary artery branch courses caudally, superimposed over the caudal left ventricular portion of the heart and extends beyond the left heart margin at approximately

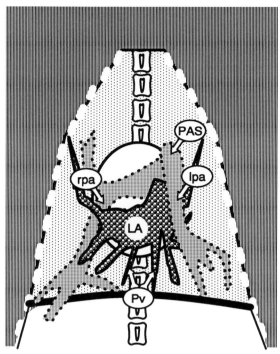
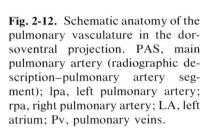

Fig. 2-12. Schematic anatomy of the pulmonary vasculature in the dorsoventral projection. PAS, main pulmonary artery (radiographic description–pulmonary artery segment); lpa, left pulmonary artery; rpa, right pulmonary artery; LA, left atrium; Pv, pulmonary veins.

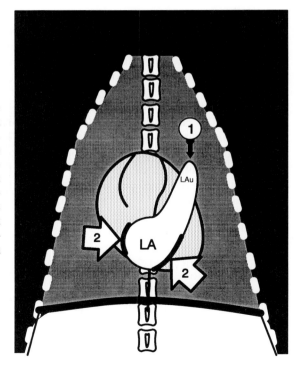

Fig. 2-13. Dorsoventral thoracic radiographic projection of the dog with severe left atrial (LA) enlargement. The left atrial auricular appendage (LAu) contributes to the cardiac silhouette at the 2 to 3 o'clock position (1). The body of the left atrium superimposed over the caudal cardiac silhouette produces a radiolucent "mach" line, a radiographic edge effect caused by an acute change in soft-tissue thickness (2).

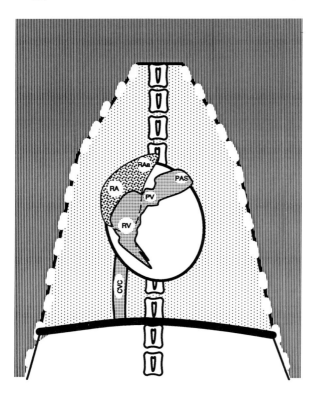

Fig. 2-14. Schematic anatomy of the chambers and outflow tract of the right side of the heart in the dorsoventral radiographic projection. RV, right ventricle; RA, right atrium; RAa, right atrial auricular appendage; PV, pulmonic valve; PAS, mainstem pulmonary artery segment; CVC, caudal vena cava.

the 4 o'clock position. The pulmonary veins are best seen as they enter the left atrium along the caudal margin of the cardiac silhouette (Fig. 2-12). Compared to the pulmonary arteries, they are clustered in a more axial position. Thus, the pulmonary arteries extend to both the cranial and caudal lung fields in a more *abaxial* position relative to the pulmonary veins.

The aortic arch is within the cranial mediastinum at the cranial heart margin and is normally not visible. The descending aorta is superimposed over the heart and extends caudally, dorsally, and medially. The left lateral margin of the aorta can be seen to the left of the vertebral column on both DV and VD views (Fig. 2-11). The caudal vena cava courses cranially from the diaphragm to the right of midline and into the right caudal margin of the heart (Fig. 2-14). This is one of the most useful landmarks for determination of proper orientation of the dorsoventral radiograph on a viewbox.

RADIOGRAPHIC INTERPRETATION

A systematic evaluation of the entire thoracic cavity involves adherence to and inclusion of the following steps with each radiographic interpretation. Abnormalities supportive of disease should be substantiated on multiple radiographic views where applicable.

   I. Evaluate the radiographs for technical quality, positioning, and proper exposure. *If the study is substandard, stop right here and repeat the radiographic study.*
  II. Determine the phase of respiration.
 III. Review the entire thoracic cavity: spine, sternum, diaphragm, thoracic wall, ribs, cranial and caudal mediastinum, conformation and position of the diaphragm.
  IV. Review the portion of the cranial abdomen included in the projection. Thoracic radiographic exposure is usually *one-half* of that required for abdominal imaging but a cursory evaluation of abdominal contrast, detail, and hepatic size (using gastric axis) can be performed.
   V. Evaluate the position, course, and diameter of the trachea and mainstem bifurcations.
  VI. Evaluate the position of the cardiac apex and caudal mediastinum.
 VII. Evaluate the size, shape, and course of the main pulmonary artery and peripheral pulmonary arteries and veins.
VIII. Evaluate the lung fields for hyper- or underinflation, and distribution and pattern of increased or decreased opacity.
  IX. Evaluate the cardiac margin (cranial, caudal, right, left, "clock position" segmentation) for enlargement, abnormal position, or conformation.

NONCARDIAC RELATED VARIABLES THAT CAN MIMIC RADIOGRAPHIC SIGNS OF CARDIAC DISEASE

CARDIAC POSITION, LATERAL PROJECTION

   I. Pulmonary pathology (such as lung consolidation, atelectasis, or pleural disease) can cause a mediastinal shift and alter the position and axis of the heart in the thoracic cavity.
  II. Mediastinal mass lesions can affect the cardiac position and axis, as well as obscure the cranial and cardiac margins when in contact with the heart, by producing a radiographic positive silhouette sign.
 III. Pneumothorax can produce disproportionate hemithoracic volume changes, altering cardiac position and axis. Pneumothorax commonly produces elevation of the cardiac apex from the sternum. This is supported by other radiographic signs of pneumothorax
     A. Premature termination of lung vasculature into the periphery of the thoracic cavity
     B. Lung lobe margin detection as it contrasts with nonparenchymal free intrathoracic gas
  IV. Sternal conformational abnormalities due to congenital defects or previous trauma can alter cardiac position and axis.

CARDIAC SIZE, LATERAL PROJECTION

   I. Younger animals appear to have larger hearts relative to their thoracic size than do mature patients.

II. The heart appears smaller on inspiration than on expiration. During expiration increased sternal contact of the right heart margin and dorsal elevation of the trachea occurs, falsely suggesting right-heart enlargement.
III. Anemic or emaciated patients often have small hearts to due to hypovolemia and are hyperinflated to compensate for hypoxemia. In deep-chested conformation breeds the cardiac apex can be elevated far enough from the sternum to mimic pneumothorax.

CARDIAC POSITION, DORSOVENTRAL/ VENTRODORSAL PROJECTION

Malposition of the Cardiac Apex to the Right or Left

I. Malposition of the heart to the right is a normal variant in the cat.
II. Uneven lung inflation secondary to disease or previous lobectomy can produce a mediastinal shift and resultant apex shift.
III. If radiographs are taken on diseased, recumbent patients or patients during or immediately following general anesthesia, hypostatic congestion and atelectasis of the dependent lung fields can produce a mediastinal shift, altering cardiac position.
IV. Pectus excavatum or "funnel chest" sternal conformation due to congenital deformities.

EVALUATION OF HEART CHAMBER ENLARGEMENT

RIGHT ATRIAL ENLARGEMENT

I. Radiographic signs
   A. Lateral projection (Fig. 2-15)
      1. Elevation of the trachea as it courses dorsally over the right atrium.
      2. Accentuation of the cranial waist. Preferential enlargement of the more dorsal margin of the cranial margin of the cardiac silhouette defines selective enlargement of the right atrial auricular appendage.
      3. Increased soft tissue opacity of the cranial aspect of the cardiac silhouette due to increased soft tissue thickness of the right atrium superimposed over the right ventricle.
   B. Dorsoventral projection (Fig. 2-16):
      1. Enlargement of the cardiac margin at 9 to 11 o'clock.
      2. Enlargement can be dramatic in severe cases (especially in the cat) and can be easily mistaken for a pulmonary or hilar mass lesion.
II. Causes of right atrial enlargement
   A. Right-heart failure
   B. Tricuspid insufficiency

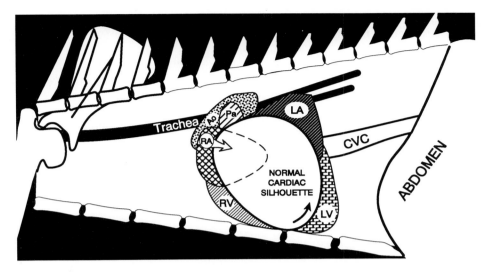

Fig. 2-15. Cardiac silhouette changes associated with vessel and chamber enlargement in the lateral thoracic radiographic projection. Ao, aortic arch; Pa, main pulmonary artery; RA, right atrium; LA, left atrium; RV, right ventricle; LV, left ventricle; CVC, caudal vena cava. *Dotted line:* area of right atrial superimposition over the right ventricle. *Curved arrow:* direction of apex location shift with right ventricular enlargement.

Fig. 2-16. Cardiac silhouette changes associated with vessel and chamber enlargement in the dorsoventral radiographic projection. Aa, aortic arch; PAS, main pulmonary artery; LAa, left atrial auricular appendage; LV, left ventricle; RV, right ventricle; RA, right atrium.

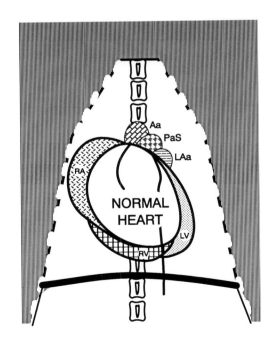

    C. Cardiomyopathy
    D. Right atrial neoplasia (e.g., hemangiosarcoma)
III. Differential diagnosis
    A. Cranial mediastinal mass
    B. Heart base neoplasia (most common in brachycephalic breeds)
    C. Tracheobronchial lymphadenopathy
    D. Superimposition of the aortic arch or main pulmonary artery
    E. Right cranial or middle lobar pulmonary alveolar consolidation or mass
       lesion

RIGHT VENTRICULAR ENLARGEMENT

I. Radiographic signs
    A. Lateral projection (Fig. 2-15)
       1. Increased sternal contact of cranial cardiac margin
       2. Elevation of the cardiac apex from the sternum
       3. Rounding of the conformation of the entire cardiac silhouette; increased
         cardiac width
       4. Disproportionate enlargement of the cranial portion of the cardiac sil-
         houette when empirically divided into its right and left chambers (Fig.
         2-17)
       5. Dorsal elevation of the caudal vena cava
    B. Dorsoventral projection (Fig. 2-16)

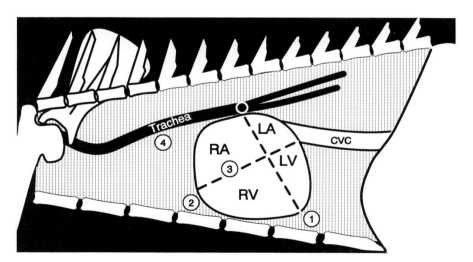

Fig. 2-17. Schematic representation of radiographic signs associated with right-sided heart enlargement in the lateral projection. (1) Dorsal lifting of apex from sternum. (2) Increased sternal contact of cranial cardiac margin. (3) Disproportionate enlargement of the cranial portion of the cardiac silhouette when empirically divided into its right and left chambers. (4) Elevation of the trachea as it courses dorsally over the right atrium. RA, right atrium; RV, right ventricle; LA, left atrium; LV, left ventricle; CVC, caudal vena cava.

    1. Cardiac silhouette enlargement at the 6 to 11 o'clock position
    2. Given the enlargement and rounded conformation of the right margin, the left margin in comparison assumes a more straightened conformation; an overall "reverse-D" conformational appearance of the cardiac silhouette results
    3. Shift of cardiac apex to the left
II. Causes of right ventricular enlargement
    A. Secondary to left-heart failure
    B. Tricuspid insufficiency
    C. Cardiomyopathy
    D. Cor pulmonale
    E. Dirofilariasis
    F. Congenital heart disease: pulmonic stenosis, patent ductus arteriosus, ventricular septal defects, tetralogy of Fallot, tricuspid valve dysplasia

LEFT ATRIAL ENLARGEMENT

I. Radiographic signs
    A. Lateral projection (Fig. 2-15)
        1. Dorsal elevation of the caudal portion of trachea and carina
        2. Disproportionate dorsal elevation of the mainstem bronchi (the two will no longer be superimposed; the left bronchus will appear more dorsal than the right bronchus)
        3. Enlargement and straightening of the caudodorsal portion of the cardiac silhouette with almost a right-angle margin conformation (Fig. 2-18); straightening of the caudal margin of the heart and loss of the caudal waist (determined by the atrioventricular junction)
    B. Dorsoventral projection (Fig. 2-16)
        1. The dog
           a) Enlargement of the atrial auricular appendage, which now produces a noticeable focal "bulge" enlargement at the 2 to 3 o'clock position (Figs. 2-13 and 2-16).
           b) A "double opacity" of the atrial body over the caudal aspect of the cardiac silhouette. The body of the left atrium superimposed over the caudal cardiac silhouette produces a radiolucent "mach" line, a radiographic edge effect caused by an acute change in soft tissue thickness (Fig. 2-13).
        2. The cat
        Enlargement of the cardiac margin at the 2 to 3 o'clock position of the silhouette.
II. Causes of left atrial enlargement
    A. Mitral insufficiency
    B. Cardiomyopathy
    C. Congenital heart disease: mitral valve dysplasia, patent ductus arteriosus, ventricular septal defects, atrial septal defects
    D. Left ventricular failure

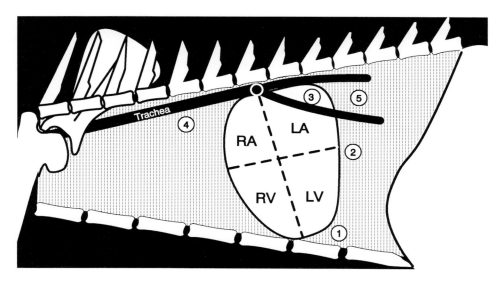

Fig. 2-18. Schematic representation of radiographic signs associated with left-sided heart enlargement in the lateral projection. *(1)* Rounding and widening of the cardiac apex conformation. *(2)* Straightening and increased vertical axis of the caudal cardiac margin. *(3)* Left atrial enlargement with characteristic right-angular caudodorsal margin conformation. *(4)* Dorsal elevation of the intrathoracic portion of the trachea, carina, and mainstem bronchi. The angle between the thoracic spine axis and trachea is diminished to the point of becoming parallel. *(5)* Separation of normally superimposed caudal mainstem bronchi. Left more dorsal in position than the right. RA, right atrium; RV, right ventricle; LA, left atrium; LV, left ventricle.

III. Differential diagnosis
  A. Hilar lymphadenopathy
  B. Pulmonary mass adjacent to hilus

Left Ventricular Enlargement

I. Radiographic signs
  A. Lateral projection (Fig. 2-15)
    1. Loss of the caudal waist
    2. Caudal cardiac margin straighter and more vertical than normal
    3. Dorsal elevation of the intrathoracic portion of the trachea, carina, and mainstem bronchi; the angle between the thoracic spine axis and trachea is diminished to the point of becoming parallel
    4. Disproportionate enlargement of the caudal portion of the cardiac silhouette when empirically divided into its right and left cardiac chambers (Fig. 2-18)
  B. Dorsoventral projection (Fig. 2-16)
    1. Rounding and enlargement of left ventricular margin
    2. Rounding and broadening of the cardiac apex conformation
    3. Shift of the cardiac apex to the right

II. Causes of left ventricular enlargement
   A. Mitral insufficiency
   B. Cardiomyopathy
   C. Congenital heart disease: patent ductus arteriosus, aortic stenosis, ventricular septal defects
   D. High-output cardiac disease: fluid overload, chronic anemia, peripheral arteriovenous fistula, obesity, chronic renal disease, hyperthyroidism

ENLARGEMENT OF THE AORTIC ARCH AND AORTA

I. Radiographic signs
   A. Lateral projection (Fig. 2-15)
      1. Widening of the dorsal aspect of the cardiac silhouette
      2. Enlargement of the craniodorsal cardiac margin
   B. Dorsoventral projection (Fig. 2-16)
      Widening and increased cranial extension of the cardiac margin between the 11 and 1 o'clock position.
II. Causes of aortic arch enlargement
   A. Patent ductus arteriosus; enlargement more abaxial (1 o'clock)
   B. Aortic stenosis with poststenotic enlargement of the aortic arch; enlargement more axial and cranial (11 o'clock)
   C. Aortic aneurysm (very rare)
III. Differential diagnosis
   A. Normal variation in some dogs
   B. Very common variant in older cats with "lazy" heart conformation; very prominent on the DV projection
   C. Cranial mediastinal mass
   D. Thymus, or the "sail-sign" in young dogs
   E. Cranial mediastinal fat in obese brachycephalic dogs

ENLARGEMENT OF THE PULMONARY ARTERY

I. Radiographic signs
   A. Lateral projection (Fig. 2-15)
      Protrusion of the craniodorsal heart border
   B. Dorsoventral projection (Fig. 2-16)
      1. Lateral bulge of the cardiac margin at 1 to 2 o'clock position
      2. Radiographically defined as the pulmonary artery segment (PAS)
II. Causes of pulmonary artery segment enlargement
   A. Dirofilariasis
   B. Pulmonary thrombosis and thromboembolism
   C. Cor pulmonale
   D. Congenital disease: pulmonic stenosis, patent ductus arteriosus, septal defects (VSD, ASD) with left to right shunting

III. Differential diagnosis
    A. Previous dirofilariasis infection and treatment
    B. Rotational (oblique) positional artifact (usually on VD projection) most
       commonly experienced with deep-chested conformation dogs

EVALUATION OF THE PULMONARY CIRCULATION

UNDERCIRCULATION

   I. Radiographic signs
    A. Lung field more radiolucent than normal due to lack of pulmonary vascular volume
    B. Hyperinflation due to hypoxemia or ventilation/perfusion mismatch
    C. Pulmonary arteries smaller than normal; may be smaller in size when compared to corresponding pulmonary veins
  II. Causes of pulmonary undercirculation
    Congenital disease: pulmonic stenosis, tetralogy of Fallot, reverse patent ductus arteriosus (right to left shunting)
 III. Differential diagnosis
    A. Emphysema, COPD
    B. Hyperinflation
    C. Pneumothorax
    D. Overexposure
    E. Pulmonary thromboembolism
    F. Hypovolemia, shock (the heart will also be smaller than normal)
    G. Hypoadrenocorticism (Addison's disease); the heart may also be smaller than normal

OVERCIRCULATION

   I. Radiographic signs
    A. Both the pulmonary arteries and veins are enlarged
    B. Arteries are frequently larger than the veins
    C. Increased pulmonary thoracic opacity because of larger vascular volume
  II. Causes of pulmonary overcirculation
    A. Dirofilariasis (arteries are larger than corresponding veins)
    B. Patent ductus arteriosus (PDA): both arteries and veins are enlarged
    C. Left-to-right shunts (VSD, ASD): both arteries an veins are enlarged
    D. Congestive heart failure: veins may be larger than arteries if mainly left sided; both arteries and veins are enlarged with concurrent left- and right-sided failure.
    E. Fluid overload
 III. Differential diagnosis

A. Underexposure
B. Expiratory phase of respiration

RADIOGRAPHIC DIAGNOSIS OF HEART FAILURE

The radiographic diagnosis of heart failure is dependent upon recognition of imbalances in the blood and fluid distribution within the body. This circulatory imbalance is the result of diminished cardiac output into the pulmonary or systemic vascular systems or reduced acceptance of blood by the failing ventricle (hypertrophy), or both. Depending on which "side" of the heart is most severely affected, blood is shifted from the systemic to the pulmonary circulation (left-heart failure) or from the pulmonary to the systemic circulation (right-heart failure).

RIGHT-HEART FAILURE

I. Physiologic phenomenon
   A. In right-sided heart failure, an inadequate right ventricular output into the pulmonary arteries exists concurrently with a reduced acceptance of blood from the systemic veins. The blood volume and pressure in the splanchnic and systemic veins are elevated. The venous congestion causes hepatomegaly.
   B. With further progression of right-sided heart failure, a progression of systemic hypertension leads to increased amounts of fluid, solutes, and protein escaping from the capillary beds of the major organs. The lymphatic circulation is overtaxed and fluid exudes into the serosal cavities, producing ascites, pleural, and even pericardial effusions.
   C. The extracardiac radiographic signs of progressively worsening right-sided failure are hepatomegaly, ascites, and then pleural effusion.
II. Radiographic signs
   A. Right-sided cardiomegaly (Figs. 2-15 to 2-17). Patients with concentric cardiac hypertrophy (e.g., pulmonic stenosis), thin-walled cardiomyopathy, or acute arrhythmias often may not have dramatic radiographic cardiomegaly. Thus, subtle cardiac silhouette changes in both the DV and lateral projections must be considered significant with supportive clinical evidence of cardiac disease.
   B. Hepatomegaly: rounded liver margin, which extends caudal to last rib; displacement of stomach caudally and to the left
   C. Ascites: abdominal distention; diffuse loss of intra-abdominal detail
   D. Pleural effusion
      1. Generalized increase in thoracic opacity
      2. Visualization of interlobar pleural fissures (see Figs. 2-4 and 2-5A)
      3. Obliteration of cardiac silhouette definition (best demonstrated on the DV projection) (see Fig. 2-5B)
      4. Separation of pulmonary visceral pleural margin away from thoracic wall (see Figs. 2-4 and 2-5)

III. Causes of pleural effusion secondary to right-heart failure
    A. Decompensated mitral and tricuspid insufficiency
    B. Decompensated pulmonic stenosis, tetralogy of Fallot
    C. Dirofilariasis (caval syndrome)
    D. Pericardial effusion with tamponade
    E. Restrictive pericarditis
IV. Differential diagnosis
    A. Pleuritis
    B. Chylothorax
    C. Hemothorax
    D. Pyothorax
    E. Hypoproteinemia
    F. Neoplasia (pleural, mediastinal, cardiac, pulmonary, primary or meta-static)

LEFT-HEART FAILURE

I. Physiologic phenomenon
    A. In left-heart failure, inadequate left ventricular output into the aorta occurs, and a diminished acceptance of blood from the pulmonary veins entering the left atrium results. This causes pulmonary venous congestion and leakage of fluid into the pulmonary interstitium, with progression to flooding of the alveoli.
    B. Clinically, this evolves as a progression of physiological events: pulmonary venous congestion, interstitial pulmonary edema, alveolar edema and lung consolidation.
II. Radiographic signs
    A. Left-sided cardiomegaly (Fig. 2-18). Patients with concentric cardiac hypertrophy (e.g., aortic stenosis), thin-walled cardiomyopathy (large and giant breed dogs), or acute arrhythmias often may not have dramatic radiographic cardiomegaly. Thus, subtle cardiac silhouette changes in both the DV and lateral projections as well as noncardiac changes (pulmonary vascular changes, pulmonary edema, etc.) must be evaluated.
    B. Pulmonary venous congestion
        1. Engorgement and distention of the pulmonary veins, especially in the hilar area as they enter the left atrium. On the DV view these are identified as the more axial of the caudal vasculature (Fig. 2-12).
        2. The diameter of the pulmonary veins is greater than that of their corresponding pulmonary arteries (best seen on the lateral projection with cranial lobar vessels) (Fig. 2-10).
        3. The radiopacity of the lung parenchyma distal and peripheral to the hilus is unchanged.
    C. Interstitial edema
        1. Diffuse increased radiopacity of the lung fields due to a hazy interstitial opacity is apparent.
        2. The margins of the pulmonary veins and arteries are indistinct due to perivascular edema. As the lung parenchyma surrounding the pulmo-

nary vasculature fills with fluid, the normal pulmonary radiographic contrast between gas (air-filled lung) and soft tissue (blood-filled vessels) is lost. Thus, the pulmonary vasculature becomes indistinct and begins to disappear in the surrounding, fluid-filled lung parenchyma.

3. In some patients, fluid accumulates around major bronchi, producing prominent peribronchial markings.

D. Alveolar edema

1. Radiographic signs

a) Fluid enters the alveolar airspaces and peripheral bronchioles, causing a coalescent fluffy alveolar infiltrate. Air bronchograms (black tubes in a white radiopaque background) and air alveolograms (lung parenchyma with the radiopacity of *liver* containing no vascular markings) are present. In the cat, cardiogenic alveolar consolidations can appear as a very well-margined, "cloudlike" conformation areas of increased pulmonary radiopacity.

b) The margins of the pulmonary vessels are usually completely obscured (see Fig. 2-3B). The alveolar infiltrate is of greatest opacity in the perihilar area, fading peripherally. In the dog, alveolar edema can be asymmetrical, with the right lung fields more severely affected than the left (best seen on the DV projection).

2. Differential diagnosis for pulmonary edema

a) Neurogenic: electrocution, head trauma, post seizure, encephalitis, brain neoplasm

b) Hyperdynamic (excessive negative intrathoracic pressures): choking, strangulation, upper airway obstructions

c) Fluid overload: overhydration

d) Toxicity

e) Systemic shock

f) Hypersensitization

g) Drowning

E. Increased bronchial markings in some cases.

F. Pleural effusion

1. In the dog, can occur only in very progressive or severe forms of left-sided heart failure; this usually indicates early concurrent left and right-sided failure.

2. In the cat, pleural effusion is very common with only left-sided heart failure; this can be separated from right-sided heart failure by the absence of accompanying hepatomegaly and ascites.

RADIOGRAPHIC DIAGNOSIS OF PERICARDIAL EFFUSION

I. Generalized enlargement of cardiac silhouette in a "basketball" conformation, with elimination of all normal cardiac margin contours on all views

II. Increased sternal contact of the cranial margin and convex bulging of the caudal margin, without the angular conformation and straightening characteristic for left atrial and ventricular enlargements (Fig. 2-19)

TABLE 2-2. SUMMARY OF RADIOGRAPHIC SIGNS OF CONGENITAL AND ACQUIRED CARDIAC DISEASE[a]

Lesion	RA	RV	LA	LV	Aorta	MPAs	PAb	PV	VC	Failure/Side	Failure/Type
Congenital defects											
Patent ductus arteriosis	N	In	In	In	In	In	In	In	N/In	Left	Volume
Pulmonic stenosis	In	In	N/De	N/De	N	In	N/De	N/De	In	Right	Pressure
Aortic stenosis	N	N/In	N/In	In	In	N	In	In	N	Left	Pressure
Ventricular septal defect	N	In	In	In	N	N/In	In	In	N/In	Left	Volume
Tetralogy of Fallot	N/In	In	N/De	N/De	N	De/N/In	De	De	N	Right	Pressure
Atrial septal defect	In	In	N/In	N	N	N/In	N/In	N/In	N/In	Left	Volume
Acquired heart disease											
Mitral insufficiency	N	N/In	In	In	N	N	N	In	N	Left	Fluid
Tricuspid insufficiency	In	In	N	N	N	N	N	N	In	Right	Fluid
Aortic insufficiency	N	N	In	In	N/In	N	N	In	N	Left	Fluid
Hypertrophic cardiomyopathy	In	In	In	In	N	N	N/In	N/In	N/In	Left > Right	Myocardial
Dilated cardiomyopathy	In	In	In	In	N	N	N/In	N/In	N/In	Right > Left	Myocardial
Pericardial effusion	In	In	In	In	N	N	N/De	N/De	In	Right	Tamponade

[a] Abbreviations: RA, right atrium; RV, right ventricle; LA, left atrium; LV, left ventricle; MPAs, main pulmonary artery segment; PAb, pulmonary artery branches; PV, pulmonary vein; VC, caudal vena cava; In, enlarged or increased; De, smaller or decreased; N, normal.

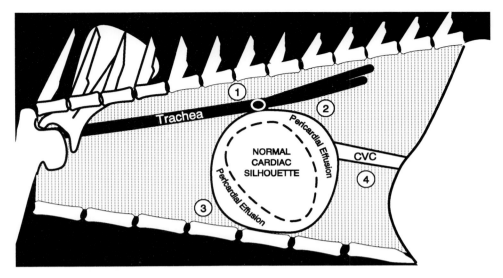

Fig. 2-19. Schematic representation of radiographic signs associated with pericardial effusion. *(1)* Dorsal elevation of the intrathoracic portion of the trachea, carina, and mainstem bronchi. The angle between the thoracic spine axis and trachea is diminished to the point of becoming parallel. *(2)* Convex enlargement of the caudodorsal cardiac margin without a "right-angle" conformation characteristic for left atrial enlargement. *(3)* Increased sternal contact of cranial margin. *(4)* Dorsal elevation and enlargement of the caudal vena cava (CVC). The cardiac silhouette takes on a smoothly contoured circular conformation with obliteration of normal cardiac contour.

III. Elevation and enlargement of the caudal vena cava
IV. Dorsal elevation of the trachea (similar to left-side enlargement)
V. Hepatomegaly, ascites, and pleural effusion secondary to cardiac tamponade (see Figs. 2-4 and 2-5)

SUMMARY

The clinician must be armed with both potential radiographic parameters and a clinically derived differential diagnostic list for cardiac disease before the radiographic image can begin to provide useful information. Table 2-2 summarizes the radiographic signs associated with congenital and acquired heart diseases. Awareness of noncardiac and artifactual conditions that can present with the same radiographic signs is also paramount to a correct diagnosis.

SUGGESTED READINGS

Buchanan JW, Bucheler J: Vertebral scale system for cardiac mensuration. Proc ACVIM, May 1991, (in press JAVMA)
Ettinger SJ, Suter PF: Canine Cardiology. WB Saunders, Philadelphia, 1970
Owens JM: Radiographic Interpretation for the Small Animal Clinician. Ralston Purina Co, St. Louis, 1982

3

Electrocardiography

Francis W. K. Smith, Jr.
Deborah J. Hadlock

INTRODUCTION

Electrocardiography is the study of myocardial function based on graphic records of the heart's electrical activity plotted over time. The electrocardiogram (ECG) is an extremely valuable test that is easy to perform and readily available to practicing veterinarians. Performing an ECG is indicated in many situations, as this test provides information that is useful in the diagnosis and management of cardiac and systemic disturbances.

INDICATIONS AND ROLE OF THE ECG IN CLINICAL PRACTICE

I. To diagnose an arrhythmia detected on physical examination.
   A. The ECG is the most sensitive test for the diagnosis of arrhythmias.
   B. An ECG should be performed on all animals with a tachycardia or brady-cardia and on all cats with any irregularity in heart rhythm. An ECG would also be recommended in any dog with an irregularity in heart rhythm that is associated with a pulse deficit or that is not associated with phases of respiration.
II. To rule out arrhythmias or conduction disturbances in patients with a history of syncope, seizures, or exercise intolerance. A postexercise ECG or Holter monitoring are sometimes needed to confirm an arrhythmia that is not present at rest.
III. To monitor effectiveness of antiarrhythmic therapy.
IV. To assess cardiac size in patients with known or suspected cardiac disease.
   A. The presence of a heart-enlargement pattern on the ECG usually correlates with cardiac chamber enlargement or hypertrophy. The more criteria for heart enlargement that are present in a patient, the more likely the heart will be enlarged.
   B. A normal ECG does not rule out heart enlargement. Thoracic radiographs and echocardiography are more sensitive tests for evaluating heart size.
V. To help individualize and monitor therapy in heart failure patients.
   A. The diagnosis of congestive heart failure (CHF) cannot be made based on an ECG alone. The presence of an arrhythmia or heart enlargement

pattern supports heart disease, but does not confirm CHF. A thoracic radiograph should be obtained along with the ECG in patients suspected of having CHF.

B. The ECG is useful in heart failure patients for the diagnosis and treatment of associated arrhythmias.

C. In patients diagnosed with CHF, follow-up ECGs are useful to follow progression of heart enlargement, arrhythmias, and to screen for digoxin toxicity in patients treated with cardiac glycosides.

VI. To evaluate patients with suspected digoxin or other cardiac drug toxicity.

VII. To screen for electrolyte disturbances, especially hyperkalemia, hypokalemia, hypercalcemia, and hypocalcemia. Although the ECG is not very sensitive or specific in diagnosing systemic disturbances, it can be useful as a rapid screening test for certain electrolyte disturbances (predominantly hyperkalemia). See Chapter 13.

VIII. To look for evidence to support a diagnosis of pericardial effusion, hypothyroidism, hyperthyroidism, and hypoadrenocorticism (Addison's disease). See Chapter 13.

PRINCIPLES OF ELECTROCARDIOGRAPHY

I. The ECG lead system is composed of positive and negative electrodes that are attached to the body and surround the heart. The ECG electrodes measure the electrical activity of the heart muscle cells during depolarization and repolarization.

II. Electrical impulses traveling toward the positive electrode cause a positive deflection. Impulses traveling away from the positive electrode cause a negative deflection and impulses traveling perpendicular to the electrode cause no deflection. The ECG tracing is the summation of all the impulses generated by all the myocytes.

III. Lead Systems (see Table 3-1 for ECG clip placement)

A. ECG electrodes are attached at multiple sites on the body to allow the electrical activity of the heart to be viewed from multiple angles. Multiple views allow greater accuracy in diagnosing complex arrhythmias and localizing problems within the heart. (See Fig. 3-1)

B. The standard leads are the bipolar limb leads I, II, III, and the augmented limb leads aVR, aVL, and aVF. The leads are recorded in the following order: I, II, III, aVR, aVL, aVF. Chest leads are sometimes used for further evaluating heart enlargement patterns. Intracardiac leads are rarely used in clinical practice.

C. Bipolar limb leads

1. Leads I, II, III are obtained by comparing electrical impulses between two electrodes placed on the limbs.

2. Lead II is the standard lead for making measurements of the P-QRS-T wave forms.

D. Augmented unipolar limb leads

1. Leads aVR, aVL, aVF are obtained by using three electrodes and

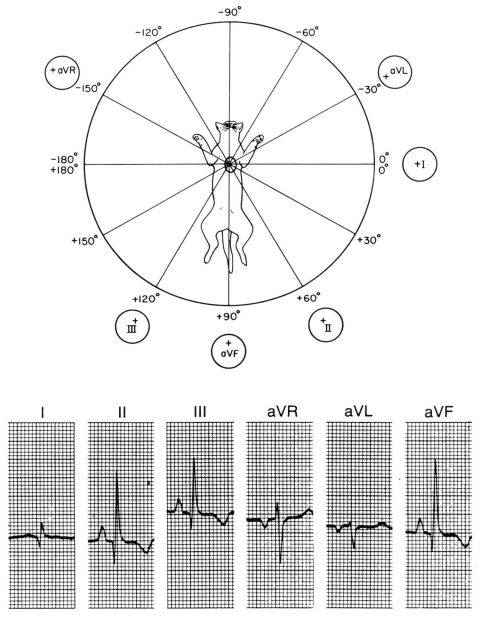

Fig. 3-1. The limb leads (I, II, III, aVR, aVL, aVF) surround the heart in the frontal plane as shown in the top part of the figure. The circled limb lead names indicate the direction of electrical activity if the QRS is positive in that lead. The mean electrical axis in this canine ECG is +90. Lead I is isoelectric. The lead perpendicular to lead I is aVF (see axis chart on top). Lead aVF is positive, making the axis +90. If lead aVF had been negative, the axis would have been −90. (From Tilley LP: Essentials of Canine and Feline Electrocardiography. 3rd Ed. Lea & Febiger, Philadelphia, 1992, with permission.)

TABLE 3-1. LEAD SYSTEMS USED IN CANINE AND FELINE
ELECTROCARDIOGRAPHY

Bipolar limb leads
    I   Right thoracic limb ($-$) compared with left thoracic limb ($+$)
   II   Right thoracic limb ($-$) compared with left pelvic limb ($+$)
  III Left thoracic limb ($-$) compared with left pelvic limb ($+$)

Augmented unipolar limb leads
    aVR Right thoracic limb ($+$) compared with average voltage of left thoracic limb and left pelvic
          limb ($-$)
    aVL Left thoracic limb ($+$) compared with average voltage of right thoracic limb and left pelvic
          limb ($-$)
    aVF Left pelvic limb ($+$) compared with average voltage of right thoracic limb and left thoracic
          limb ($-$)

Unipolar precordial chest leads plus exploring electrode located as follows
    CV_5RL (rV_2)   Right fifth intercostal space near the sternum
    CV_6LL (V_2)   Left sixth intercostal space near the sternum
    CV_6LU (V_4)   Left sixth intercostal space near the costochondral junction
    V_{10} Over the dorsal process of the seventh thoracic vertebra

Base apex bipolar lead
    Record in lead I position on ECG machine with leads placed as follows
        LA electrode over left sixth intercostal space at costosternal junction
        RA electrode over spine of right scapula near the vertebra

comparing the signal at the ($+$) limb with the average of the two other limbs ($-$).

    2. Augmented unipolar leads are helpful in calculating the mean electrical axis.

  E. Unipolar precordial chest leads
    1. Chest leads are obtained by adding a unipolar ($+$) exploring electrode attached at various places on the chest in order to encircle the heart in the sagittal or horizontal plane.
    2. Chests leads are helpful in evaluating heart enlargement patterns and identifying P waves not visible in the standard limb leads.
    3. The chest leads are recorded using the V position on the ECG machine.

  F. Base-apex bipolar lead
    1. A bipolar lead, like leads, I, II, and III. The two leads are placed over the left apex and right side of the neck, instead of on the limbs.
    2. Lead frequently used for rhythm analysis in horses.

TECHNIQUE FOR RECORDING AN ELECTROCARDIOGRAM

  I. Place the animal in right lateral recumbency. This is important for accurate evaluation of the ECG wave forms and determining the heart axis. If the animal is dyspneic and restraint may be dangerous to the patient, a rhythm strip can be obtained with the animal in any comfortable position. A standard right lateral ECG can then be performed later, when the animal is stable.

II. Part the hair and attach the ECG electrodes to the skin, just proximal to the elbows and stifles, and wet with alcohol. If there is excessive baseline motion associated with respiration, move the thoracic limb leads distal to the elbow to minimize electrode movement.

III. Hold the limbs perpendicular to the long axis of the patient and parallel to the floor. If the limbs are not parallel, the mean electrical axis will be altered.

IV. Record approximately three to four complexes in each of the six limb leads at 25 mm/sec and then run a long lead II strip at 50 mm/sec. Push the standardization button during the recording.

V. Chest leads can be obtained using the V lead while keeping the limb leads attached.

CARDIAC CONDUCTION

The ECG records the electrical activity of the heart. Electrical impulses originate in specialized pacemaker tissue in the sinus node of the right atrium. The impulse rapidly traverses the atrium, causing atrial contraction, and then slows as it passes through the AV node. Electrical activity then rapidly passes through the bundle of His, the anterior and posterior branches of the left bundle branches, the right bundle branch, and the terminal Purkinje fibers. The interventricular septum, left ventricular, and right ventricular myocardium are then activated (Fig. 3-2).

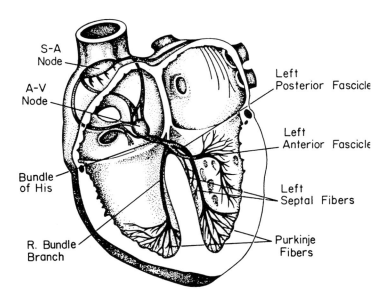

Fig. 3-2. Anatomy of the cardiac conduction system. (From Tilley LP: Essentials of Canine and Feline Electrocardiography—Interpretation and Treatment. Lea & Febiger, Philadelphia, 1985, with permission.)

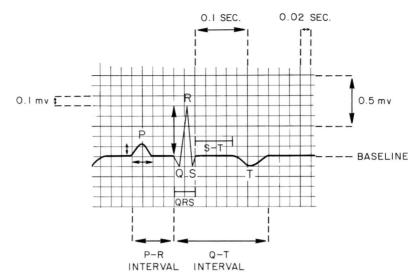

Fig. 3-3. Closeup of a normal feline lead II P-QRS-T complex with labels and intervals. Measurements for amplitude (millivolts) are indicated by positive (+) and negative (−) movement; time intervals (hundredths of a second) are indicated from left to right. Paper speed, 50 mm/s; sensitivity 1 cm = 1 mV. (From Tilley LP: Essentials of Canine and Feline Electrocardiography–Interpretation and Treatment. Lea & Febiger, Philadelphia, 1985, with permission.)

ECG WAVEFORMS (FIG. 3-3)

    I. The *P wave* reflects atrial depolarization. Note the height and width of the P wave.

    II. The *PR interval* is the time for conduction of the impulse from the SA node to the AV node and delay of the impulse in the AV node, His bundle, bundle branches, and Purkinje system. The PR interval is measured from the beginning of the P wave to the beginning of the QRS complex.

    III. The *QRS complex* indicates ventricular myocardial depolarization. Note the height and width of the QRS components.

    IV. The *Q wave* is associated with depolarization of the interventricular septum and is identified as the first negative deflection following the P wave.

    V. The *R wave* is associated with depolarization of the ventricles from the endocardium to the epicardium. The R wave is identified as the first positive deflection in the QRS complex.

    VI. The *S wave* is associated with depolarization of the basal portions of the ventricular free wall and septum. The S wave is identified as the first negative deflection following the R wave in the QRS complex. When there is a negative QRS without any positive component, this is referred to as a QS wave.

    VII. The *ST segment* is measured from the end of the S wave to the beginning of the T wave. Evaluate the degree of elevation or depression from the baseline.

VIII. The *T wave* indicates ventricular repolarization. Note the absolute height and relative height compared to the R wave.

IX. The *QT interval* indicates ventricular systole. The QT interval is measured from the beginning of the Q wave to the end of the T wave.

EVALUATING THE ELECTROCARDIOGRAM

I. Always evaluate the ECG from left to right.

II. Identify and label the ECG waveforms (P-QRS-T).

III. Calculate the approximate heart rate (HR) by counting the number of RR intervals in 3 seconds (2 sets of time markers at 50 mm/s) and multiplying by 20.

IV. Measure the height and width of the complexes. Determine the PR and QT intervals and evaluate the ST segment.

V. Determine the mean electrical axis. The easiest way to approximate the axis is to identify the isoelectric lead (sum of the positive and negative deflections of the QRS complex closest to zero). Then determine the perpendicular lead and evaluate that lead to see if the complexes are positive or negative. The axis is in the direction of the main deflection (Fig. 3-1). If all leads are isoelectric, an axis can not be determined in the frontal plane.

VI. Determine the rhythm.

VII. Compare the heart rate, rhythm, and sizes of the complexes to the normal values (Table 3-2).

EVALUATING THE ECG WAVEFORMS

Abnormalities Involving the P Waves

I. Atrial Enlargement Patterns

A. The P wave reflects atrial depolarization and is therefore used to assess atrial size.

B. Right atrial enlargement is supported by taller than normal P waves in lead II (Dog > 0.4 mV; Cat > 0.2 mV). See Fig. 3-4A.

C. Left atrial enlargement is supported by wider than normal P waves in lead II (Dog & Cat > 0.04 sec; Giant breed dogs > 0.05 s). P waves may also be notched. Notching of the P waves, without an increased width, does not support left atrial enlargement (Fig. 3-4B).

II. Absence of P waves

A. P waves are not present or visible in lead II in all cases. If P waves can not be seen, yet a sinus rhythm is suspected, check the other standard leads. If there is still no evidence of a P wave, obtain a chest lead. P waves are often visible in the chest leads, even when not visible in the limb leads.

B. The differential diagnosis for absence of P waves includes atrial standstill,

TABLE 3-2. NORMAL CANINE AND FELINE ECG VALUES[a]

	Canine	Feline
Heart Rate (HR)	Puppy: 70–220 bpm Toy breeds: 70–180 bpm Standard: 70–160 bpm Giant breeds: 60–140 bpm	120–240 bpm
Rhythm	Sinus rhythm Sinus arrhythmia Wandering pacemaker	Sinus rhythm
P Wave		
Height	Maximum: 0.4 mV	Maximum: 0.2 mV
Width	Maximum: 0.04 s (Giant breeds 0.05 s)	Maximum: 0.04 s
PR Interval	0.06–0.13 sec	0.05–0.09 s
QRS		
Height	Large Breeds: 3.0 mV maximum[b] Small Breeds: 2.5 mV maximum	Maximum: 0.9 mV
Width	Large Breeds: 0.06 s maximum Small Breeds: 0.05 s maximum	Maximum: 0.04 s
ST Segment		
Depression	no more than 0.2 mV	none
Elevation	no more than 0.15 mV	none
QT Interval	0.15–0.25 s at normal HR	0.12–0.18 s at normal HR
T Waves	May be positive, negative, or biphasic Amplitude range ± 0.05–1.0 mV in any lead Not more than 1/4 of R wave amplitude	Usually positive and < 0.3 mV
Electrical Axis	+40 to +100	0 ± 160
Chest Leads		
CV$_5$RL (rV$_2$)	T positive; R < 3.0 mV	
CV$_6$LL (V$_2$)	S < 0.8 mV; R < 3.0 mV	R < 1.0 mV
CV$_6$LU (V$_4$)	S < 0.7 mV; R < 3.0 mV	R < 1.0 mV
V$_{10}$	QRS negative; T negative except in Chihuahua	T negative. R wave/Q wave < 1

[a] Measurements are made in lead II unless otherwise stated.
[b] Not valid for thin, deep-chested dogs under 2 years of age.

silent atrium, and atrial fibrillation. These conditions are discussed later in this chapter.

III. Variation in the height of the P waves is seen with a wandering sinus pacemaker and atrial or junctional premature complexes.

Abnormalities of the PR Interval

I. Shortened PR intervals are associated with either increased levels of sympathetic tone or an accessory pathway that bypasses the AV node.

II. Prolonged PR intervals define first-degree AV block.

III. Variation in the PR interval in normally conducted beats is seen with varying levels of vagal tone. Dissociation of sinus and ventricular activity, as seen in ventricular tachycardia and AV block, will also cause variation in the PR interval.

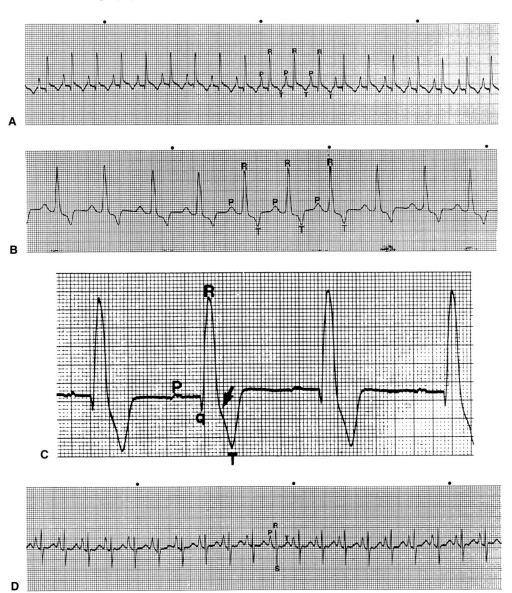

Fig. 3-4. Abnormalities in ECG waveforms. **(A)** Tall P waves in a dog with chronic bronchitis; **(B)** wide P waves in a dog with mitral valve disease; **(C)** tall and wide QRS with ST slurring in a doberman pinscher with dilated cardiomyopathy; **(D)** tall P waves and deep S waves in a cat with pulmonic stenosis; **(E)** electrical alternans in a German shepherd with pericardial effusion; **(F)** ST elevation in a dog with myocardia hypoxia under anesthesia; **(G)** ST depression in a dog with hypokalemia; **(H)** tall spiked T waves in a cat with hyperkalemia due to urethral obstruction. (*Figure continues.*)

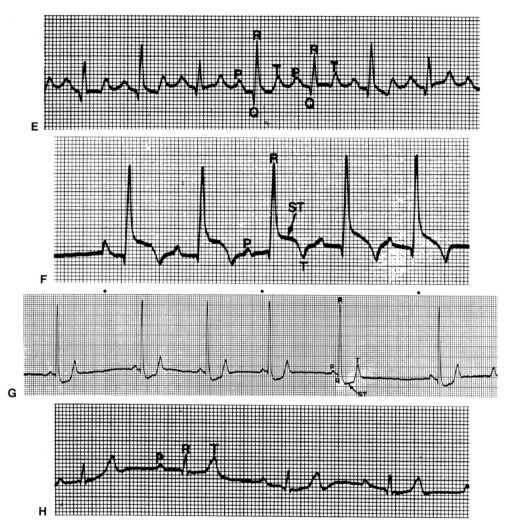

Fig. 3-4. (*Continued*).

Abnormalities of the QRS Complexes

   I. Ventricular enlargement patterns
      A. The QRS complexes reflect septal, left ventricular and right ventricular depolarization. Therefore, they are useful in evaluating ventricular size.
      B. Left ventricular enlargement criteria (Fig. 3-4C)
         1. Increased amplitude of the R waves
            a) Dog
               (1) R greater than 3.0 mV (2.5 mV in small breeds) in leads II, aVF, CV_6LU (V_4), CV_6LL (V_2) and CV_5RL (rV_2)
               (2) R greater than 1.5 mV in lead I
               (3) Sum of R wave amplitude in leads I and aVF greater than 4.0 mV
            b) Cat
               (1) R > 0.9 mV in lead II
               (2) R > 1.0 mV in CV_6LL (V_2) and CV_6LU (V_4)
               (3) R wave/Q wave > 1.0 in lead V_{10}
         2. QRS duration greater than 0.06 seconds (large dog), 0.05 seconds (small dog), or 0.04 seconds (cat)
         3. ST slurring or coving (ST segment does not flatten out at baseline)
         4. Left axis orientation (dog < +40; cat < 0)
      C. Right ventricular enlargement criteria (Fig. 3-4D)
         1. Increased amplitude of S waves
            a) Dog
               (1) S wave in leads I, II, III and aVF
               (2) S wave in lead I > 0.05 mV
               (3) S wave in lead II > 0.35 mV
               (4) S wave in lead CV_6LL (V_2) > 0.8 mV
               (5) S wave in lead CV_6LU (V_4) > 0.7 mV
            b) Cat
               (1) S wave in leads I, II, III and aVF
               (2) Prominent S waves in CV_6LL (V_2) and CV_6LU (V_4)
         2. T wave positive (except in Chihuahua) in V_{10}
         3. W-shaped QRS complex in V_{10} (dog)
         4. R:S ratio < 0.87 in CV_6LU (V_4)
         5. Right axis orientation (dog > +100; cat > +160)
  II. Differentials for wide QRS complexes
         1. Left ventricular enlargement
         2. Bundle branch blocks
         3. Ventricular premature complexes or ventricular escape beats
 III. Electrical Alternans (Fig. 3-4E)
      A. Electrical alternans is a pattern of alternating configurations of the ECG complexes. The most common pattern is a variation in the height of the QRS complexes (taller:shorter).
      B. Electrical alternans may be associated with pericardial effusion, pleural effusion, supraventricular tachycardia and alternating bundle branch block.
      C. Electrical alternans is not present in all cases of pericardial effusion.
      D. Electrical alternans is sometimes confused with ventricular bigeminy.

With ventricular bigeminy, the alternating height of the QRS complexes is due to the alternating rhythm of a sinus beat and a ventricular premature complex.

IV. Small Complexes
   A. Low amplitude complexes (R wave amplitude < 0.5 mV in lead II in dogs) may be a normal variant and can be associated with pericardial effusion, pleural effusion, pulmonary edema, hypothyroidism, obesity, pneumothorax, hypoalbuminemia, and any cause of severe myocardial damage and loss of muscle mass.
   B. Small complexes are frequently seen as a normal variant in cats.

Abnormalities of the ST Segment

I. ST Elevation (Fig. 3-4F)
   A. ST segment elevation in the dog is defined as an elevation of greater than 0.15 mV in leads II, III, aVF or those with dominant R waves. Any elevation of the ST segment in cats is abnormal.
   B. ST segment elevation is seen with myocardial hypoxia, pericardial effusion and pericarditis. Digitalis toxicity can cause ST segment elevation in cats. Transmural myocardial infarction causes ST segment elevation in leads overlying the infarcted myocardium.
II. ST Depression (Fig. 3-4G)
   A. ST segment depression in the dog is defined as a depression of greater than 0.2 mV in leads II, III, aVF or those with dominant R waves. Any depression of the ST segment in cats is abnormal.
   B. ST segment depression is seen with myocardial hypoxia, hyperkalemia or hypokalemia, and digitalis toxicity. Subendocardial myocardial infarction causes ST segment depression in leads overlying the infarcted myocardium.
   C. Pseudodepression due to prominent T_a waves (atrial repolarization), caused by atrial disease or tachycardia also causes ST segment depression.
III. Miscellaneous ST changes
   A. ST segment changes can occur secondary to bundle branch blocks, myocardial hypertrophy and ventricular premature complexes. The changes in the ST segment are in opposite direction from the main QRS deflection. The ST segment change in these conditions is often one of slurring or coving of the S wave into the T wave.
   B. Artifact related to baseline motion
   C. Normal variant

Abnormalities of the QT Interval

I. QT interval changes are relatively nonspecific. The QT interval is inversely related to the heart rate; it is shorter with more rapid heart rates. As a rule of thumb, the QT interval should be less than ½ the preceding RR interval.

II. QT prolongation is associated with hypokalemia, hypocalcemia, hypothermia, quinidine administration, interventricular conduction disturbances that are associated with prolongation of the QRS complexes, bradycardia, ethylene glycol toxicity, strenuous exercise, and central nervous system disturbances.

III. QT shortening is associated with hypercalcemia, hyperkalemia, and digitalis.

Abnormalities Involving the T Waves

I. T wave changes are relatively nonspecific. In dogs, the T wave should not be more than $\frac{1}{4}$ the height of the associated R wave (Q wave, if Q larger than R), or amplitude ± 0.5 to 1.0 mV in any lead.

II. In most leads, T waves may be positive, negative, or biphasic, but should not change polarity on serial electrocardiograms. T waves should be positive in CV_5RL in dogs over 2 months of age and should be negative in V_{10}, except in the Chihuahua.

III. Large T waves can be seen with myocardial hypoxia, interventricular conduction disturbances, ventricular enlargement, and in animals with heart disease and bradycardia.

IV. Large and sharply pointed T waves are associated with hyperkalemia (Fig. 3-4H).

V. Small, biphasic T waves can be seen with hypokalemia.

VI. Nonspecific T wave changes can be seen secondary to metabolic disturbances (hypoglycemia, anemia, shock, fever), drug toxicity (digitalis, quinidine, procainamide), and neurologic disease.

VII. T wave alternans (alternating positive and negative T waves) has been reported secondary to hypocalcemia, high levels of circulating catecholamines, and sudden increase in sympathetic tone.

ARRHYTHMIAS AND CONDUCTION DISTURBANCES

I. Definition

An arrhythmia is any disturbance in the normal rhythm of the heart. Irregularities in rhythm are due to abnormalities in impulse formation, conduction, or both. These abnormalities can occur within the sinus node, atria, AV node, bundle branches, and ventricles. See Table 3-3 for the classification of arrhythmias used for this chapter.

II. Systematic approach to arrhythmia recognition

A. Determine atrial (P waves) and ventricular (QRS complexes) rates. They should be the same and within the established range for the species and breed.

B. Determine if P waves are present.

1. Is there a P wave related to each ventricular complex? If not, an arrhythmia or conduction disturbance is present.

2. Does the P wave precede or follow the QRS complex? If P waves follow

TABLE 3-3. CLASSIFICATION OF CARDIAC ARRHYTHMIAS

Normal sinus impulse formation
    Normal sinus rhythm
    Sinus arrhythmia
    Wandering sinus pacemaker
Disturbances of sinus impulse formation
    Sinus arrest
    Sinus bradycardia
    Sinus tachycardia
Disturbances of supraventricular impulse formation
    Atrial premature complexes
    Atrial tachycardia
    Atrial flutter
    Atrial fibrillation
    Atrioventricular junctional rhythm
Disturbances of ventricular impulse formation
    Ventricular premature complexes
    Ventricular tachycardia
    Ventricular asystole
    Ventricular fibrillation
Disturbances of impulse conduction
    Sinoatrial block
    Persistent atrial standstill ("silent" atrium)
    Atrial standstill (hyperkalemia)
    Ventricular pre-excitation
    First-degree AV block
    Second-degree AV block
    Complete AV block (third degree)
    Bundle branch blocks
Disturbances of both impulse formation and impulse conduction
    Sick sinus syndrome
    Ventricular pre-excitation and the Wolff-Parkinson White (WPW) syndrome
    Atrial premature complexes with aberrant ventricular conduction
Escape rhythms
    Junctional escape rhythms
    Ventricular escape rhythms (idioventricular rhythm)

the QRS complex, the animal probably has junctional or ventricular premature complexes.

3. Are there any P waves with no subsequent QRS complexes? If so, the animal has either an AV nodal conduction disturbance or blocked atrial premature complexes.

C. Determine the PP intervals.

1. Are they regular? If so, the rhythm is sinus rhythm or junctional.

2. Are they regularly irregular and varying with respiration? If so, the rhythm is a sinus arrhythmia.

3. Are there long pauses between some of the P waves to suggest sinus arrest or sinus block?

4. Are they regular with some coming early? If so, the animal has atrial premature complexes.

D. Determine the PR interval.

1. Is it constant? Variable PR intervals can be seen with increased vagal tone and arrhythmias that result in AV dissociation.

2. Is the duration normal? If shortened, the animal may have pre-excita-

tion. If prolonged, the AV node may be diseased or conduction slowed from high vagal tone or drugs such as digoxin.
  E. Determine the width of QRS complexes.
    1. Is it normal?
    2. Are all QRS complexes identical and normal in contour? If not, the animal probably has a ventricular arrhythmia or intermittent bundle branch block.
    3. Are there any QRS complexes without P waves? If so, do they appear after a pause, suggesting an escape beat, or prematurely, suggesting a ventricular premature complex?
  F. Determine the RR intervals.
    1. Irregularly irregular intervals are generally abnormal.
    2. Regular intervals do not rule out an arrhythmia. Ventricular tachycardia and atrial tachycardia are generally regular.
  G. Note morphology, frequency, and repetitiveness of any premature beats.

Normal Sinus Impulse Formation

  I. Normal sinus rhythm
    A. Definition: Regular impulse formation beginning in the sinus node at frequencies between 60 and 180 bpm in the adult dog and between 120 and 240 bpm in the cat. Normal heart rate ranges vary some in dogs depending on age and breed. See Table 3-2 for more detailed normal rate ranges.
    B. ECG features (Fig. 3-5A): The rhythm is regular with RR interval variation less than 10 percent. A QRS complex is associated with each P wave.
    C. Sinus nodal discharge rate varies significantly and depends on many factors, including age, physical activity, and autonomic tone. Vagal stimulation decreases spontaneous discharge rate and predominates over steady sympathetic stimulation.
  II. Sinus arrhythmia
    A. Definition: Variation in sinus rhythm related to respiration and resulting from vagal tone inhibition. Heart rate increases with inspiration and decreases with expiration. The slowing-speeding pattern can be striking in some patients.
    B. ECG features: Same as for sinus rhythm except RR interval variation is greater than 10 percent.
    C. Causes: Normal variant in dogs associated with changes in vagal tone. Conditions that increase vagal tone (respiratory disease, some neurologic diseases, some gastrointestinal diseases, pressure on vagus) will increase irregularity of rhythm.
    D. Significance: Normal in dogs; unusual rhythm in congestive heart failure; generally abnormal in cats.
  III. Wandering sinus pacemaker
    A. Definition: Site of impulse formation shifts within the SA node or to an atrial focus or AV node.
    B. ECG features: P wave changes configuration and sometimes direction

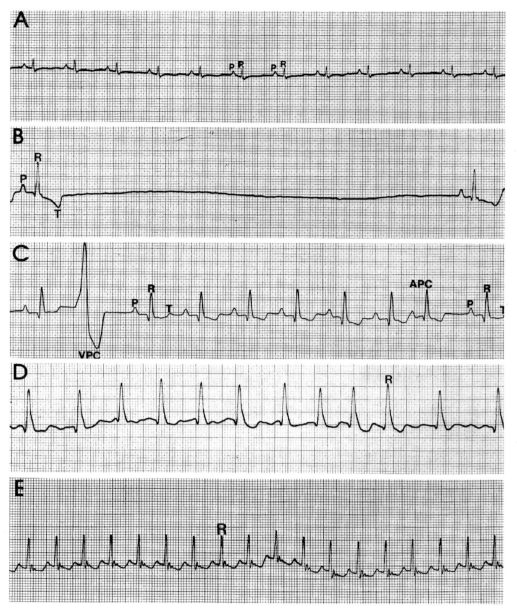

Fig. 3-5. Common arrhythmias in the dog and cat. Lead II rhythm strips, paper speed of 50 mm/sec; 1 cm = 1 mV. **(A)** Sinus rhythm in the cat; **(B)** sinoatrial block or arrest (sick sinus syndrome) in the miniature schnauzer; **(C)** atrial and ventricular premature complexes in a dog; **(D)** atrial fibrillation in a dog; **(E)** supraventricular tachycardia in a cat with hyperthyroidism; **(F)** ventricular pre-excitation in a cat; **(G)** second-degree AV block in a dog; **(H)** complete AV block in a dog; **(I)** ventricular tachycardia in a dog; **(J)** ventricular fibrillation in a dog. (Modified from Tilley LP, Miller MS: Antiarrhythmic drugs and management of cardiac arrhythmias. In Kirk RW (ed): Current Veterinary Therapy. WB Saunders, Philadelphia, 1985, with permission.) (*Figure continues.*)

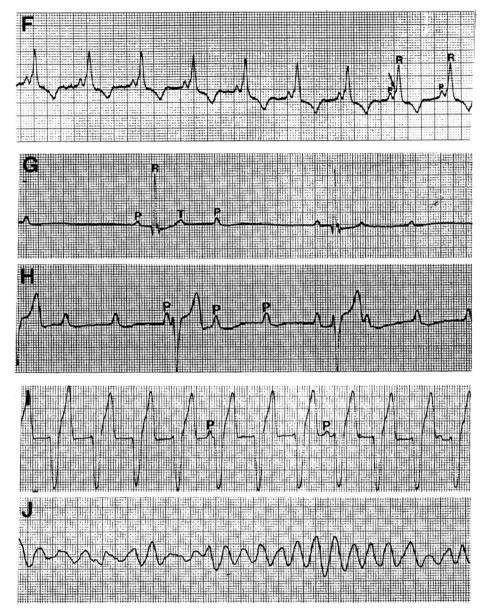

Fig. 3-5. (*Continued*).

indicative of change of site of pacing stimulus. May have no P wave if it "wanders" into junctional tissue.

C. Significance: Generally normal variation in dogs, often associated with sinus arrhythmia.

DISTURBANCES OF SINUS IMPULSE FORMATION

I. Sinus arrest
 A. Definition: Prolonged failure of sinus node automaticity.
 B. ECG features (Fig. 3-5B): Entire P-QRS-T complex dropped, resulting in RR interval greater than twice the normal interval; junctional or ventricular escape beats may occur. Sometimes indistinguishable from sinus block on surface ECG.
 C. Causes: Vagal stimulation, certain drugs, sick sinus syndrome (SSS)
 D. Significance: Not of clinical importance unless associated with signs of decreased cardiac output (exercise intolerance, weakness, collapse).
II. Sinus bradycardia
 A. Definition and ECG features: A regular sinus rhythm with a heart rate below 70 bpm in the dog (60 bpm in giant breeds) and below 120 bpm in the cat.
 B. Causes
  1. Physiologic: increased vagal tone, conditioned athletes
  2. Drugs: propranolol, digitalis, some anesthetics (xylazine, acepromazine)
  3. Pathologic: hypothermia, hypothyroidism, hyperkalemia, SSS, increased intracranial pressure
 C. Significance: None unless associated with clinical signs of weakness or collapse.
III. Sinus tachycardia
 A. Definition and ECG features: A regular sinus rhythm with a heart rate above 160 bpm in adult dogs (220 bpm in puppies, 180 bpm in toy breeds, and 140 bpm in giant breeds) and above 240 bpm in cats.
 B. Causes
  1. Physiologic: exercise, pain, restraint
  2. Drugs: atropine, epinephrine, bronchodilators
  3. Pathologic: fever, shock, hyperthyroidism, anemia, hypoxia, congestive heart failure
 C. Significance: Underlying cause should be identified and corrected or treated. Treatment of sinus tachycardia with antiarrhythmic drugs is generally limited to patients in CHF.

DISTURBANCES OF SUPRAVENTRICULAR IMPULSE FORMATION

I. Atrial Premature Complexes (APCs)
 A. Definition: Premature atrial beats that originate outside the SA node and disrupt the normal sinus rhythm for one or more beats.

B. ECG features (Fig. 3-5C)
   1. Ectopic P' wave is premature; its configuration often differs from sinus P waves.
   2. QRS complex is premature and its configuration usually normal.
   3. If premature impulse arrives at the ventricles at a time when they are refractory to depolarizing excitation, a nonconducted (blocked) APC occurs; no QRS follows the P wave, which is usually identified in the ST segment or T wave of the preceding beat.
   4. May originate from multiple sites; multifocal APCs.
   5. A noncompensatory pause generally follows APCs, resulting in normal RR interval between the APC and subsequent beat.
C. Causes: Cardiomyopathy, valvular heart disease, atrial neoplasia, chronic obstructive pulmonary disease (COPD), hypoxia, autonomic influence.
D. Significance: Incidental or may herald a more serious arrhythmia to follow.

II. Atrial Tachycardia
A. Definition: A paroxysmal supraventricular tachycardia where the P wave configuration differs from the sinus P waves
B. ECG features
   1. Rate is rapid.
   2. Atrial beats tend to occur regularly.
   3. Ventricular depolarization generally follows the usual pathways; QRS morphology is normal.
   4. In multifocal atrial tachycardia, rhythm is irregular.
   5. Onset usually sudden, often initiated by an APC.
      Note: Not always an abnormality of impulse formation, may be result of an AV nodal re-entry mechanism (conduction abnormality).
C. Causes: Stress, hypoxia, hypokalemia, primary cardiac problems (including congenital heart disease), cardiomyopathy, valvular heart disease, Wolff-Parkinson-White Syndrome, hyperthyroidism, systemic hypertension, cor pulmonale, digitalis.
D. Significance: Depends on severity of signs and symptoms. Can cause exercise intolerance, weakness, and collapse.

III. Atrial Flutter
A. Definition: Rapid atrial rate of greater than 250 bpm where atrial repolarization is altered, resulting in bidirectional saw-toothed atrial complexes, designated as F waves. Ventricular rate depends on degree of physiologic AV block present.
B. Causes: Valvular disease, cardiomyopathy, digitalis; rarely occurs in absence of organic heart disease.
C. Significance: The more rapid the ventricular rate, the more serious the hemodynamic consequences; can be difficult to differentiate from atrial fibrillation.

IV. Atrial fibrillation
A. Definition: Numerous unorganized ectopic foci in the atria discharge impulses at very high rates causing uncoordinated activity of the atria and loss of effective muscular propulsive movement (''atrial kick'').

    B. ECG features (Fig. 3-5D)
       1. Atrial complexes appear as erratic f (fibrillatory) waves.
       2. The f waves create continuous, irregular undulations of the baseline.
       3. Ventricular response irregularly irregular and generally rapid.
    C. Causes: Cardiac valve disorders, cardiomyopathy, CHF, thyrotoxicosis, congenital heart disease, certain drugs.
    D. Significance: Loss of effective atrial pumping action, reducing cardiac efficiency and cardiac output as much as 15 to 30 percent.
  V. Junctional premature complexes
    A. Definition: Abnormal acceleration of automaticity produces an early beat in the AV junction
    B. ECG features
       1. P wave occurs before, during, or after QRS complex.
       2. QRS complex premature but normal morphology.
    C. Causes: Same as APCs
    D. Significance: Same as APCs
 VI. Junctional tachycardia
    A. Definition: Ectopic focus in the AV junction acts as the primary pacemaker
    B. ECG features
       1. P waves usually inverted.
       2. P waves may precede, be superimposed on, or follow the QRS complex.
       3. Heart rate over 60 bpm (term *enhanced AV junctional rhythm* used for rates greater than 60 but less than 100 bpm).
    C. Causes: Most common is digitalis toxicity, CHF, infarction, or inflammatory disease of the heart.
 VII. Supraventricular tachycardia
    A. Definition: Term applied to rapid rates when sinus tachycardia, atrial tachycardia, and AV junctional tachycardia may be difficult to distinguish.
    B. ECG features (Fig. 3-5E)
       1. P waves blend with T waves.
       2. QRS configuration is normal.

DISTURBANCES OF IMPULSE CONDUCTION

  I. Sinoatrial block
    A. Definition: Sinus node discharges but impulse is blocked and dissipates within the sinus node itself.
    B. ECG features (Fig. 3-5B): Absence of an entire P-QRS-T complex; subsequent beats pick up without change to cadence.
    C. Causes: Vagal stimulation, certain drugs, SSS
    D. Significance: Generally none unless associated with symptoms of decreased cardiac output.
  II. Atrial standstill (hyperkalemia)
    A. Definition: Inhibition of atrial myocardial depolarization secondary to hyperkalemia ($K+ > 8.5$ mEq/L).

B. ECG features: Disappearance of P waves with a slow idioventricular rhythm characterized by wide and bizarre QRS complexes

C. Causes: Addison's disease, anuric or oliguric renal failure, uncontrolled diabetic ketoacidosis, metabolic acidosis, urethral obstruction, ruptured bladder

D. Comment: Distinguish from "silent atrium" (persistent atrial standstill)—a diffuse myocardial disorder associated with various types of muscular dystrophy in dogs (most common in the English springer spaniel) and cardiomyopathy in cats

II. Ventricular pre-excitation syndrome

  A. Definition: An atrial bypass tract outside the AV junction connects the atrium to the ventricle or bundle of His, short-circuiting the AV node, which results in premature activation of the ventricles. Conduction occurs through both the bypass tract and the AV node simultaneously. Conduction can be antegrade or retrograde through the bypass tract and AV node (Table 3-4).

  B. ECG features (Fig. 3-5F)

    1. Abnormally short PR interval.

    2. If the bypass tract circumvents both the AV node and the bundle of His, early activation of the ventricles causes a slurring of the QRS (delta wave). Patients with Wolff-Parkinson-White Syndrome usually have delta waves when not tachycardic.

  C. Causes: Congenital, feline hypertrophic cardiomyopathy (HCM).

  D. Significance: No clinical consequence unless tachycardia develops. Not all patients with pre-excitation have tachycardic episodes.

III. First-degree AV block

  A. Definition: Delayed conduction velocity through the AV node

  B. ECG: Prolongation of the PR interval; in the dog greater than 0.13 seconds, in the cat greater than 0.09 seconds

  C. Causes: Drug therapy, chronic degenerative disease of the conduction system, electrolyte imbalance, vagal stimulation

  D. Significance: None but may be harbinger of a more serious form of conduction disorder.

TABLE 3-4. SUMMARY OF PRE-EXCITATION SYNDROME

Cardiac Sequence	Mechanism	ECG
1. Sinus impulse	Normal	—
2. Atrial depolarization	Normal	Normal P wave
3. AV node accessory pathways	Relatively rapid conduction, skirting the A-V nodal system	Short PR interval
4. Early ventricular depolarization	One ventricle activated early	Initial QRS slurred (delta wave) (∴ widened QRS)
5. Retrograde conduction from ventricles to atria	Atrial re-entry impulse	Tendency to supraventricular paroxysmal arrhythmias
6. Late ventricular depolarization	Fusion between normal and anomalous ventricular activation	Delay, often with altered direction, of terminal QRS

IV. Second-degree AV block
    A. Definition: Intermittent failure or disturbance of AV conduction, resulting in absence of ventricular activation
    B. ECG features: One or more P waves not followed by QRS complexes
    C. Various forms
        1. Mobitz Type I (Wenckebach): progressively increasing or decreasing PR intervals interrupted by periodic blocked sinus beats
        2. Mobitz Type II (Fig. 3-5G)
            a) Conducted beats have a constant PR interval until a dropped beat occurs without warning.
            b) May have a fixed ratio of atrial to ventricular contractions, i.e., 2:1, 3:2. Advanced second-degree AV block occurs when two or more consecutive P waves are blocked.
    D. Causes: May be normal, increased vagal tone, fibrosis, certain drugs (digoxin, beta-blockers, calcium channel blockers, xylazine), electrolyte imbalances
    E. Significance: Mobitz Type II is often associated with organic disease of the conduction pathways. May progress to complete heart block.
 V. Third-degree AV block (complete heart block)
    A. Definition: All atrial impulses are blocked at the AV junction, and the atria and ventricles beat independently. A secondary "escape" pacemaker site (junctional or ventricular) stimulates the ventricles.
    B. ECG features (Fig. 3-5H)
        1. No relation between P waves and QRS complexes.
        2. QRS complex configuration depends on location of subsidiary pacemaker origin.
        3. Ventricular rate is generally slow and less than the sinus rate.
    C. Causes: Digitalis toxicity, infiltrative disease, neoplasia, amyloid, idiopathic fibrosis, infectious disease such as Lyme disease, hyperkalemia
    D. Significance: Frequently associated with signs of weakness, lethargy, and syncope. If symptomatic, a permanent cardiac pacemaker is required
VII. Left bundle branch block (LBBB)
    A. Definition: A conduction delay or block in both the left posterior and left anterior fascicles of the left bundle. A supraventricular impulse activates the right ventricle first through the right bundle branch. Left ventricle is activated late.
    B. ECG features
        1. QRS prolonged (greater than 0.08 seconds in the dog, greater than 0.06 seconds in the cat).
        2. QRS wide and positive in Leads I, II, III and aVF
        3. May be confused with ventricular ectopic beats
        4. Must differentiate from left ventricular enlargement
    C. Causes: Cardiomyopathy, congenital defects, neoplasia, trauma, fibrosis
    D. Significance: Does not cause hemodynamic compromise but is an indication of extensive disruption of the conduction pathways because of the large size of the thick left bundle branch

VIII. Left anterior fascicular block (LAFB)
  A. Definition: Block in conduction through the left anterior fascicle of the left bundle branch, altering activation sequence in the left ventricle
  B. ECG features
    1. QRS width normal
    2. Left axis deviation (Dog < +40, Cat < 0)
    3. Small q and tall R in leads I and aVL (small q not essential)
    4. Deep S wave in leads II, III, and aVF (exceeding the R wave)
  C. Causes
    1. Associated conditions: Hypertrophic cardiomyopathy, causes of left ventricular hypertrophy or hyperkalemia, ischemic cardiomyopathy, and cardiac surgery
    2. Must differentiate from left ventricular enlargement, altered position of the heart within the thorax, hyperkalemia, and ventricular pre-excitation
  D. Significance: Not associated with clinical signs
IX. Right bundle branch block (RBBB)
  A. Definition: A block in the right bundle branch resulting in late depolarizing of the right ventricle
  B. ECG
    1. QRS wide as in LBBB.
    2. QRS complexes have large, wide S wave in Leads I, II, III and aVF
  C. Causes: May be normal, congenital heart disease, valvular disease, cardiac neoplasia, Chagas disease, heartworm, acute pulmonary embolism, hypokalemia
  D. Significance: Does not cause hemodynamic problems; more vulnerable to adverse physiologic and pathologic factors than LBBB because of its smaller size. (Note: Block in all three major ventricular pathways results in complete AV block)

DISTURBANCES OF VENTRICULAR IMPULSE FORMATION

I. Ventricular Premature Complexes (VPCs)
  A. Definition: An ectopic beat originating in the ventricles and occurring earlier than the normally expected beat, often followed by a compensatory pause. The compensatory pause following the VPC allows the next sinus beat to occur where it would have occurred without the VPC. This is in contrast to the noncompensatory pause following APCs.
  B. Terminology
    1. Unifocal: arising from same ectopic focus
    2. Multifocal (multiform): arising from two different ventricular sites—a more ominous sign
    3. Interpolated: occurring without interfering with the normal cardiac cycle
    4. Fusion beat: an impulse from the SA node and a late VPC simultaneously activate the ventricles

    C. ECG features (Fig. 3-5C)
      1. No P wave associated with VPC
      2. QRS wide and bizarre
      3. Altered ST segment and T wave form
    D. Causes: Cardiac including CHF, cardiomyopathy, neoplasia, traumatic myocarditis, inherited in young German shepherds, idiopathic in boxers; secondary to hypoxia, anemia, uremia, gastric dilatation volvulus, pancreatitis, Lyme disease; drugs (digitalis, atropine, anesthetics)
    E. Significance
      1. May be none depending on how well the ventricle functions and how long the arrhythmia lasts
      2. Decreased cardiac output because of decreased filling time for the ventricles
      3. Generally more serious if occurs in presence of heart disease
      4. VPC patterns that require special attention
        a) Couplet or pair is two VPCs; a salvo or run is three VPCs or more
        b) Bigeminy: every other beat is a VPC
        c) Multiform
        d) R-on-T phenomenon: VPC falls on preceding beat's T wave; occurs during the cardiac cell's relative refractory (vulnerable) period, which increases risk for development of ventricular tachycardia or fibrillation
  II. Ventricular tachycardia
    A. Definitions: Runs of ventricular premature complexes occurring in succession at a rate usually above 100 bpm. Accelerated idioventricular rhythm used when rate is greater than 50 bpm and less than 100 bpm. May be intermittent or sustained.
    B. ECG features (Fig. 3-5I)
      1. P waves are not associated with QRS complexes.
      1. P waves usually not visible; if seen are normal.
      2. QRS complex wide and bizarre.
    C. Causes: Same as for VPCs
    D. Significance: Usually a manifestation of significant organic heart disease. May be life threatening. The reduction in cardiac output, resulting from the arrhythmia, depends on the heart rate and condition of the heart.
 III. Ventricular flutter
    A. Definition: An extremely rapid form of ventricular tachycardia with a regular up and down wavy pattern; often appears as transient state between ventricular tachycardia and ventricular fibrillation
    B. ECG features
      1. No P waves
      2. QRS indistinct, usually wide and continuous in a zigzag pattern
      3. ST segment and T waves not discernible
    C. Causes: Same as VPCs, R-on-T phenomenon
    D. Significance: life threatening
 IV. Ventricular fibrillation
    A. Definition: Rapid, disorganized depolarization of the ventricles characterized by a lack of organized electrical impulse, conduction, and ventricular contraction

B. ECG features (Fig. 3-5J)
  1. P, QRS, T not discernible
  2. Wavy undulating baseline
     a) Large waves indicate coarse fibrillation
     b) Small waves indicate fine fibrillation.
C. Causes: Shock, anoxia, electric shock, electrolyte imbalance, hypothermia, untreated ventricular tachycardia
D. Signs: Loss of consciousness; absent pulse, heart sounds, and blood pressure; dilated pupils
E. Significance: Unless converted to a higher order of rhythm, death will ensue

V. Ventricular asystole (arrest or standstill)
  A. Definition: A total absence of ventricular electrical activity
  B. ECG features
    1. P waves may or may not be present.
    2. QRS-T is absent.
  C. Causes: Severe metabolic disturbance, acute respiratory failure, extensive myocardial damage
  D. Significance: Represents a dying heart unless CPR successful

DISTURBANCES OF BOTH IMPULSE FORMATION AND IMPULSE CONDUCTION

I. Sick sinus syndrome (SSS)
  A. Definition: Term applied to a syndrome that encompasses a number of sinus nodal abnormalities, including sinus bradycardia, sinus arrest, sinoatrial block, alternating bradycardia-tachycardia, and combinations of SA or AV conduction disturbances; more than one of these may be recorded from the same patient on different occasions
  B. Common in miniature schnauzers, cocker spaniels, dachshunds, pugs, and West Highland white terriers; most common in older females
  C. Causes: Ischemia, inflammation, fibrosis, metastatic disease, idiopathic, hereditary
  D. Symptoms: Lethargy, weakness, syncope

II. Pre-excitation with re-entrant tachycardia (Wolff-Parkinson-White syndrome)
  A. Definition: A re-entrant supraventricular tachycardia that results from a circuit developing between the ventricular bypass tract and the AV node. Conduction can occur retrograde or antegrade through the AV node.
  B. ECG features
    1. Antegrade conduction through the AV node results in a narrow, complex tachycardia with the complexes looking like supraventricular complexes.
    2. Retrograde conduction through the AV node results in a wide, complex tachycardia that could be confused for ventricular tachycardia.
  C. Causes: Same as pre-excitation.
  D. Significance: Tachycardia can cause weakness and collapse.

III. Atrial premature complexes with aberrant conduction
  A. Aberrant conduction occurs when a premature beat fails to conduct through a bundle branch that is in an absolute or relative refractory period.
  B. Aberrant conduction is more common at slower heart rates. Aberrant complexes usually have a right bundle branch block pattern, because of the longer refractory period of the right bundle branch cells.
  C. Aberrant beats are frequently confused for VPCs. An aberrantly conducted beat will have an associated P wave with a normal or slightly prolonged PR interval. VPCs do not have associated P waves with consistent PR intervals. Determine if the pause following the premature complex has a compensatory (VPC) or noncompensatory (APC) pause.

Escape Rhythms

  I. Junctional escape beat
  A. Definition: With depression of sinus impulse formation (or conduction), a latent automatic focus in the AV junction initiates a late-appearing impulse
  B. ECG features: P waves inverted, occurring before or after the QRS complex, hidden in the QRS complex, or absent
  C. Significance: Serve as safety feature, should never be suppressed
 II. Junctional rhythm (nodal)
  A. Definition: Junctional escape beats occur in succession if sinus node slowing is sustained or if sinus arrest occurs
  B. ECG features: Generally occur at a rate of 40 to 60 bpm unless accelerated
  C. Causes: Digitalis toxicity, hypoxia, vagal stimulation
  D. Significance: Underlying cause should be treated
III. Ventricular escape beat
  A. Definition: Complex that arises after failure of supraventricular pacemaker drive, or from failure of transmission of a supraventricular impulse to the ventricles
  B. ECG features
    1. Occurs after prolonged pause
    2. P waves usually not present
    3. QRS altered contour and duration
  C. Significance: Compensatory mechanism—do not suppress; hemodynamic state may be altered secondary to slow rate with signs of decreased cardiac output
IV. Ventricular escape rhythm (idioventricular rhythm)
  A. Definition and ECG features: Series of ventricular escape complexes occurring at a regular interval, with a rate of less than 60 bpm in dogs and 100 bpm in cats
  B. Significance: Same as ventricular escape beats

Miscellaneous

  I. Cardiopulmonary arrest
  A. Definition: Abrupt cessation of cardiac output with subsequent loss of effective tissue perfusion.

B. ECG features
1. Ventricular fibrillation
2. Ventricular flutter (pulseless)
3. Ventricular asystole
4. Electromechanical dissociation: recognizable QRS complexes with absence of arterial pulses and blood pressure
C. Causes: anesthetics; toxemia; CNS trauma; acid-base, electrolyte, and autonomic imbalances; respiratory failure due to airway obstruction, suffocation, severe respiratory disease; cardiovascular collapse

II. Artificial pacemaker
A. Definition: Electronic impulse provided by an artificial pacemaker that protects against excessive slowing of the heart beat
B. ECG features: Pacemaker impulse appears as a vertical line (pacemaker spike); capture occurs when followed by a wide, bizarre QRS complex (ventricular pacing)
C. Indications: SSS, advanced second-degree or complete heart block, persistent atrial standstill

III. Other complex rhythms (see Suggested Readings)
A. Parasystole: A parallel pacemaker that operates independently but concurrently with the dominant rhythm. The dominant rhythm is usually sinus while the parasystolic rhythm may be of atrial, junctional, or ventricular origin.
B. Ashman's phenomenon: Tendency of premature supraventricular beats to have aberrant ventricular conduction when a short cycle follows a long one. May be confused with pathologic ectopic beats and treated inappropriately with antiarrhythmic drugs.

SUGGESTED READINGS

Bonagura JD: Cardiovascular diseases. In Sherding RG (ed): The Cat, Diseases and Clinical Management. Churchill Livingstone, New York, 1989

Braunwald E (ed): Heart Disease: A Textbook of Cardiovascular Medicine. 4th Ed. WB Saunders, Philadelphia, 1992

Edwards NJ: Bolton's Handbook of Canine and Feline Electrocardiography. 2nd Ed. WB Saunders, Philadelphia, 1987

Ettinger SJ, Suter PF: Canine Cardiology. WB Saunders, Philadelphia, 1970

Fox PR (ed): Canine and Feline Cardiology. Churchill Livingstone, New York, 1988

Hamlin RL (ed): Efficacy of Cardiac Therapy. Vet Clin North Am (Small Anim Pract) 21:5. WB Saunders, Philadelphia, 1991

Harpster NK: The cardiovascular system. In Holzworth J (ed): Diseases of the Cat, Medicine and Surgery. WB Saunders, Philadelphia, 1987

Jaffee AS (Chairman): Textbook of Advanced Cardiac Life Support. American Heart Association, 1987

Morgan RV (ed): Handbook of Small Animal Practice. 2nd Ed. Churchill Livingstone, New York, 1992

Murtaugh RJ, Kaplan PM: Veterinary Emergency and Critical Care Medicine. Mosby-Year Book, St. Louis, 1992

Phillips RE, Feeney MK: The Cardiac Rhythms. 2nd Ed. WB Saunders, Philadelphia, 1980

Tilley LP: Essentials of Canine and Feline Electrocardiography. 3rd Ed. Lea & Febiger, Philadelphia, 1992

Tilley LP, Miller MS, Smith FW, Jr: Canine and Feline Cardiac Arrhythmias: Self-Assessment. Lea & Febiger, Philadelphia, 1993

4

Echocardiography and Doppler Ultrasound

Rosemary A. Henik

INTRODUCTION

Echocardiography, or cardiac ultrasound, has been used clinically in veterinary medicine for approximately 15 years to noninvasively evaluate cardiac anatomy and function. Conventional echocardiographic modalities include both two-dimensional and M-mode echo. Two-dimensional (2-D) echocardiography is used to qualitatively assess the heart and pericardial space, and M-mode echocardiography provides quantitative information in systole and diastole and permits indices of myocardial function to be calculated.

Although anatomic information is obtained with conventional echo, valvular or shunting lesions, especially if mild, cannot be documented or quantitated without invasive diagnostic studies such as cardiac catheterization. Doppler echo identifies blood flow direction, velocity, and turbulence, and permits quantitative analysis of valvular regurgitation, valvular stenosis, and shunts.

All 3 modalities of echocardiography that will be discussed (M-mode, 2-D, and Doppler) are used in concert to both diagnose cardiac disease and monitor response to therapy. Their utility depends on accurate assessment of the patient's history, physical examination, thoracic radiographs, and other diagnostic tests. In addition, the experienced echocardiographer with a thorough understanding of cardiac anatomy, cardiac diseases of dogs and cats, and supplemental diagnostic tests will gain the most benefit from the echocardiographic examination.

ECHOCARDIOGRAPHIC DISPLAYS

I. Two-dimensional (2-D) echocardiography, also known as real-time echocardiography, sector scanning, or cross-sectional echocardiography, records a planar image of the heart.
   A. Advantages
      1. It provides an anatomically correct and easily understood view of the heart, and anatomic relationships between structures are readily defined.
      2. The identification of masses, valves, great vessels, and wall motion abnormalities are more readily appreciated using 2-D compared with M-mode echocardiography.

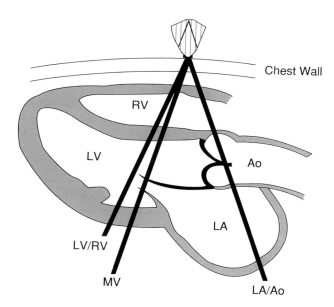

Fig. 4-1. Schematic drawing of a two-dimensional echocardiographic view of the heart in the right parasternal long-axis plane, demonstrating the placement of the cursor for M-mode measurements. Left ventricular (LV) and right ventricular (RV) wall and lumen measurements are made with the cursor in the LV/RV position. Mitral valve (MV) measurements are made with the cursor in the MV position, and aortic (Ao) and left atrial (LA) measurements are made in the LA/Ao position.

3. It allows superior evaluation of the right ventricle, right atrium, and left atrium compared with M-mode.
4. It is more sensitive and specific for diagnosing pericardial effusion and cardiac tamponade than M-mode echocardiography.
5. It facilitates cursor placement for M-mode echocardiographic quantitation (Fig. 4-1).

B. Disadvantages
1. The interfaces between various tissue densities (e.g., fluid and muscle) are not as sharply delineated with 2-D compared with M-mode echocardiography, and therefore measurement of wall thickness is more difficult.
2. Accurate end-systolic and end-diastolic chamber and wall dimensions are often difficult to determine, since multiple cardiac cycles are not seen on the oscilloscope simultaneously.

II. M (Motion)-mode echocardiography displays signals caused by echogenic tissues at known depths, and gives an "ice-pick" view of the heart. Time on the X-axis is plotted against points of varying intensity or brightness on the Y-axis as a result of reflection from tissue interfaces.

A. Advantages
1. Quantitative measurements of chamber dimensions, wall thicknesses, and valvular motion are performed in M-mode.

    2. Functional indices, such as shortening fraction, can be calculated from dimension measurements.

    3. Wall and chamber interfaces are more easily delineated than with 2-D echocardiography.

    4. Multiple cardiac cycles are viewed simultaneously.

  B. Disadvantages

    1. Anatomic relationships between chambers and vessels may be difficult to define.

    2. Discrete lesions may not be visualized, since the ultrasound beam is localized to a small region of the heart.

III. Doppler echocardiography measures the direction and velocity of red blood cells moving through the heart and great vessels, and differentiates laminar from nonlaminar flow. The Doppler effect, as it relates to echocardiography, states that when red blood cells are moving relative to a stationary receiver (the transducer), the frequency of sound reflected by the red blood cells will change in proportion to their velocity and direction. If red blood cells move toward the transducer, the frequency of the reflected ultrasound signal increases, and if away, the frequency decreases. This change in frequency is the basis of the Doppler principle and is termed the Doppler frequency shift (Doppler shift).

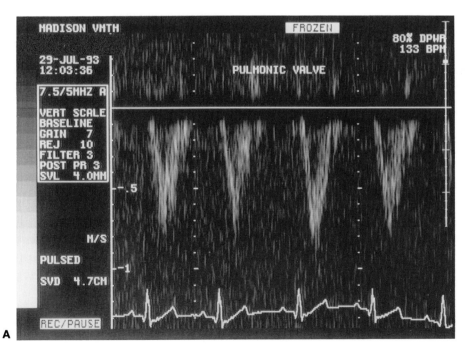

Fig. 4-2. (A) Spectral pulsed-wave Doppler display of laminar blood flow distal to the pulmonic valve in a normal dog obtained from a right parasternal short-axis view. A clearly defined envelope is created as blood cells accelerate and decelerate together in normal pulsatile flow. (*Figure continues.*)

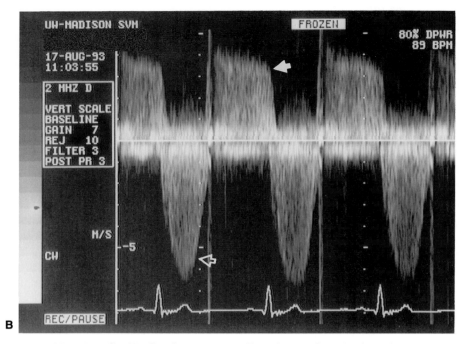

Fig. 4-2. (*Continued*). **(B)** Continuous wave Doppler tracing obtained from a subcostal view in a rottweiler puppy with both severe aortic stenosis *(open arrow)* and aortic insufficiency *(closed arrow)*. Spectral dispersion is created by red blood cells moving at different velocities, and is characteristic of both continuous wave Doppler and turbulent blood flow in pulsed-wave Doppler. High-velocity flow occurs as blood moves through the narrowed orifice, and results in a systolic pressure gradient across the aortic valve of 160 mmHg in this patient. (*Figure continues.*)

Blood flow velocity can be calculated from the Doppler equation: $V = (\Delta f \times c)/(2f_0 \times \cos\theta)$, where V is the velocity of blood flow (in m/s), Δf is the change in frequency (in Hz), c is a constant (velocity of sound in soft tissue: 1.54 m/s), f_0 is the transmitted frequency of ultrasound, and θ is the angle between the ultrasound beam and the flow of blood in the heart or vessel. Velocity of blood flow over time is presented as a spectral display (Fig. 4-2), with blood flow toward the transducer displayed above baseline, and blood flow away from the transducer displayed below baseline. Maximum pressure gradients across shunts and stenotic valves can be calculated from velocity measurements using a modification of the Bernoulli equation: Pressure gradient = 4(maximum velocity)^2.

A. Advantages
1. Quantitative information regarding pressure gradients across stenotic valves and regurgitation across insufficient valves is obtained.
2. Shunting lesions can be documented and quantitated even if they are too small to be visualized.
3. Overestimation of blood velocity (and therefore pressure gradients) will not occur.

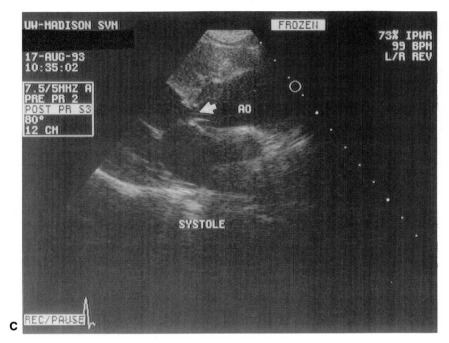

Fig. 4-2. (*Continued*). (C) Two-dimensional right parasternal long-axis view of the aortic outflow tract in the dog mentioned above, showing a dramatically reduced left ventricular outflow tract in systole due to subvalvular narrowing (*closed arrow*) and primary valvular dysplasia. AO, aorta.

B. Disadvantages

1. Parallel alignment with blood flow is necessary during Doppler interrogation; therefore, the 2-D image of the heart (which is best achieved with perpendicular alignment with tissue interfaces) is usually poor.

2. The true pressure gradient across the valve or lesion will be underestimated with Doppler as the angle of interrogation increases relative to alignment with blood flow. If the angle of incidence between the direction of blood flow and the ultrasound beam (θ) is less than or equal to 20 degrees, velocity is underestimated by less than 6 percent.

C. Modalities

1. Pulsed-wave (PW) Doppler (including color flow imaging) transmits ultrasound waves at a given frequency to a designated point (sample volume or range gate) from the transducer. The time between bursts of ultrasound waves (pulse repetition frequency) is determined by the distance from the transducer to the sample volume. PW Doppler allows a specific area of the heart or a great vessel (e.g., proximal pulmonary artery) to be examined for abnormalities of blood flow velocity, direction, or turbulence.

    a) PW Doppler is unable to measure high-velocity blood flow. For a given frequency transducer and depth of examination, there is a maximum velocity, or Nyquist limit, that can be accurately deter-

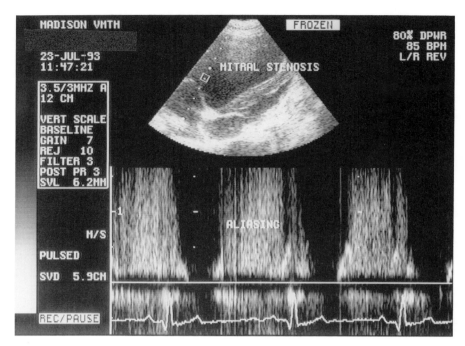

Fig. 4-3. Pulsed-wave Doppler display of a dog with mitral stenosis and increased diastolic velocity from the left atrium to the left ventricle. Aliasing results from high-velocity flow that exceeds the capability of the pulsed-wave transducer, and results in signals both above and below baseline. Neither blood flow direction nor velocity can be determined from this tracing.

mined. The maximum velocity that can be measured occurs when the Doppler shift exceeds one half of the pulse repetition frequency.

b) Aliasing, or velocity ambiguity, occurs if the maximum velocity that can be measured by the PW transducer is exceeded. Aliasing does not allow determination of blood flow direction or velocity; the signal is displayed as a band both above and below baseline (Fig. 4-3).

2. High pulse repetition frequency (High PRF) Doppler functions similar to pulsed-wave Doppler but uses multiple range gates. Multiple range gates permit higher velocity flow to be measured compared with single-gated PW Doppler.

3. Continuous wave (CW) Doppler uses a split-crystal transducer that simultaneously transmits and receives. Sound is reflected from all of the depths through which the ultrasound beam travels, and the heart can be scanned very quickly for abnormal flow signals (either in velocity or direction). CW Doppler has a very high velocity limit compared with pulsed-wave Doppler, but is unable to localize an abnormal signal along the sound beam (range ambiguity).

4. Color flow (CF) imaging is a form of PW Doppler echo that integrates

anatomic 2-D or M-mode images with blood flow. CF Doppler has multiple range gates, compared to PW Doppler echo which has a single range gate.

Color flow systems commonly have three types of CF Doppler maps: red/blue, enhanced, and velocity/variance. Blood flow moving toward the transducer is shown in red and blood flow away from the transducer is blue. Enhanced color signifies faster blood flow, and darker color indicates slower blood flow. Variance is shown in green and indicates turbulence (multiple velocities and directions of blood flow). *Since CF Doppler echo is a form of PW Doppler it is prone to aliasing, which is displayed as red/blue reversal.*

IV. Contrast echocardiography uses agents that produce an abrupt increase in the intensity of reflected echoes received by the transducer, and is used most commonly to demonstrate right-to-left cardiac shunts.

   A. Agents that have been used to create echo targets include the patient's blood, 0.9% NaCl, indocyanine green dye, or 5% dextrose solution.

   B. Microcavitation, or microbubbles, in the injected solution produce clouds of echoes that may persist for more than 10 seconds. The microcavitation is cleared by the lungs; therefore, peripheral injection of contrast will only result in left heart or aortic opacification if a right-to-left shunt is present.

   C. The chambers that are opacified vary depending on the level of the shunt.

   1. Right-to-left atrial shunting causes dye to appear in the left atrium, left ventricle, and aorta, as well as the right atrium and right ventricle.

   2. Right-to-left ventricular shunting leads to opacification of the right atrium, right ventricle, left ventricle, and aorta.

   3. Right-to-left PDA results in opacification of the right atrium, right ventricle, and descending aorta, but not the left atrium or left ventricle.

INDICATIONS FOR ECHOCARDIOGRAPHY

Due to the expense of echocardiographic equipment, the procedure continues to be a second step or referral procedure in the diagnosis of congenital or acquired cardiac disease. Echocardiographic findings are best interpreted in light of an accurate history and physical examination, in addition to high-quality dorsoventral or ventrodorsal and lateral chest radiographs.

Other tests that may be indicated prior to echocardiography include an electrocardiogram, measurement of systemic arterial blood pressure, or selected blood tests (including packed cell volume to determine if anemia or polycythemia is present, serum creatinine, electrolytes (especially potassium), digoxin concentration, or thyroxine concentration).

Certain cardiovascular diseases, such as mitral insufficiency due to endocardiosis in small breed dogs, can be managed properly based on the results of the physical examination, thoracic radiographs, and selected serum chemistry tests (e.g., creatinine, potassium). A low sodium diet with vasodilator and diuretic therapy can be instituted when clinical signs become apparent, and the results of echocardiography usually will not dictate alternate therapy.

Other patients, such as cats with cardiomegaly who are not hypertensive or hyperthyroid, or animals with congenital heart disease, have cardiovascular disease that cannot be definitively diagnosed by physical examination, radiography, or electrocardiography. Therefore, accurate identification of the underlying abnormality with cardiac ultrasound is essential in order to institute correct medical or interventional therapy.

   I. Patients in whom echocardiography is indicated early in the diagnostic evaluation for proper management
     A. Animals with suspected congenital heart disease
     B. Animals without a cardiac murmur but with polycythemia or cyanosis
     C. Large breed dogs with an acquired murmur (whether symptomatic or not)
     D. Cats with an acquired murmur who are not hypertensive or hyperthyroid
     E. Animals with evidence of left-sided (pulmonary edema) or right-sided (pleural effusion, jugular venous distention, ascites) congestive heart failure
     F. Animals with cardiac arrhythmias without an identifiable cause (e.g., secondary to trauma or electrolyte imbalance)
     G. Animals with suspected pericardial disease or cardiac neoplasia
     H. Animals with suspected bacterial endocarditis
  II. Patients who usually can be managed adequately without an initial echocardiogram
     A. Small breed dogs with mitral valvular regurgitation
     B. Hypertensive or hyperthyroid cats
     C. Dogs with heartworm disease

ECHOCARDIOGRAPHIC EQUIPMENT

   I. Transducers of various frequencies, usually 3.5 to 7.5 megahertz (MHz; equal to 1,000,000 cycles/s), are needed to perform high-quality echocardiograms in veterinary patients since a wide range of body weights and chest configurations exist.
     A. Higher frequency transducers (e.g., 7.5 MHz) permit better resolution of small structures; however, they have less penetrating ability. They are used for echocardiographic examinations in cats, puppies, and small breed dogs. Lower frequency transducers (e.g., 3.5 MHz) provide greater depth of penetration but less well-defined images, and are used for echo examinations in large breed dogs. Transducers with variable frequencies are also available with certain echocardiograph machines.
     B. Most transducers have dual M-mode and 2-D capabilities. The addition of PW and CW Doppler capabilities to conventional echo transducers allows multiple functions to be performed by a single transducer.
  II. The echocardiographic images (M-mode, 2-D, or Doppler) are displayed on an oscilloscope screen and can be recorded on videotape or printed on paper or special radiographic film.
 III. Many echocardiographs are equipped with cardiac analysis programs that allow the clinician to enter wall thickness, chamber dimension, and valvular motion measurements. With this information, ratios, thickening fractions, shortening fractions, and other parameters are automatically calculated by

the machine's software and displayed on the oscilloscope. The cardiac volume calculations that are performed by echocardiographic software were created for human beings, and are not reliable for veterinary patients.

IV. ECG electrodes and lead wires are integrated with the echocardiographic display so that cardiac electrical activity can be correlated with chamber and wall dimensions in systole and diastole.

THE ECHOCARDIOGRAPHIC EXAMINATION

I. Patient preparation and positioning
   A. It is usually not necessary to shave the patient's hair prior to echocardiographic examination except in some dogs with heavy haircoats. The hair should be wetted with alcohol over the echocardiographic window (usually located at the right fourth to fifth intercostal space), followed by the application of liberal amounts of coupling gel.
   B. Electrocardiographic leads should be attached so that cardiac electrical activity can be correlated with chamber and wall dimensions in systole and diastole. Single-use patch electrodes applied to the metacarpal and metatarsal pads result in excellent electrocardiographic tracings and avoid the necessity of shaving the patient's hair. Alternatively, alligator clip or plate electrodes can be used for electrocardiography.
   C. Positioning the animal in lateral recumbency on a cutaway table so that the transducer is placed beneath the animal will minimize lung interference, position the heart closer to the transducer, and enhance image quality. Alternatively, animals can be placed in left lateral recumbency on a standard table and the echocardiographic window can be approached from above.
      1. If necessary, the patient can stand throughout the echocardiographic examination, although patient movement and increased respiratory effort are common and the examination is more difficult.
      2. In unsedated cats that detest restraint in lateral recumbency with ECG electrodes attached, the echocardiographic examination can be performed with the cat in sternal recumbency in the examiner's lap.
II. Effects of selected drugs and fluid therapy on echocardiographic measurements
   A. Sedation is not required nor is it desirable except in uncooperative patients. If chemical restraint is needed, light tranquilization is generally sufficient.
      1. Dogs: buprenorphine (0.0075 to 0.01 mg/kg IV) with acepromazine (0.03 mg/kg IV)
      2. Cats: ketamine (2.0 to 4.0 mg/kg IV) with midazolam (0.2 mg/kg IV) or acepromazine (0.1 mg/kg IM)
   B. If sedation is used, the influence of the drug(s) on heart rate, chamber dimensions, and functional indices compared to the unsedated state must be considered in interpretation.
      1. Pentobarbital or other myocardial depressants may result in a slow

heart rate, increased ventricular chamber dimensions, and reduced shortening fraction.

2. Ketamine will increase heart rate and may result in decreased left atrial dimension, decreased left ventricular diastolic dimension, increased septal and left ventricular posterior wall diastolic thicknesses, and reduced shortening fraction.

3. Oxymorphone should be avoided prior to echocardiographic examination since it will increase ventilatory drive and produce excessive lung interference.

4. Acute volume loading may result in increased ventricular diastolic dimensions and reduced ventricular wall thicknesses.

III. Imaging planes

   A. An imaging plane that transects the left ventricle parallel to the long axis of the heart from apex to base is called a long-axis plane.

   B. A plane that transects the left ventricle or aorta perpendicular to the long axis of the heart is called a short-axis plane.

IV. Image orientation

   A. The index mark of the 2-D transducer, which marks the edge of the imaging plane, should be oriented to indicate the part of the cardiac image that will appear on the right side of the image display.

   B. The transducer index mark should then be pointed either toward the base of the heart (long-axis views) or cranially toward the patient's head (short-axis views).

   C. The images should be displayed so that the transducer artifact and near-field echoes appear at the top and the far-field echoes toward the bottom of the display.

V. Three transducer locations or "windows" result in consistent cardiac imaging planes, and are recommended for 2-D echocardiographic examinations.

   A. The right parasternal location is between the right third and sixth intercostal space (usually fourth to fifth) between the sternum and costochondral junctions.

      1. Two long-axis views are usually obtained: a four-chamber view with the cardiac apex (ventricles) displayed to the left and the base (atria) to the right (Fig. 4-4A), while the second view shows the left ventricular outflow tract, aortic valve, and aortic root (Fig. 4-4B).

      2. Right parasternal short-axis views include the ventricular apex, papillary muscles, chordae tendineae, mitral valve, and aortic valve (Fig. 4-5). As the transducer is directed from apex to base, the images should be displayed so that the right ventricle is in the near field, and the right heart encircles the left ventricle and aorta clockwise (right ventricular outflow tract and pulmonic valve to the right).

   B. The left caudal (apical) location is between the fifth and seventh intercostal spaces, as close to the sternum as possible.

      1. The left apical 2-chamber view is obtained with the beam plane perpendicular to the long axis of the body, parallel to the long axis of the heart, and with the transducer index mark pointing toward the heart base (dorsal). The left atrium, mitral valve, and left ventricle are visualized (Fig. 4-6A). Slight counterclockwise rotation of the transducer

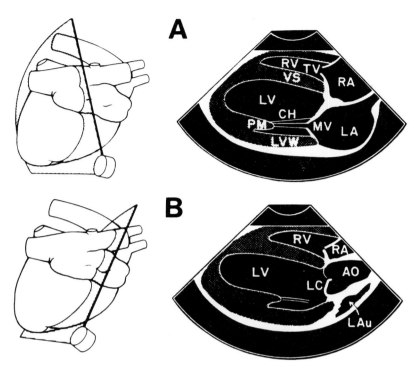

Fig. 4-4. Long-axis views obtained from the right parasternal transducer location. The diagrams on the left illustrate the heart viewed from the right side and the orientation of the ultrasound beam transecting the heart. The diagrams on the right illustrate the echocardiographic images corresponding to the imaging planes shown on the left. **(A)** Long-axis 4-chamber view. **(B)** Long-axis view of the left ventricular outflow tract. RV, right ventricle; TV, tricuspid valve; VS, ventricular septum; RA, right atrium; LV, left ventricle; CH, chordae tendineae; PM, papillary muscle; MV, mitral valve; LA, left atrium; LVW, left ventricular wall; AO, aorta; LC, left cusp (aortic valve); LAu, left auricle. (From Thomas WP: Two-dimensional, real-time echocardiography in the dog. Vet Radiol 25:50, 1984, with permission.)

results in a long-axis view of the left ventricle, outflow tract, aortic valve, and aortic root (Fig. 4-6B).

2. Left apical four-chamber views are obtained with the beam placed into a right-cranial to left-caudal orientation and directed dorsally toward the heart base. The image shows the ventricles in the near field, closest to the transducer, and the atria in the far field, with the heart oriented vertically (Fig. 4-6C).

3. Slight cranial tilting of the beam from the four-chamber view brings the LV outflow tract into view, and a "five-chamber" view, including all four cardiac chambers, both AV valves, and the aortic valve and proximal aorta, may be visualized.

C. The left cranial (base) parasternal location is between the left third and

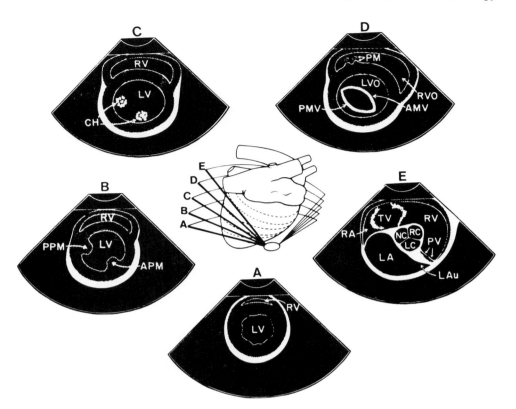

Fig. 4-5. Short-axis views obtained from the right parasternal location. The diagram in the center illustrates the beam orientations used to obtain images at five levels of the left ventricle. The corresponding images are shown clockwise from the bottom. **(A)** Apical level. **(B)** Papillary muscle level. **(C)** Chordal level. **(D)** Mitral valve level (diastole). **(E)** Aortic valve level (diastole). Abbreviations: RV, right ventricle; LV, left ventricle; CH, chordae tendineae; PM, papillary muscle; LVO, left ventricular outflow tract; PMV, posterior (parietal) mitral valve cusp; RVO, right ventricular outflow tract; AMV, anterior (septal) mitral valve cusp; PPM, posteromedial (dorsal) papillary muscle; APM, anterolateral (ventral) papillary muscle; PV, pulmonic valve; TV, tricuspid valve; RA, right atrium; LA, left atrium; NC, noncoronary or septal cusp (aortic valve); RC, right cusp (aortic valve); LC, left cusp (aortic valve); LAu, left auricle. (From Thomas WP: Two-dimensional real-time echocardiography in the dog. Vet Radiol 25:50, 1984, with permission.)

fourth intercostal spaces between the sternum and costochondral junctions.

1. The long-axis views are obtained with the beam plane oriented parallel to the long axis of the body and to the long axis of the heart, allowing the left ventricular outflow tract, aortic valve, and ascending aorta to be viewed. The right ventricular outflow tract, aortic valve, and ascending aorta are visualized better than the corresponding left apical view. Angling of the beam ventral to the aorta produces an oblique view of the left ventricle and the right atrium, tricuspid valve, and

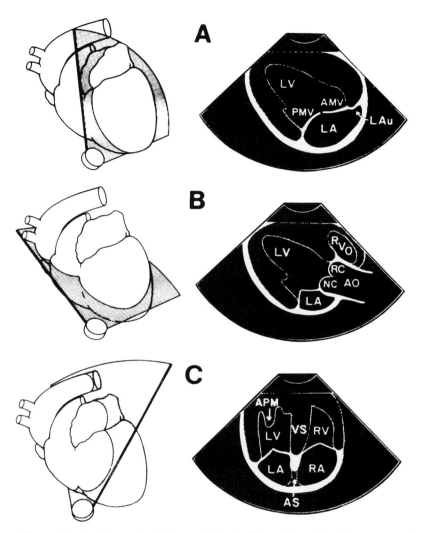

Fig. 4-6. Views obtained from the left caudal (apical) location. The diagrams on the left illustrate the heart viewed from the left side with the approximate transducer and echo beam orientations. The corresponding echocardiographic images are shown on the right. **(A)** Long-axis two-chamber view of the left atrium and ventricle. **(B)** Long-axis view of the left ventricular outflow region. **(C)** Four-chamber view. LV, left ventricle; AMV, anterior (septal) mitral valve cusp; PMV, posterior (parietal) mitral valve cusp; LA, left atrium; LAu, left auricle; RVO, right ventricular outflow tract; NC, noncoronary or septal cusp (aortic valve); RC, right cusp (aortic valve); AO, aorta; APM, anterolateral (ventral) papillary muscle; VS, ventricular septum; RV, right ventricle; RA, right atrium; AS, atrial septum. (From Thomas WP: Two-dimensional, real-time echocardiography in the dog. Vet Radiol 25:50, 1984, with permission.)

inflow region of the right ventricle. Angling of the transducer and beam plane dorsal to the aorta produces a view of the right ventricular outflow tract, pulmonary valve, and pulmonary artery.

2. A short-axis view of the aortic root encircled by the right heart is obtained with the beam plane oriented perpendicular to the long axis of the body and to the long axis of the heart. The right ventricular inflow region is displayed to the left and the outflow region and pulmonary artery to the right.

M-MODE ECHOCARDIOGRAPHIC ANATOMY AND INTERPRETATION

An electrocardiogram is obtained with the M-mode echocardiogram so that valvular and wall motion can be correlated with cardiac electrical activity. Diastolic measurements are obtained at the onset of the Q wave, and systolic measurements are obtained when maximum posterior interventricular septal motion excursion occurs.

Measurements obtained during or immediately after arrhythmias should be avoided, since lumen and wall dimensions will be altered, as will cardiac function. Similarly, pericardial effusion causes abnormalities of ventricular filling and wall motion, resulting in unreliable measurements.

I. Mitral valve (MV) view
  A. The mitral valve consists of the extension of the endocardial layer of the left atrial wall and the lateral posterior wall of the aortic root.
  B. The septal (anterior) leaflet can be recognized echocardiographically by its double or biphasic kick (Fig. 4-7). The maximum excursion of the leaflet should be used for recording purposes.
    1. Maximum anterior excursion of the valve (from D point to E point) occurs in early ventricular diastole and corresponds to rapid ventricular filling.
    2. As the left ventricle (LV) fills rapidly with blood from the left atrium (LA), the valve drifts closed (F point).
    3. The second peak, which occurs with reduced amplitude (A point), results from atrial contraction at end-diastole, just after the P wave of the ECG.
      a) The A point height is affected by end-diastolic pressure. Increased end-diastolic pressure causes increased A point height (e.g., congestive heart failure due to dilated cardiomyopathy; Fig. 4-8), while unloading agents (vasodilators) cause A point height to decline.
      b) A points may not be seen in tracings of animals with high heart rates (e.g., cats; Fig. 4-9).
      c) A points will be absent in tracings from animals with atrial fibrillation (E to F point to systole)
      d) isolated A points on the M-mode tracing can be seen after each P wave of the ECG with 2° or 3° AV block
    4. Rapid posterior movement to C point coincides with mitral valve closure (first heart sound) and the onset of systole (QRS complex).

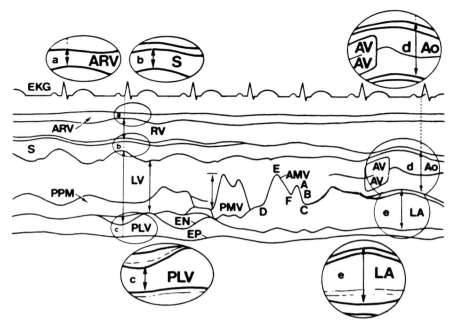

Fig. 4-7. Diagrammatic echocardiographic sweep shows the recommended criteria for measurement superimposed upon the structures. Diastolic measurements are made at the onset of the QRS complex of the ECG, cavities and walls are measured at the level of the chordae below the mitral valve. The illustration and the elliptical inserts a, b, c, d, and e illustrate the leading edge method, as well as measurements using the thinnest continuous echo lines. ARV, right ventricular anterior wall; RV, right ventricle; LV, left ventricle; PLV, posterior left ventricular wall; S, septum; PPM, papillary muscle; AMV and PMV, anterior and posterior mitral valve leaflets; A, B, C, D, E, and F = point of mitral valve motion; EN, endocardium; EP, epicardium; AV, aortic valve leaflet; Ao, aorta; LA, left atrium. The extra line in insert B that is excluded from the septal measurement represents a portion of tricuspid valve apparatus. (From Sahn DJ et al: Recommendations regarding quantitation in M-mode echocardiography: Results of a survey of echocardiographic measurements. Circulation 58:1072, 1978, with permission.)

     5. There normally is a straight line between A and C points, but in situations of elevated LV end-diastolic pressure there may be an interruption in the descent, called the B bump.

  C. During systole the closed leaflets move anteriorly in a smooth, continuous manner as a result of left ventricular emptying.

  D. Echocardiographic abnormalities of MV motion and structure

     1. Severe MV insufficiency may cause systolic fluttering of the septal leaflet.

     2. Aortic insufficiency results in diastolic fluttering of the MV.

     3. Systolic anterior motion (SAM) of the MV may occur in hypertrophic cardiomyopathy. SAM is characterized by movement of the MV leaflets toward the IVS shortly after the onset of systole, with return to

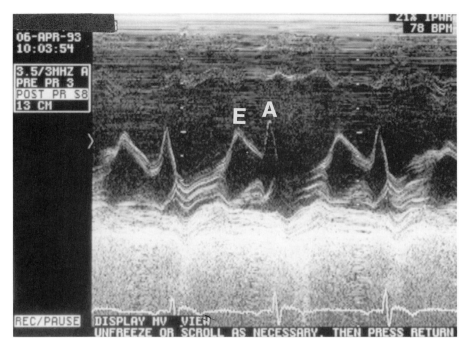

Fig. 4-8. M-mode echocardiographic tracing at the level of the mitral valve in a doberman pinscher with dilated cardiomyopathy. The mitral valve A point is increased relative to the E point as a result of increased end-diastolic pressure and low transvalvular flow.

normal position just before the onset of diastole (Fig. 4-10). It suggests that the MV apparatus may contribute to dynamic outflow obstruction.

   4. MV may appear thickened in patients with endocardiosis, congenital mitral valve dysplasia, or endocarditis.
   5. MV prolapse is characterized by "buckling" of the valve leaflet into the left atrium during systole.
   6. Ruptured chordae tendineae result in a flail MV, with movement of the entire valve leaflet into the left atrium during systole.
   E. Anterior leaflet D-E excursion (mm) and D-E slope (mm/s) suggest the volume of blood flowing between the LA and LV. The D-E slope is decreased with low flow states and low cardiac output. The mitral valve A point may be accentuated with a decreased D-E slope, since atrial systole is responsible for more LV filling in low flow states (Fig. 4-8).
   F. E point-septal separation (EPSS) is the distance in millimeters between the mitral valve E point and the IVS. When the ejection fraction is decreased, there is an increased distance between MV E point and the IVS (Fig. 4-11). Excursion of mitral valve E point correlates with flow through the valve. A decreased stroke volume leads to decreased amplitude of the MV E point (e.g., dilated cardiomyopathy). Increased EPSS may also be seen as a result of intrinsic valvular disease. Excursion of the mitral valve leaflet is physically limited in mitral stenosis, and a regurgitant jet of aortic insufficiency may also limit excursion of the MV leaflet.

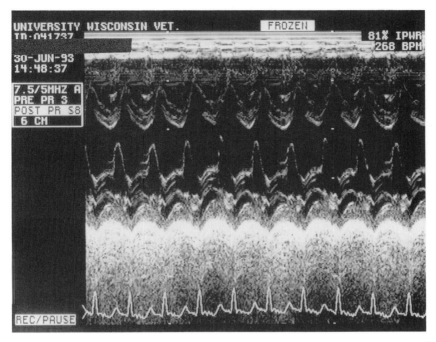

Fig. 4-9. M-mode echocardiographic tracing at the level of the mitral valve in a female kitten with patent ductus arteriosus. The mitral valve A point is not present due to elevated heart rate.

    G. E-F slope is measured in mm/s and represents the rate of LA emptying; it is also known as the diastolic closure velocity. Dysplasia and stenosis of the mitral valve, resulting in a stiffened valve, and hypertrophic cardiomyopathy, resulting in a stiff LV, may be associated with a decreased E-F slope and correlate with a decreased LV filling rate. However, the E-F slope may also be decreased with pulmonary hypertension without LV or valvular alterations.

  II. Left atrial and aortic view

    A. Left atrial (LA) diameter

      1. The LA is the chamber posterior to the aortic root and can be recognized by its immobile posterior wall. LA dimension should be measured at end-systole, which occurs during maximum anterior wall excursion (see Fig. 4-7). It is measured by "leading edge" methodology, from the anterior (inner) edge of the posterior aortic wall to the anterior edge of the left atrial wall.

      2. Enlargement of the LA may be seen in association with mitral valve insufficiency or stenosis, hypertrophic cardiac disease (primary or secondary), dilated cardiomyopathy, or congenital left-to-right shunts (e.g., PDA, VSD, or ASD).

    B. Aortic root diameter

      1. The base of the aorta is called the aortic root and contains three valve

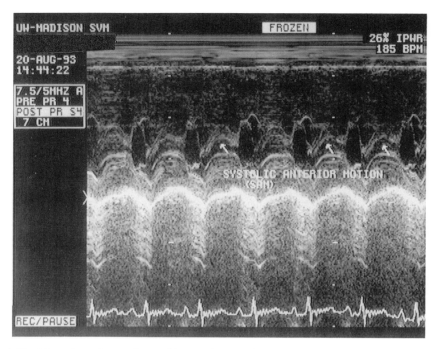

Fig. 4-10. M-mode echocardiographic tracing at the level of the mitral valve in a male domestic shorthair cat with hypertrophic cardiomyopathy. Systolic anterior motion of the mitral valve is present, and is characterized by movement of the mitral valve leaflets toward the interventricular septum shortly after the onset of systole. Systolic anterior motion may contribute to dynamic outflow obstruction.

cusps. Two cusps are seen during M-mode echocardiography: right coronary and noncoronary. The aortic root is recognized echocardio-graphically by parallel movement of the walls, which move anteriorly in systole and posteriorly in diastole. The septal leaflet of the mitral valve blends into the posterior aortic wall at the same time the IVS blends into the anterior aortic wall.

2. The aortic root should be measured at end-diastole at the onset of the QRS complex since expansion of the aortic root in systole may increase diameter (see Fig. 4-7). Aortic root diameter is measured from the anterior portion of the anterior aortic wall to the inner or anteriormost boundary of the posterior aortic wall, where two aortic cusps are visualized.

3. The aortic root diameter may be decreased in any cardiac disease that results in low cardiac output (e.g., dilated cardiomyopathy, severe mitral insufficiency). Aortic root diameter may be increased in tetralogy of Fallot as a result of increased blood flow through the aorta.

4. Subaortic stenosis causes LV outflow tract (LVOT) narrowing, resulting in an LVOT:aortic root ratio of less than one. Normal LVOT and aortic root diameters are equal.

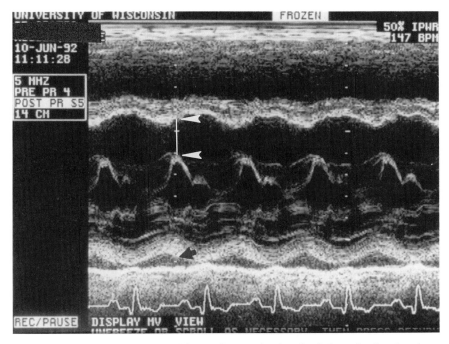

Fig. 4-11. M-mode echocardiographic tracing at the level of the mitral valve in a male Labrador retriever with dilated cardiomyopathy. Increased mitral valve E point to septal separation (EPSS) is present *(arrowheads)* due to reduced ejection fraction. A small amount of pericardial effusion *(arrow)* is also present.

   C. Left atrial to aortic root ratio (LA:Ao)
      1. Increased LA:Ao usually reflects LA enlargement, and may result from mitral valve insufficiency or stenosis, hypertrophic cardiac disease, dilated cardiomyopathy, or congenital left-to-right shunts.
      2. Right-to-left shunts that bypass the left atrium (e.g., tetralogy of Fallot) will result in decreased LA:Ao.
   D. Echocardiographic abnormalities of aortic valve motion and structure
      1. The aortic cusps separate and remain parallel to each other throughout systole, and close abruptly at the end of ventricular ejection. Aortic cusp separation is measured as the distance between the edge of the anterior aortic valve leaflet and the edge of the posterior aortic valve leaflet in early systole, but is rarely obtained in veterinary patients due to inadequate visualization of both aortic cusps.
      2. Aortic cusp separation varies with arrhythmias depending on the preceding R-R interval. Short R-R intervals caused reduced ventricular filling and decreased-to-absent aortic cusp separation and LV ejection time, resulting in pulse deficits. Early systolic closure of the aortic cusps may suggest reduced ventricular function, reduced forward stroke volume, or LV outflow obstruction (e.g., subaortic stenosis). Aortic cusp separation will be reduced if the cusps are thickened due to aortic valve dysplasia or endocarditis.

3. Abnormalities associated with aortic valve endocarditis include irregular thickening of the valve, multiple linear echoes in the aortic root, diastolic prolapse of the aortic vegetation, or diastolic fluttering of a torn aortic valve. In addition, left ventricular dilation, diastolic fluttering of the mitral valve, premature closure of the mitral valve, and left ventricular hyperkinesia may result from aortic valve insufficiency due to endocarditis.

4. Diastolic fluttering of the aortic cusps may be noted with aortic valve insufficiency. Systolic fluttering of the aortic cusps may be a normal variation or occur with high blood flow.

E. Systolic time intervals (STI) include the pre-ejection period (PEP), left ventricular ejection time (LVET), and total electromechanical systole (QAVC). STI measure sequential phases of LV systole, and provide a noninvasive indication of global LV performance.

STI correlate well with invasively derived ejection fraction, cardiac output, and stroke volume. Changes seen with STI are nonspecific however, because they are affected by myocardial contractility, heart rate, and loading conditions. As a result, STI provide a quantitative evaluation of overall LV performance, reflecting the combined influence of intrinsic disease, compensatory mechanisms, and pharmacologic intervention. Aortic valve opening and closing must be clearly visualized with the electrocardiogram during M-mode echocardiography in order to measure STI, and a trace speed of 100 mm/s and average of 10 consecutive beats are advised for increased accuracy.

1. PEP is measured echocardiographically from the onset of ventricular electrical activity (Q wave) to the onset of mechanical activity (opening of the aortic valve cusps; Fig. 4-12). PEP appears to be a sensitive indicator of myocardial performance in some dogs and cats.

2. Left ventricular ejection time (LVET) is the total time that the aortic leaflets are open during systole (Fig. 4-12), and is inversely related to heart rate. In the cat, the aortic leaflets may be difficult to visualize and LVET may be measured from the first anterior motion of the LV posterior wall to the point of its peak excursion. Left ventricular ejection time index (LVETI) corrects for alterations in heart rate, and can be calculated using two formulas.
   a) Dogs: LVET + (0.55 × heart rate)
   b) Cats: LVET + (0.4 × heart rate)

3. Total electromechanical systole (QAVC) is the interval from the onset of the QRS complex to the closure of the aortic valve. It is the sum of the left ventricular ejection time plus the pre-ejection period (LVET + PEP).

4. PEP/LVET is a derivative of STI, and was developed to diminish heart rate dependency of LVET; it also combines pre-ejection and ejection phase indices into one indicator of myocardial performance. PEP/LVET can detect LV dysfunction when either PEP or LVET (or both) are normal. PEP/LVET appears to be a sensitive indicator of myocardial performance in veterinary patients.

5. The velocity of circumferential fiber shortening (Vcf) is a derivative

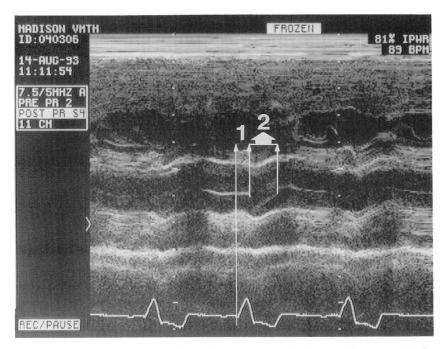

Fig. 4-12. M-mode echocardiographic tracing at the level of the aortic root and left atrium in a 6-month-old male springer spaniel with pulmonic stenosis. The pre-ejection period (PEP) (time between arrows indicated by 1) is measured echocardiographically from the onset of the QRS complex to the onset of mechanical activity (opening of the aortic valves). The left ventricular ejection time (LVET) (time between arrows indicated by 2) is the total duration that the aortic leaflets are open during systole. Ideally, systolic time intervals such as PEP and LVET should be measured using a trace speed of 100 mm/s and averaging 10 consecutive beats.

    of STI and reflects the rate of LV shortening. It is calculated by subtracting the LV internal dimension at systole (LVID$_s$) from the LV internal dimension at diastole (LVID$_d$) and dividing this number by the product of LVET and LVID$_d$.

6. Expected findings in STI associated with diminished LV performance include prolongation of PEP, increased PEP/LVET, abbreviation of LVET, subnormal Vcf, and normal QAVC. PEP prolongation can be attributed to the diminished rate of LV systolic pressure rise, while LVET is decreased due to reduced fiber shortening.

III. Left ventricular view

In the healthy animal, the LV internal dimension (LVID) is three to four times larger than the RV internal dimension (RVID). Measurements of right and left ventricular internal dimensions and walls are made at the level of the chordae tendinae, as opposed to the ventricular apex (where lumen diameter is decreased) or papillary muscles (where wall thickness is increased).

The indices of LV function calculated from left ventricular measurements include: percentage of left ventricular wall thickening, percentage of interven-

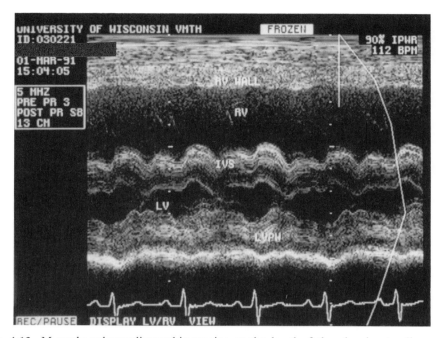

Fig. 4-13. M-mode echocardiographic tracing at the level of the chordae tendineae in a
male Labrador retriever with chronic heartworm disease. The right ventricular lumen (RV)
is increased, and the right ventricular wall (RV wall) is hypertrophied. Paradoxic septal
motion is present, and is characterized by rapid anterior septal movement during systole.
It is seen with diseases causing right ventricular volume or pressure overload. IVS, interventricular septum; LV, left ventricular lumen; LVPW, left ventricular posterior wall.

tricular septal thickening, shortening fraction, and velocity of circumferential
fiber shortening.
A. RVID should be measured only when the right side of the septum and the
   endocardium of the RV anterior wall are clearly visualized in the plane
   passing through the LV at the chordal level. RVID should be measured
   at end-diastole (onset of the QRS complex), and ideally, at end-expiration,
   since RV filling is enhanced during inspiration (see Fig. 4-7).
   1. RVID will be increased with tricuspid insufficiency, pulmonic stenosis,
      cor pulmonale, atrial septal defect, ventricular septal defect, or heart-
      worm disease (Fig. 4-13).
   2. RV wall hypertrophy will accompany diseases of pressure overload,
      including pulmonic stenosis, right-to-left shunts (e.g., tetralogy of Fal-
      lot), and pulmonary hypertension associated with heartworm disease
      (Fig. 4-13).
B. The interventricular septum (IVS) is continuous with the anterior wall of
   the aorta as the heart is scanned from apex to base. Septal motion reflects
   filling and depolarization patterns of the left and right ventricles. The
   echocardiographer should be aware of the continuity of the septum to

detect septal defects or abnormal relationships between the septum and other cardiac structures (e.g., over-riding aorta in tetralogy of Fallot).

1. Interventricular septal diastolic thickness (IVS_d) is measured at the onset of the QRS complex, from the anterior edge of the left ventricular side of the IVS to the anterior edge of the right ventricular side of the IVS (see Fig. 4-7). Interventricular septal systolic thickness (IVS_s) is measured at the point of maximum posterior excursion of the IVS (nadir of septal motion). The percent change or thickening fraction of the IVS is calculated from the formula: (IVS systolic thickness − IVS diastolic thickness)/IVS systolic thickness × 100.

2. Hypertrophy of the IVS is defined as excessive diastolic thickness.

3. IVS may be hypertrophied in pressure-overload diseases that affect the left ventricle (e.g., subaortic stenosis) or right ventricle (e.g., pulmonic stenosis). In some patients with hypertrophic cardiomyopathy or systemic hypertension, the septum may hypertrophy more than the free wall, either diffusely or focally. If the septal diastolic thickness to LVPW diastolic thickness is greater than or equals 1.3:1, asymmetric septal hypertrophy is present.

4. In conditions of LV volume overload without myocardial disease, such as mitral regurgitation, septal motion is hyperkinetic and recognized echocardiographically as marked anterior (i.e., toward the transducer) movement during early diastole as a result of excessive blood flowing into the LV.

5. RV volume or pressure overload may be associated with reduced or paradoxical septal motion (PSM). PSM is characterized by rapid anterior septal movement during systole, and septal movement that is parallel with LVPW motion (Fig. 4-13). Calculation of accurate LVID or LV shortening fraction is not possible if PSM is present.

   a) 2-D echocardiographic assessment of septal motion in pure RV volume overload (e.g., tricuspid insufficiency) shows septal flattening on the cross-sectional view during diastole; however, the normal circular appearance of the LV returns during systole.

   b) Conditions of advanced RV pressure overload characterized by RV pressures that exceed LV pressures during both systole and diastole result in a flattened septum on the 2-D cross-sectional view throughout the cardiac cycle (Fig. 4-14).

6. Septal "drop-out" is characterized by the disappearance of echoes as IVS is scanned from apex to base, and may occur with large septal defects.

7. Septal thickening may be decreased with dilated cardiomyopathy, fibrosis, or infarction.

C. The LVPW is measured at the chordal level using the thinnest continuous lines, from the anterior edge of the pericardium to the anterior edge of the LVPW endocardium (see Fig. 4-7). Discontinuous lines anterior to the LVPW result from reflection of chordae tendineae. Diastolic thickness of the LVPW ($LVPW_d$) is measured at the onset of the QRS complex, and systolic thickness of the LVPW ($LVPW_s$) is measured at the point of maximum anterior excursion of the LVPW. The percent change or thickening fraction of the LVPW is calculated from the formula: (LVPW

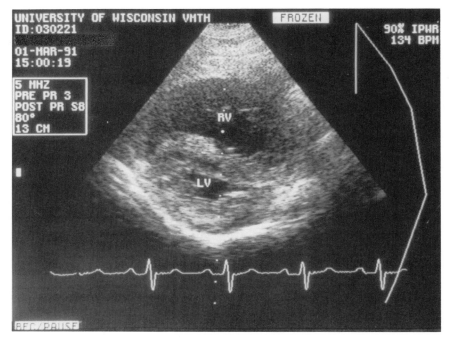

Fig. 4-14. Two-dimensional cross-sectional echocardiographic display at the level of the chordae tendineae in a male Labrador retriever with chronic heartworm disease. The right ventricular lumen (RV) is increased, and the right ventricular wall is hypertrophied as a result of pulmonary hypertension and right ventricular pressure overload. Paradoxic septal motion is present, and is characterized by a flattened interventricular septum on the two-dimensional cross-sectional view. When right ventricular pressure exceeds left ventricular pressure the septum is pushed toward the left ventricle. LV, left ventricular lumen.

systolic thickness − LVPW diastolic thickness) / LVPW systolic thickness × 100.

1. Hypertrophy is defined as excessive thickness of the $LVPW_d$. Hypertrophy may occur in hypertrophic cardiomyopathy, subaortic stenosis, hyperthyroidism, systemic hypertension, and infiltrative myocardial disease.

2. The thickening fraction of the LVPW may be increased in early endocardiosis, hypertrophic cardiomyopathy, hyperthyroidism, systemic hypertension, and other diseases of LV volume overload (e.g., PDA).

3. The thickening fraction of the LVPW may be decreased with dilated cardiomyopathy, infarction or fibrosis of the LVPW, tetralogy of Fallot, or right-to-left PDA.

D. LVID is measured from the anterior edge of the LVPW to the anterior edge of the left ventricular side of the IVS (see Fig. 4-7). The diastolic dimension ($LVID_d$) is measured at the onset of the QRS complex, and the systolic dimension ($LVID_s$) is measured from the IVS at peak posterior motion to the anterior edge of the LVPW, as long as septal motion is normal. If septal motion is abnormal (e.g., paradoxical septal motion), $LVID_s$ is measured at the peak anterior motion of the left ventricular posterior wall to the IVS. The shortening fraction (SF; also known as fractional shortening or percent change in diameter) of the LVID is calculated from the formula: $(LVID_d - LVID_s) / LVID_d \times 100$.

1. The septum is usually depolarized a few milliseconds before the LVPW, resulting in earlier maximum posterior movement of the IVS compared with maximum anterior motion of the LVPW.
2. LVID increases in diseases that cause volume overload, including mitral insufficiency, dilated cardiomyopathy (Fig. 4-15), aortic insufficiency, left-to-right shunts, and high-output states (e.g., anemia, fever, hyperthyroidism).
3. LVID may be decreased in volume depletion (e.g., hypoadrenocorticism, severe dehydration) or inadequate return of blood to the LV (e.g., severe right-heart disease or pericardial effusion).
4. Shortening fraction is a commonly used index of cardiac performance; however, it is assumed that wall motion, which may be assessed with 2-D echocardiography, is uniform. The heart must be viewed perpen-

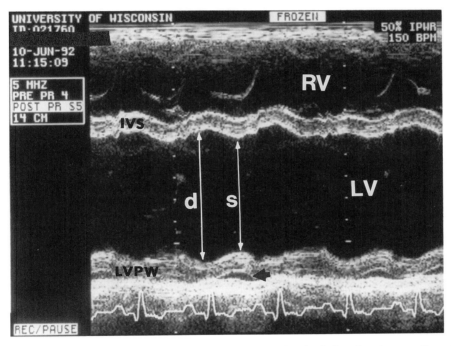

Fig. 4-15. M-mode echocardiographic tracing at the level of the chordae tendinae in a male Labrador retriever with dilated cardiomyopathy. The right ventricular (RV) and left ventricular (LV) internal dimensions are increased in both systole (s) and diastole (d) due to volume overload. Interventricular septal (IVS) and left ventricular posterior wall (LVPW) thickening are reduced, and shortening fraction is severely decreased. Minimal pericardial effusion *(arrow)* is also present.

dicular to the transducer to obtain an accurate minor dimension (cross section) and SF.

    a) SF may be increased in early mitral insufficiency, hypertrophic cardiomyopathy, thyrotoxic heart disease, or systemic hypertension.

    b) SF may be decreased in dilated cardiomyopathy (Fig. 4-15), PDA, infarction, and severe volume overload (e.g., advanced mitral insufficiency).

  5. Ventricular volumes may be calculated from M-mode measurements; however, assumptions regarding ventricular geometry may contribute to unreliable volume calculations. Formulas assume that the two short axes of the LV are equal and approximated by the LVID, and the long axis of the LV is twice the length of the short axes. Actually the shape of the LV is irregular, and the LV walls may not contract uniformly. Discretion must be used by the echocardiographer to avoid overinterpretation of echocardiographic findings.

IV. Pericardial effusion is characterized by an echo-free space between the left and right ventricular walls and pericardium (Fig. 4-16). Its presence is easier

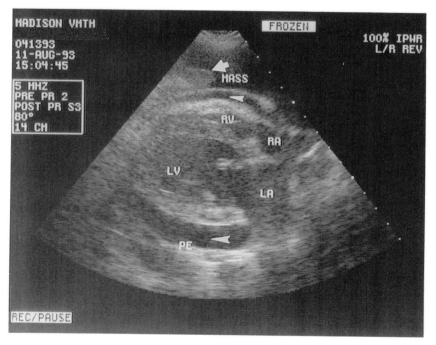

Fig. 4-16. Two-dimensional right parasternal long-axis echocardiographic display in a 10-year-old female spayed Shetland sheepdog-cross dog with a 5-month history of pericardial effusion (PE) with secondary pleural effusion and ascites. A mass *(arrow)* is visible outside the pericardial sac, and a small amount of pericardial effusion *(arrowheads)* is present after pericardiocentesis. Exploratory thoracotomy revealed multiple hemorrhagic masses, and a partial pericardectomy was performed. Histopathology of the masses showed chronic fibrosing pericarditis with multifocal hematomas of the pericardial sac. Mitral valve endocardiosis is also present, characterized echocardiographically by thickened and nodular mitral valves. RA, right atrium; RV, right ventricle; LA, left atrium; LV, left ventricle.

to recognize with 2-D echocardiography; however, M-mode echocardiography shows a hypoechoic area posterior to the LVPW that increases in size with ventricular systole (see Figs. 4-11 and 4-15).

A. Pericardial effusion, unlike pleural effusion, only extends to the level of the left atrium when the heart is scanned from apex to base.

B. Changes in position of cardiac structures on the M-mode echocardiogram correlate with swinging of the heart in the pericardial sac, and are responsible for the electrocardiographic finding of electrical alternans.

C. If significant pericardial effusion is present, measurement of SF is unreliable due to abnormal septal motion and decreased left ventricular size. Other M-mode findings with pericardial effusion include reduced RV and LA dimensions.

D. Cardiac tamponade is recognized on 2-D echocardiography by diastolic collapse of the right atrium, and may be difficult to appreciate on M-mode echocardiography.

NORMAL ECHOCARDIOGRAPHIC MEASUREMENTS AND ALTERATIONS WITH CARDIOVASCULAR DISEASE

Tables have been established for M-mode echocardiographic measurements in dogs based on body weight (Table 4-1) and in cats based on awake versus sedated

TABLE 4-1. NORMAL CANINE ECHOCARDIOGRAPHIC VALUES[a,b]

Wt (kg)	3	5	7	10	15	20	25	30	35	40	50
$LVID_d$ (mm)	24.6 (6.2)	27.4 (5.2)	30.0 (4.5)	32.7 (3.5)	37.1 (2.4)	41.4 (2.2)	44.8 (2.9)	48.3 (3.9)	51.7 (5.0)	54.8 (6.1)	60.7 (8.3)
$LVID_s$ (mm)	13.6 (5.5)	16.0 (4.7)	17.9 (4.0)	20.6 (3.1)	24.3 (2.1)	28.0 (2.0)	31.0 (2.5)	33.9 (3.4)	36.9 (4.5)	39.6 (5.4)	44.6 (7.4)
$LVPW_d$ (mm)	5.0 (2.1)	5.4 (1.7)	5.7 (1.5)	6.2 (1.2)	6.8 (0.8)	7.4 (0.7)	7.9 (1.0)	8.4 (1.3)	8.9 (1.7)	9.3 (2.0)	10.2 (2.8)
$LVPW_s$ (mm)	7.2 (1.7)	7.9 (1.6)	8.4 (1.4)	9.2 (1.3)	10.2 (1.1)	11.3 (1.1)	12.1 (1.2)	13.0 (1.3)	13.8 (1.5)	14.5 (1.7)	16.0 (2.2)
IVS_d (mm)	5.8 (2.1)	6.2 (1.7)	6.5 (1.5)	7.0 (1.2)	7.6 (0.8)	8.2 (0.7)	8.7 (0.9)	9.2 (1.3)	9.7 (1.7)	10.2 (2.0)	11.0 (2.7)
IVS_s (mm)	9.8 (2.6)	10.2 (2.2)	10.4 (2.0)	10.9 (1.7)	11.5 (1.2)	12.3 (1.1)	13.0 (1.5)	13.9 (2.3)	14.6 (2.6)	15.4 (3.5)	—
LA (mm)	12.7 (5.3)	14.0 (4.5)	15.0 (3.8)	16.3 (3.0)	18.3 (2.0)	20.2 (1.9)	21.8 (2.4)	23.3 (3.3)	24.8 (4.3)	26.2 (5.2)	28.8 (7.1)
Ao (mm)	13.8 (3.6)	15.3 (3.0)	16.4 (2.6)	18.1 (2.0)	20.4 (1.4)	22.8 (1.3)	24.6 (1.6)	26.4 (2.2)	28.3 (2.9)	30.0 (3.5)	33.1 (4.8)

Abbreviations: $LVID_d$, Left ventricular internal dimension at end diastole; $LVID_s$, left ventricular internal dimension at end systole; $LVPW_d$, left ventricular posterior wall at end diastole; $LVPW_s$, left ventricular posterior wall at end systole; IVS_d, interventricular septum at end diastole; IVS_s, interventricular septum at end systole; LA, left atrium (systole); Ao, aortic root (diastole).

[a] Fractional shortening: 28% to 40%; mitral valve E point to septal separation: <5 to 6 mm.

[b] Mean value given, ± SD in parenthesis below.

(From Ware WA: Diagnostic tests for the cardiovascular system. p. 13. In Nelson RW, Couto CG (eds): Essentials of Small Animal Internal Medicine. Mosby-Year Book, St. Louis, 1992, with permission, and with data from Bonagura JD, O'Grady MR, Herring DS: Echocardiography: principles of interpretation. Vet Clin North Am 15:1177, 1985.)

TABLE 4-2. NORMAL FELINE ECHOCARDIOGRAPHIC VALUES

Parameter	Range (Unsedated)[a] (n = 30)	Range (Sedated with Ketamine)[b] (n = 30)
RVID$_d$ (mm)	2.7–9.4	1.2–7.5
LVID$_d$ (mm)	12.0–19.8	10.7–17.3
LVID$_s$ (mm)	5.2–10.8	4.9–11.6
SF (%)	39.0–61.0	30–60
LVPW$_d$ (mm)	2.2–4.4	2.1–4.5
LVPW$_s$ (mm)	5.4–8.1	—
IVS$_d$ (mm)	2.2–4.0	2.2–4.9
IVS$_s$ (mm)	4.7–7.0	—
LA (mm)	9.3–15.1	7.2–13.3
Ao (mm)	7.2–11.9	7.1–11.5
LA/Ao	.95–1.65	.73–1.64
EPSS (mm)	−0.17–0.21	—
PEP (s)	—	.024–.058
LVET (s)	0.10–0.18	.093–0.176
PEP/LVET	—	.228–.513
Vcf (circumf/s)	2.35–4.95	2.27–5.17

Abbreviations: RVID$_d$, right ventricular internal dimension at end diastole; LVID$_d$, left ventricular internal dimension at end diastole; LVID$_s$, left ventricular internal dimension at end systole; SF, shortening fraction; LVPW$_d$, left ventricular posterior wall at end diastole; LVPW$_s$, left ventricular posterior wall at end systole; IVS$_d$, interventricular septum at end diastole; IVS$_s$, interventricular septum at end systole; LA, left atrium (systole); Ao, aortic root (end diastole); EPSS, E point to septal separation; PEP, pre-ejection period; LVET, left ventricular ejection time; Vcf, velocity of circumferential fiber shortening.
[a] Data from Jacobs, 1985.
[b] Data from Fox, 1985.

states (Table 4-2). Expected values in dogs based on body weight alone are most likely simplistic and a presumptive approach, since differences in M-mode measurements vary with breed. Similarly, the echocardiographic measurement ranges in cats presume no breed variation, which will most likely be proved false as additional information is collected. Reference tables for cats also assume standard body size in cats (a "per cat" approach), and information regarding changes in cardiac size in growing kittens is lacking.

I. Echocardiographic factors in dogs affected by breed
   A. Evaluation of echocardiographic measurements in Pembroke Welsh corgis, miniature poodles, Afghan hounds, and golden retrievers have shown that for all measurements except RVID, means were significantly different among breeds after differences in weight were taken into account.
   B. As more data becomes available in veterinary patients, breed will be considered in establishing echocardiographic measurement reference ranges.
II. Echocardiographic factors in dogs affected by growth
   A. Although body weight has been used to determine echocardiographic reference ranges in dogs, sequential echocardiographic examinations in growing pups have shown that cardiac measurements increase in a curvilinear fashion relative to body weight.
   B. Sixteen English pointers were echoed at 1, 2, 4, and 8 weeks of age and

TABLE 4-3. DOPPLER-DERIVED PEAK VELOCITIES IN NORMAL DOGS

Valve	Transducer Site	PW or CW	Peak Velocity (M/S)	Sedation	Body Weight (kg)	Reference	n
AoV*	Left apical	PW	1.06 ± .21	Acepromazine .02 mg/kg IV	5–48	Brown, 1991	28
	Left apical	PW	1.19 ± .18	?	?	Gaber, 1987	28
	Left apical	CW	1.18 ± .11	None	3–41	Yuill, 1991	20
	Subcostal	CW	1.7	None	?	Sisson, 1992	
PV	Right parasternal SA	PW	0.84 ± .17	Acepromazine .02 mg/kg IV	5–48	Brown, 1991	28
	Lt or Rt parasternal SA	PW	1.00 ± .15	?	?	Gaber, 1987	28
	Lt cranial parasternal LA	CW	0.98 ± .09	None	3–41	Yuill, 1991	20
	Right parasternal SA	CW	0.96 ± .10	None	3–41	Yuill, 1991	19
MV	Left apical	PW	0.71 ± .07	?	≤10	Gaber, 1987	15
	Left apical	PW	0.81 ± .14	?	≥19	Gaber, 1987	13
	Left apical	CW	0.86 ± .10	None	3–41	Yuill, 1991	20
TV	Left apical	PW	0.49 ± .11	?	≤10	Gaber, 1987	15
	Left apical	PW	0.63 ± .18	?	≥19	Gaber, 1987	13
	Left apical	CW	0.69 ± .08	None	3–41	Yuill, 1991	20

Abbreviations: SA, short axis; LA, long axis; PW, pulsed wave; CW, continuous wave; AoV, aortic valve; PV, pulmonic valve; MV, mitral valve; TV, tricuspid valve; ?, not listed; n, number of dogs evaluated.
* Subcostal view using dedicated CW probe best for aortic outflow gradients.

103

TABLE 4-4. CONVENTIONAL AND DOPPLER ECHOCARDIOGRAPHIC ALTERATIONS IN CONGENITAL HEART DISEASE

	RV Wall	RVIDd	IVS$_d$	LVPW$_d$	LVID$_d$	FS	Ao	LA	Additional Echocardiographic Findings
Valvular Defects									
Aortic stenosis	N	N	↑	↑	→	N	N↑	N↑	Echo-dense proliferation in LVOT; CW systolic aortic flow velocity > 1.7 M
Pulmonic stenosis	↑	↑	↑	N	N→	N↓	N	N	PSM may be present; ↑ systolic flow velocity across pulmonic valve
Tricuspid dysplasia	N	↑	N	N	N→	N↓	N	N	PSM may be present; TV may be displaced apically
Mitral dysplasia	N	N	N	N	↑	N↑	N→	↑	↓ EF slope and ↑ LV inflow velocity if MV stenotic
Left-to-Right Shunts									
Atrial septal defect	N	↑	N	N	N	N	N	↑	↑ flow velocity across atrial septum in systole & diastole; echo "dropout"
Patent ductus arteriosus	N	N	N	N	↑	→	N↑	↑	Diastolic PA flow; continuous flow in ductus
Ventricular septal defect	N	↑	N	N	↑	N↓	N	↑	Echo "drop-out" of IVS; ↑ flow velocity across ventricular septum
Right-to-Left Shunts									
Atrial septal defect	↑	↑	N	N	N↑	N↓	N	↑	Contrast echo: RA to LA clouding; Echo "drop-out" of atrial septum
Patent ductus arteriosus	↑	↑	↑	N	→	→	→	→	Contrast echo: clouding of RA, RV, and descending aorta
Tetralogy of Fallot	↑	↑	↑	N	→	→	N↑	→	Contrast echo: clouding of RA, RV, and aorta; discontinuity of IVS and aorta
Ventricular septal defect	↑	↑	↑	N	↑	→	N↑	→	Contrast echo: RV to LV outflow clouding; echo "drop-out" of IVS

Abbreviations: LV, left ventricle; RV, right ventricle; RVIDd, right ventricular internal dimension at end diastole; IVS, interventricular septum at end diastole; LVPW, left ventricular posterior wall at end diastole; LVID$_d$, left ventricular internal dimension at end diastole; SF, shortening fraction; Ao, aortic root; LA, left atrium; LVOT, left ventricular outflow tract; PSM, paradoxical septal motion; TV, tricuspid valve; PA, pulmonary artery; RA, right atrium; CW, continuous wave Doppler; N, normal; ↑, increased; ↓, decreased.

TABLE 4-5. M-MODE AND 2-D ECHOCARDIOGRAPHIC ALTERATIONS IN ACQUIRED HEART DISEASE

	RV Wall	RVID$_d$	IVS$_d$	LVPW$_d$	LVID$_d$	SF	Ao	LA	Additional M-mode or 2-D Findings
Dilated cardiomyopathy	N↓	↑	N↓	N↓	↑	↓	N↓	↑	Reduced wall thickening
Hypertrophic cardiomyopathy	N↑	N↓	N↑	N↑	N↓	N↑	N	↑	Focal septal hypertrophy may be present
Intermediate cardiomyopathy	N↑	N↑	N↑	N↑	N↑	N↓	N	↑	Focal septal hypertrophy may be present
Mitral regurgitation	N	N	N↑	N↑	↑	↑N↓	N↓	↑	Increased SF early in disease, N → ↓ later
Tricuspid regurgitation	N↑	↑	N↑	N	N	N	N	N	Usually accompanies mitral value insufficiency
Pericardial effusion	N	→	N	N	→	→	→	→	Collapse of RA wall occurs with tamponade; Abnormal septal motion; echo-free space between pericardium and LVPW
Hypothyroidism	N	N	N	N	N^a	→↓	N	N	Prolonged PEP
Hyperthyroidism	N↑	N↑	N↑	N↑	N↑	N↑	N	↑	Myocardial failure may develop with severe disease
Heartworm disease	↑	↑	↑	N	N↓	N↓	N	N	Echodense worm mass or linear echoes may be associated with TV; PSM may be present
Systemic hypertension	N	N	N↑	N↑	N	N	N	↑	Focal or diffuse septal hypertrophy may be present

Abbreviations: RV, right ventricle; RVID$_d$, right ventricular internal dimension at end diastole; IVS$_d$, interventricular septum at end diastole; LVPW$_d$, left ventricular posterior wall at end diastole; LVID$_d$, left ventricular internal dimension at end diastole; SF, shortening fraction; Ao, aortic root; LA, left atrium; RA, right atrial; PEP, pre-ejection period; TV, tricuspid value; PSM, paradoxical septal motion; N, normal; ↑, increased; ↓, decreased.
^{a} Systolic LVID increased.

105

at 3, 6, 9, and 12 months of age. Left atrial, aortic, left and right ventricular chamber dimensions, septal, and LV free wall measurements were best predicted by indexing echocardiographic measurements to body weight[1/3]. Shortening fraction and left atrial to aortic ratio decreased slightly but significantly as body weight increased.

III. Doppler-derived peak velocities in normal dogs (Table 4-3)
IV. Conventional and Doppler echocardiographic alterations in congenital heart disease (Table 4-4)
 V. M-mode and 2-D echocardiographic alterations in acquired heart disease (Table 4-5)

CONCLUSION

In summary, M-mode, 2-D, and Doppler echocardiography give the clinician an opportunity to noninvasively and accurately investigate cardiovascular disease in small animal patients. Echocardiographic findings, in conjunction with the physical examination and results of thoracic radiographs, electrocardiography, blood pressure measurement, and selected blood tests, enable accurate diagnosis and proper management of animals with cardiac disease.

SUGGESTED READINGS

Brown DJ, Knight DH, King RR: Use of pulsed-wave Doppler echocardiography to determine aortic and pulmonary velocity and flow variables in clinically normal dogs. Am J Vet Res 52:543, 1991

Feigenbaum H: Echocardiography. 4th Ed. Lea & Febiger, Philadelphia, 1986

Fox PR, Bond BR, Peterson ME: Echocardiographic reference values in healthy cats sedated with ketamine hydrochloride. Am J Vet Res 46:1479, 1985

Gaber CE: Normal pulsed Doppler flow velocities in adult dogs (abstract). p. 923. Am Coll Vet Intern Med, 1987

Jacobs G, Knight DH: M-Mode echocardiographic measurements in nonanesthetized healthy cats: Effects of body weight, heart rate, and other variables. Am J Vet Res 46: 1705, 1985

Moise NS: Echocardiography. p. 113. In Fox PR (ed): Canine and Feline Cardiology. Churchill Livingstone, New York, 1988

Moise NS: Doppler echocardiographic evaluation of congenital cardiac disease. J Vet Intern Med 3:195, 1989

Morrison SA, Moise NS, Scarlett J et al: Effect of breed and body weight on echocardiographic values in four breeds of dogs of differing somatotype. J Vet Intern Med 6:220, 1992

Sahn DJ, DeMaria A, Kisslo J, Weyman A: Recommendations regarding quantitation in M-mode echocardiography: Results of a survey of echocardiographic measurements. Circulation 58:1072, 1978

Sisson D: Fixed and dynamic subvalvular aortic stenosis in dogs. p. 760. In Kirk RW, Bonagura JD (eds): Current Veterinary Therapy XI. WB Saunders, Philadelphia, 1992

Sisson D, Schaeffer D: Changes in linear dimensions of the heart, relative to body weight, as measured by M-mode echocardiography in growing dogs. Am J Vet Res 52:1591, 1991

Thomas WP, Gaber CE, Jacobs G et al: Recommendations for standards in transthoracic two-dimensional echocardiography in the dog and cat. J Vet Intern Med 7:247, 1993

Thomas WP: Two-dimensional, real-time echocardiography in the dog. Vet Radiol 25:50, 1984

Ware WA: Diagnostic tests for the cardiovascular system. p. 13. In Nelson RW, Couto CG (eds): Essentials of Small Animal Internal Medicine. Mosby-Year Book, St. Louis, 1992

Yuill CDM, O'Grady MR: Doppler-derived velocity of blood flow across the cardiac valves in the normal dog. Can J Vet Res 55:185, 1991

5

Special Diagnostic Techniques for Evaluation of Cardiac Disease

John E. Rush

INTRODUCTION

In most clinical cases, the standard diagnostic tests (electrocardiography, echocardiography, and thoracic radiography) described in the previous chapters will provide adequate information to establish a definitive diagnosis and permit initiation of therapy. In selected cases, however, the cause of the clinical signs is still unclear after initial testing and further diagnostic procedures are required. Although the availability of many of the diagnostic techniques described in this chapter is limited to university or referral private practice settings, some of the tests described, such as serologic testing, pericardiocentesis, and postexercise electrocardiography, are relatively simple and do not require additional equipment; their use need not be limited to cardiologists.

When considering the use of special diagnostic techniques, the status of the patient and the potential morbidity or mortality of the technique must be considered. Noninvasive diagnostic techniques are generally preferred, especially in critically ill animals. For example, in most clinical situations, echocardiography would be preferable to nonselective angiography, as the latter technique carries a greater potential for complication. In addition to equipment limitations and considerations of risk, financial constraints often preclude use of the most sophisticated diagnostic techniques (e.g., invasive electrophysiologic studies or nuclear magnetic resonance imaging). For each special diagnostic test, the indications and technique, clinical utility, and limitations of risk and economy are discussed. Alternative tests that might give similar information are mentioned where appropriate.

CONTINUOUS IN-HOSPITAL ELECTROCARDIOGRAPHIC MONITORING

I. Indications
  A. Hospitalized patients in which knowledge of cardiac rate and rhythm will aid or improve case management
    1. Primary cardiac diseases
    2. Severe systemic diseases

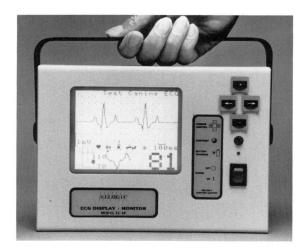

Fig. 5-1. ECG/Respiratory EC-60 Monitor with direct applications to veterinary use. This unit provides continuing monitoring on species with a wide range of heart rates (up to 900 beats/minute). Data stored in memory can be reviewed with a three or six lead trace sent to a compatible printer for hard copy. Other features include an ECG display screen for monitoring, together with alarm settings, indication of respiration, large heart rate numerals, and trend graph reflecting stored data. (Courtesy of Silogic Design, England and Stewartstown, PA. 800-765-5093).

    B. Patients with cardiac arrhythmias to evaluate arrhythmia resolution or deterioration and/or to assess the response to therapy

    C. Animals requiring potent positive inotropes (dopamine, dobutamine, or amrinone) can be monitored for the development of tachycardia or arrhythmia.

    D. Patients with trauma, shock, gastric dilation and volvulus, neurologic injury, and splenic masses often develop cardiac arrhythmias and may benefit from continuous ECG monitoring.

    E. Other critically ill animals that may be at risk for cardiopulmonary arrest should be continuously monitored for the development of cardiac arrhythmias.

    F. Animals with syncope of unknown etiology may be monitored to obtain an ECG diagnosis at the time of the syncopal episode.

 II. Technique

    A. An ECG monitor with oscilloscope is required (Fig. 5-1).

    B. The ECG signal is transmitted from the patient to the monitor via a cable (hardwire) or by telemetry. The lead wires (typically 3 in number) to the cable or telemetry box are connected to the patient via disposable, adherent ECG electrode patches.

    C. The ECG electrode patches are usually placed such that a transthoracic lead system is recorded with the positive lead at the left apex of the heart and the negative lead at the right base; the ground can be placed anywhere on the chest. Some veterinarians prefer to place the electrodes on the limbs. Regardless of placement, the hair must be clipped and the skin cleaned with alcohol and thoroughly dried before placement of the electrode patches. There must be adequate skin contact for good recordings, since the ECG electrode patches will not stay adhered if the skin is not well prepared. An unreadable or isoelectric ECG tracing may be improved with repositioning of the electrodes.

    D. The aforementioned technique will provide a continuous screen-display of the ECG. Many options are then available. Hard copy ECG recordings are highly useful for subsequent analysis, as is the ability to "freeze" the ECG tracing on the screen. Computer programs that analyze the recorded ECG have been developed for use in humans, although in many cases these programs do not accurately interpret canine ECGs.

III. Clinical utility

This technique is highly useful for demonstration of infrequent or dynamic changes in cardiac rhythm and is easy to perform.

IV. Limitations, risks, and costs

A. Limitations include the need to replace dislodged electrodes and mild patient discomfort when the electrodes are removed. Acetone aids in removal of the adhesive electrode patches.

B. Risks are minimal, although some animals require an Elizabethan collar to guard against patient chewing or destruction of the cable.

C. ECG monitoring devices can be purchased for $1,000 to $10,000 and the charge for daily monitoring is typically $10 to $50.

V. Alternative tests

Serially recorded ECG rhythm strips at 4- to 6-hour intervals provide some information, but can miss clinically important changes in heart rate and rhythm.

SPECIAL PROVOCATIVE ELECTROCARDIOGRAPHIC TECHNIQUES

I. Indications

Special provocative ECG techniques, such as ECG recording during vagal maneuver and postexercise ECG recordings, are useful in the evaluation of animals with syncope, collapse, or exercise intolerance when the baseline ECG fails to yield a diagnosis. An ECG recorded during a vagal maneuver is also useful to help differentiate supraventricular tachycardia from sinus tachycardia in animals who have narrow-complex tachycardia (i.e., not ventricular in origin).

II. Technique

A. Vagal maneuver

A vagal maneuver with ECG recording may be performed with a standard electrocardiograph or while performing continuous ECG monitoring. The patient is placed in a comfortable position, usually sternal recumbency. A vagal maneuver with simultaneous ECG recording is performed with either firm ocular pressure or carotid sinus massage. For carotid sinus massage, the patient's head is turned slightly to the left and the right side of the neck, near the angle of the mandible to behind the larynx, is repeatedly massaged in a cranial to caudal fashion. The pressure on the carotid sinus must be quite firm for an appropriate response.

B. Post-exercise ECG recordings

Post-exercise ECG recordings are performed, immediately after exercise, usually in dogs. The type and duration of exercise has not been standardized for veterinary patients.

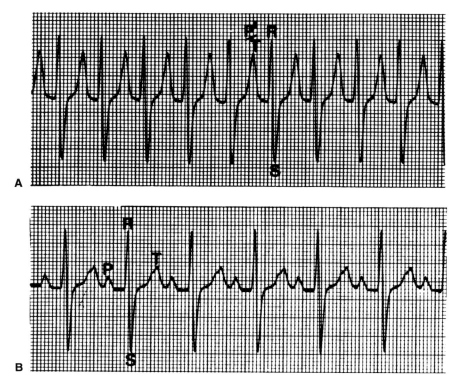

Fig. 5-2. Value of vagal stimulation by ocular pressure for the analysis and temporary treatment of a tachycardia in a dog. **(A)** Before ocular pressure; **(B)** after ocular pressure. The P and T waves easily can be seen. This response most often favors a diagnosis of supraventricular tachycardia. The atrial ectopic complexes (P′) are superimposed on the T waves of the previous complexes (P′/T) in Fig. A. (From Tilley L: Essentials of Canine and Feline Electrocardiography. 3rd Ed. Lea & Febiger, Philadelphia, 1992, with permission.)

III. Clinical utility

    In selected patients these techniques can provide a definitive ECG diagnosis or clarify the cause of syncope.

    A. Vagal maneuver

        The typical response of sinus tachycardia to a vagal maneuver is a mild slowing of the heart rate with resumption of sinus tachycardia following termination of carotid sinus pressure. When a narrow-complex tachycardia is abruptly terminated by a vagal maneuver, then the rhythm diagnosis of supraventricular tachycardia is clear and additional drug therapy may not be required (Fig. 5-2). Some dogs with a presenting complaint of syncope develop profound sinus arrest after vagal stimulation, which presumably results from exaggerated reflex responses that contribute to the development of bradycardia at the time of syncope.

    B. Post-exercise ECG recordings

        This test is most frequently used to evaluate dogs with aortic stenosis.

Evaluation of the recordings for profound ST segment depression or the development of cardiac arrhythmias may help quantify the degree of cardiac insufficiency. Those with ST segment changes or ventricular arrhythmias may be at risk for sudden death and may benefit from treatment with beta-blockers or calcium channel blockers. The technique may also be useful in evaluation of dogs presented for evaluation of exercise intolerance of unknown cause. Cardiac arrhythmias that are not identified on a resting ECG are occasionally discovered on a postexercise ECG.

IV. Limitations, risks, and costs
   A. Vagal maneuvers are difficult to perform in a manner that yields reliable and consistent results. In addition, while an abrupt termination of tachycardia may obviate the need for further therapy, the lack of response to a vagal maneuver supplies little additional information with respect to patient management.
   B. Ocular pressure, which seems less effective than carotid sinus massage, should not be performed in patients with ocular disease or increased intraocular pressure.
   C. Excessive cardiac slowing following a vagal maneuver, with resultant hypotension and collapse, is uncommon.
   D. These techniques are inexpensive and can be performed in most practices with the facilities for electrocardiography.

V. Alternative tests
   Holter monitor recordings, which provide a continuous ECG recording, can provide similar information but are more expensive and more difficult to perform.

CONTINUOUS AMBULATORY ELECTROCARDIOGRAPHY OR HOLTER MONITOR RECORDING

I. Indications
   Holter monitor recordings are indicated in animals with syncope, collapse, or exercise intolerance of undetermined origin after ECG, echocardiographic, and radiographic studies have been performed. Holter monitor recordings may also be indicated to evaluate the need for therapy, or the response to therapy, in animals with ventricular arrhythmias (Fig. 5-3). Holter recordings are also useful for evaluation of pacemaker malfunction.

II. Technique
   A. Recorder
      1. The recorder is a durable, lightweight device that continuously records the ECG on a reel-to-reel tape or, more commonly, a standard cassette tape.
      2. The unit is battery powered.
      3. Most have a depressible "event" marker button with which the owner can mark the tape at the time of collapse, drug administration, and other occurrences.
   B. Lead systems
      1. Most recorders have five lead wires to provide recording of two transthoracic leads with one lead wire as a ground.

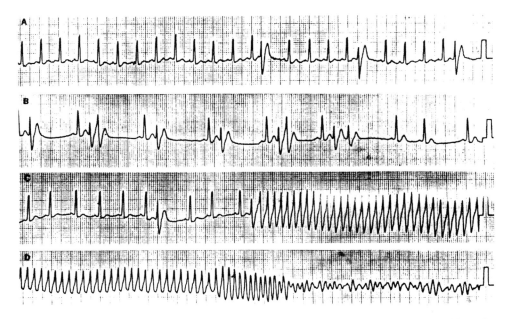

Fig. 5-3. Electrocardiographic tracings taken during a continuous (Holter) recording of a doberman pinscher with dilated cardiomyopathy during: walking outdoors (**A**); sleeping (**B**); unobserved (**C**) and (**D**). Isolated ventricular premature complexes (VPCs) are seen in Fig. A, repetitive VPCs (R on T wave) in Fig. B, and sustained ventricular tachycardia in Fig. C that degenerated into ventricular flutter and then fibrillation. (From Rush JE, Keene BW: ECG of the Month. J Am Vet Med Assoc, 194:52, 1989, with permission.)

    2. The leads are positioned on the thorax such that QRS complex on the recorded ECG is at least 1 mV tall.

    3. The positive electrodes are usually placed on the left side of the thorax.

C. Electrodes

    1. The electrodes are disposable, adhesive patches.

    2. The hair must first be clipped and the skin cleaned with alcohol or acetone.

    3. After the skin is dry, the electrodes are firmly placed on the skin.

    4. Lead dislodgement, a common cause of recording failure, is often due to inadequate skin preparation.

    5. Mild skin abrasion may improve electrode adhesion.

D. Patient application

    1. Once the electrodes are in place and the leads are connected, the size of the QRS complex is evaluated on a separate ECG machine.

    2. The recording is initiated and the recorder is carried by the patient in a backpack or is affixed to the animal with adhesive bandages.

E. Owner instructions

    1. The owners are instructed to keep a diary of the patient's activities.

    2. Owners should also be instructed to depress the event marker button any time the animal collapses during the recorded period.

    3. The recording time is typically a minimum of 24 hours and owners are instructed to return for removal of the recorder at that time.

  F. Analysis
   1. Computer analysis is performed after the recording is completed. The computerized scanner provides information on the minimum and maximum heart rates, frequency of ventricular arrhythmia, and periods of bradycardia.
   2. Pertinent hard copy ECG recordings are usually provided with the analysis.

III. Clinical utility

Holter monitor recording can be extremely useful in selected patients. The diagnostic yield can be low, however, and may only provide useful information that results in a change in therapy in 20 to 50 percent of recorded patients.

IV. Limitations, risks, and costs
  A. Several limitations are evident, including availability of the recorder and computer analysis, lead dislodgement that results in recording failure, and limitations of computer analysis. Some companies will send the recorder to veterinary practices by overnight delivery and provide analysis within a few days. Many of the computer analysis systems, however, are designed to interpret human ECGs and will "read" sinus arrhythmia as atrial premature depolarizations or bradycardia/tachycardia syndrome. Sinus tachycardia is often reported as supraventricular tachycardia. The reports and interpretations by human ECG analysts must be evaluated in light of the patient's clinical signs. The monitor can be time consuming to put on correctly, especially if the technique is performed infrequently.
  B. The risks are minimal, although lead removal at the end of the recording period can cause some patient discomfort and local skin irritation.
  C. Costs are typically $100 to $400 for recording and interpretation.

V. Alternative testing

See Continuous in-house electrocardiographic monitoring.

NONINVASIVE BLOOD PRESSURE MEASUREMENT

 I. Indications

Measurement of arterial blood pressure is indicated in animals with left ventricular hypertrophy of unknown cause, cats with retinal hemorrhages or detachments, animals with renal failure or adrenal disease, and patients in shock or those that are critically ill.

 II. Technique

Noninvasive blood pressure measurement can be accomplished using either the oscillometric or the Doppler technique.
  A. Oscillometric technique (Critikon-type)
   1. Uses a single cuff and a machine that automatically inflates and deflates the cuff.
   2. Place cuff around the rear limb, tail, or forelimb.
   3. Heart rate, systolic, diastolic, and mean blood pressure are reported.
  B. Doppler technique (Parks)
   1. Uses amplification of a Doppler shift from a transducer, which is usually placed over the tibial artery on the metatarsus.

    2. Ultrasonic gel is used to provide good contact between the skin and the transducer. An inflatable cuff, attached to a pressure manometer, is manually inflated proximal to the transducer until the Doppler sound disappears.

    3. The pressure is slowly reduced in the cuff until the Doppler sound returns; this value is reported as the systolic blood pressure. The diastolic pressure is estimated by a change in the character of the sound, although this change in tone is often difficult to appreciate.

III. Clinical utility

These techniques are extremely useful for a variety of settings in which either hypertension or hypotension is suspected. Blood pressure measurement allows rational choices to be made with respect to the need for and efficacy of antihypertensive therapy. Drug-induced hypotension, which may occur following initiation of vasodilator therapy, can be confirmed if suspected. The presence of hypotension and need for additional blood volume resuscitation or inotropic pressor support can be readily identified in critically ill patients.

IV. Limitations, risks, and costs

    A. The oscillometric technique often underestimates the blood pressure by 5 to 20 mmHg or more. While both techniques require an appropriately sized cuff, the oscillometric technique is more highly dependent on correct cuff size for accurate measurement than the Doppler technique. Despite these limitations, the oscillometric technique is easier to perform and is usually preferred in the intensive care setting where serial blood pressure measurements are desired to evaluate the response to fluid and/or drug therapy.

    Although the Doppler technique is somewhat more labor intensive, the measurement of systolic blood pressure is very accurate. Therefore, for a single blood pressure measurement the Doppler technique is usually preferred.

    Using either technique, normal values must be established for each individual clinic. Blood pressure varies widely depending upon the degree of patient excitement and presence or absence of sedation. Most patients with clinically significant disease resulting from systemic hypertension have a systolic blood pressure in excess of 170 mmHg.

    B. The risks are minimal.

    C. The Parks Medical instrument ($500 to $750) is less expensive than the Critikon unit ($4,000 to $5,000).

V. Alternative testing

    A. Digital palpation of the femoral or tibial arterial pulses may provide some indication of low blood pressure, but is totally ineffective for evaluating hypertension. When the femoral pulse is weak and the tibial pulse cannot be palpated, the mean arterial pressure is often less than 60 mmHg.

    B. Invasive blood pressure measurement.

INVASIVE BLOOD PRESSURE MEASUREMENT

I. Indications

Invasive blood pressure measurement is indicated when an extremely accurate measurement of blood pressure is required. This technique is usually limited to critically ill patients and/or research settings when serial blood pressure measurements are required.

II. Technique

Catheterization of any systemic artery will permit blood pressure measurement, although the tibial artery over the metatarsus and the femoral artery are most frequently used.

Most commonly, an over-the-needle intravenous catheter is advanced through the skin and subcutaneous tissues toward the artery until the hub of the catheter has a flash of arterial blood. The catheter is then advanced into the artery, the line is flushed, and the catheter is connected to a transducer through pressure tubing. The catheter is affixed to the skin with suture and/or adhesive tape or glue. The arterial line must be flushed frequently with heparinized saline to provide accurate blood pressure readings.

III. Clinical utility

Invasive blood pressure measurement provides a very accurate assessment of blood pressure. This degree of accuracy, however, is rarely needed in most clinical settings and this technique is seldom used in situations other than intensive care units.

IV. Limitations, risks, and costs

A. Arterial catheters require significant technical skill for placement and appropriate facilities for continuous monitoring. This technique is typically limited to those clinics with 24-hour nursing care and intensive patient monitoring capabilities. Transducers and a method for oscilloscopic or digital display of the blood pressure are also required.

B. Recognized risks include arterial thrombosis, catheter-related sepsis, inadvertent arterial injections, and catheter dislodgement with hematoma formation.

C. Invasive blood pressure measurement involves moderate expense in addition to the intensive monitoring requirements. The transducers and oscilloscopic devices can be obtained for as little as $2,000; however, many of the newer devices have multiple capabilities (ECG, invasive pressure monitoring, temperature, noninvasive blood pressure, pulse oximetry, etc.) and cost as much as $40,000.

V. Alternative testing

See Noninvasive blood pressure measurement

PHONOCARDIOGRAPHY AND AUSCULTATION AIDS

I. Indications

Phonocardiography is indicated when a pictographic display of the auscultatory findings is desired. The relationship of the auscultatory findings to the ECG/cardiac cycle can be accurately determined so that uncertain auscultatory findings can be accurately characterized (i.e., S_3 gallop versus midsystolic click). Auscultation aids can be used to amplify the cardiac sounds or record and replay the auscultatory findings at a slower speed.

II. Technique

The transducer is placed over areas of interest for auscultation.

    A. For phonocardiography, the heart sounds are displayed and recorded on paper or oscilloscope during simultaneous recording of the electrocardiogram.

    B. The findings are amplified and/or recorded on tape for the auscultatory aids.

III. Clinical utility

These techniques are highly useful as teaching tools for auscultation. The auscultation aids, which amplify the heart sounds, have additional utility for individuals with diminished auditory perception.

IV. Limitations, risks, and costs

    A. Phonocardiography requires appropriate equipment for detection, amplification, and simultaneous display of the heart sounds and ECG. The use of these techniques can be time consuming; however, for teaching auscultation phonocardiography is an invaluable tool.

    B. The risks are minimal to nonexistent.

    C. Equipment costs for phonocardiography and auscultatory aids are highly variable.

V. Alternative techniques

Instructional tapes of recorded heart sounds can be used as teaching tools.

NONSELECTIVE ANGIOCARDIOGRAPHY

I. Indications

Nonselective angiocardiography is indicated to identify congenital and acquired abnormalities of intracardiac or intravascular blood flow. Abnormalities of the veins and structures on the right side of the heart (right atrium, right ventricle, pulmonary arteries) are most readily identified by this technique. Nonselective angiography is useful to establish a diagnosis of heartworm in cats when laboratory findings are inconclusive. Additionally, this technique is useful to confirm thromboembolism of the renal arteries in cats with cardiomyopathy and anuria.

II. Technique

    A. Nonselective angiocardiography may require sedation or a light plane of anesthesia.

    B. A short, large-bore (18-gauge or larger) catheter is placed intravenously, preferably in the jugular vein.

    C. The animal is placed in the most appropriate position for opacification of desired structures (i.e., lateral recumbency for most congenital and acquired defects, sternal for a dorsoventral view to visualize pulmonary arteries).

    D. A large bolus of contrast is rapidly injected intravenously. The dose of contrast material is typically 0.75 cc to 1.5 cc of contrast/kg body weight. Alternatively, the dose of iodine to be administered may be calculated using 400 mg of iodine/kg body weight as the desirable dose.

    E. Depending on the structures of interest and the performance of the cardiovascular system, radiographic exposures are obtained 2 to 8 seconds after the injection is initiated. Shorter times should be used for evaluation of the right heart and pulmonary arteries, longer times for evaluation of structures on the left side of the heart and/or animals with heart failure and slow circulation times. Techniques to obtain rapid sequential exposures using a tunnel system have been described (Owens et al, 1977).

III. Clinical utility

In the absence of echocardiography, nonselective angiocardiography is a reasonable alternative technique to evaluate lesions that involve the right side of the heart in smaller patients. Occasionally, nonselective angiocardiography is used when echocardiography fails to identify the area of interest and cardiac catheterization is not an option due to poor patient condition or lack of appropriate facilities.

IV. Limitations, risks, and costs

A. Due to contrast dilution, nonselective angiocardiography, especially for evaluation of structures on the left side of the heart, is most successful in animals weighing less than 30 to 40 pounds. Adequate opacification of structures of interest can be difficult, especially without a pressure injector. The exact timing for appropriate exposures is difficult to predict and several exposures are often required. Complex cardiac malformations are difficult to appreciate with nonselective angiocardiography. For these reasons, nonselective angiocardiography often yields inconclusive findings.

B. Recognized complications that may result from intravenous contrast agents include transient hypotension, cardiac arrhythmias, nephrotoxicity (especially in animals with pre-existing renal dysfunction), and allergic reactions including fever, urticaria, or laryngeal edema. Hyperosmolar contrast agents may worsen pre-existing heart failure.

C. The costs of nonselective angiocardiography are less than those of selective cardiac catheterization and are often comparable to or slightly more expensive than echocardiography.

V. Alternative techniques

Where available, echocardiography should almost always be performed prior to nonselective angiocardiography. When echocardiography fails to identify the cause of the problem, selective cardiac catheterization is usually preferred over nonselective angiocardiographic studies. Computed tomography and nuclear magnetic resonance imaging may provide similar information.

CARDIAC CATHETERIZATION

I. Indications

Many procedures fall within the category of cardiac catheterization, including balloon valvuloplasty, cardiac pacing, and endomyocardial biopsy. Standard cardiac catheterization procedures for evaluation of congenital or acquired diseases typically include measurement of intracardiac pressures, blood oximetry, and selective angiocardiography. Indications for cardiac catheterization include certain congenital heart defects (i.e., pulmonic or aortic stenosis, ventricular septal defect, or complex congenital defects), high-grade atrioventricular block or persistent atrial standstill, and suspected myocarditis.

II. Technique

A. Cardiac catheterization usually requires anesthesia.

B. Surgical preparation of the neck for catheterization of the jugular vein and carotid artery, or of the inguinal region for catheterization of the femoral artery and vein.

C. Vascular access can be obtained with an incision down to the blood ves-

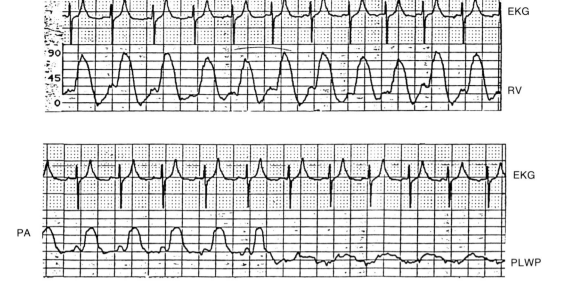

Fig. 5-4. Pressure tracings from a selective catheterization of the right ventricle and pulmonary artery. The right ventricular pressures are 88/15 mmHg (normal = 15–28/0–6 mmHg). The pulmonary arterial pressure is 84/30 mmHg (normal = 15–25/10–16 mmHg), and the pulmonary capillary wedge pressure is 15 mmHg (normal = 3–14 mmHg). The findings confirm pulmonary hypertension and provide a basis for initiation of drug therapy (diltiazem) in an attempt to reduce pulmonary arterial pressures. RV = right ventricle, PLWP = pulmonary capillary wedge pressure, PA = pulmonary artery.

sels, or with a percutaneous catheter introducer system using a modified Seldinger technique.

D. Catheters are advanced under fluoroscopic guidance, or by recognition of pressure wave forms, to the cardiac chambers of interest.

E. Intravascular pressures are recorded from chambers of interest to determine whether stenoses are present and to determine whether congestive heart failure is present or imminent (Fig. 5-4). The pressures are typically recorded before and after therapeutic interventions, such as balloon valvuloplasty, to quantify postprocedural improvements in hemodynamics.

F. Oximetry: Blood samples are obtained to measure oxygen saturation for calculation of shunt fraction in animals with atrial or ventricular septal defects.

G. Angiocardiography: Radiopaque contrast material is injected through the catheter(s) located at the appropriate areas of interest and the image is recorded on VCR tape, radiographic film, or cineangiography, or is digitally stored for digital subtraction angiographic techniques (Figs. 5-5 and 5-6).

H. Cardiac output may be determined using thermodilution (injection of a specific quantity of saline or dextrose that has a known temperature). The resulting drop in blood temperature is calculated as the cardiac output by using a cardiac-output computer.

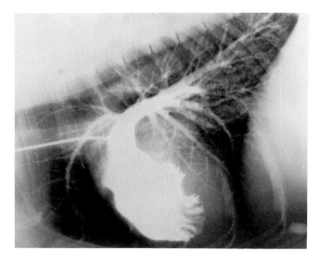

Fig. 5-5. Normal right ventriculogram obtained by selective catheterization.

    I. Additional techniques that may be performed include balloon valvuloplasty or balloon angioplasty, endomyocardial biopsy, and cardiac pacing.

III. Clinical utility

Cardiac catheterization is invaluable in certain cases when the diagnosis is still in question following ECG, thoracic radiographs, and echocardiography. For stenotic valvular lesions (i.e., pulmonic ± aortic stenosis) balloon valvuloplasty provides a less invasive alternative to surgery for relief of the obstruction. Cardiac catheterization is also a valuable research tool for evaluation

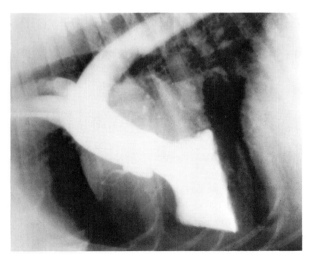

Fig. 5-6. Normal left ventriculogram obtained by selective catheterization.

of vascular patency, hemodynamic responses to new cardiovascular drugs, and new catheterization techniques.

IV. Limitations, risks, and costs
   A. Cardiac catheterization is limited to university practice and a few private referral institutions. The techniques can be time consuming, especially if not performed on a routine basis.
   B. Procedural success and patient risk are related to operator skill. Patient risk is also a function of the technique involved and the patient's clinical status. Patients with severe heart failure are at higher risk of complications resulting from either anesthesia or catheterization. Balloon valvuloplasty carries a higher risk than isolated right heart catheterization to determine cardiac output or pulmonary capillary wedge pressure. In addition to the previously mentioned complications of IV radiopaque contrast material, surgical or cardiovascular infection, cardiac arrhythmias, air embolism, vascular thrombosis or thromboembolism, and vascular perforation are recognized complications. With appropriate case selection and operator skill, the morbidity for cardiac catheterization should be less than 10 percent and the mortality less than 2 percent.
   C. Cardiac catheterization is an expensive procedure, typically ranging from $500 to $2,000.

ENDOMYOCARDIAL BIOPSY

I. Indications
   Endomyocardial biopsy is indicated in animals suspected of having myocarditis as well as other metabolic, biochemical, or nutritional defects that cause or result from cardiac dysfunction.

II. Technique
   A. A bioptome is passed through a sheathed introducer into the jugular vein and advanced into the right ventricle.
   B. Multiple small myocardial biopsy samples are sequentially obtained from the interventricular septum or the right ventricle.

III. Clinical utility
   Histopathologic myocardial lesions can be detected through the use of this technique. Myocarditis may be present in some animals with high-grade AV block or dilated cardiomyopathy, although the therapeutic implications of this inflammation are unclear at this time. Similarly, several dogs with dilated cardiomyopathy have been shown to have myocardial carnitine deficiency, although not all cases have responded dramatically to carnitine supplementation. Therefore, much debate about the clinical utility of this technique exists. Further developments in the analysis of myocardial biopsies for defects in metabolism or immunologic testing may expand the role for endomyocardial biopsy beyond its current use as a research tool.

IV. Limitations, risks, and costs
   A. The technique is limited to universities and a few referral practices.
   B. The risks are the same as those listed for cardiac catheterization. Transient ventricular arrhythmias at the time of biopsy are common, but rarely

problematic. Perforation of the right ventricle with resulting cardiac tamponade is another potential complication.

C. The expense may range from $250 to $1,000.

V. Alternative techniques

There are currently no techniques that give similar information.

SEROLOGIC TESTING

I. Indications

Animals with clinical signs suggestive of myocardial dysfunction resulting from infectious or immune-mediated etiologies.

A. Dogs with high grade atrioventricular block with a history of tick exposure in a Lyme endemic region (*Borrelia* titer).

B. Animals with right-sided heart failure from Mexico, southern Texas, or other areas where Chagas disease is endemic (Trypanosome titer).

C. Animals with heart failure or arrhythmias and additional evidence of immune-mediated disease (anti-nuclear antibody titer).

D. Cats with myocardial dysfunction and fever, pneumonia, neurologic disease, chorioretinitis or other clinical signs compatible with toxoplasmosis (toxoplasmosis titer).

II. Technique

Serum should be submitted to a laboratory that has the appropriate facilities to perform serologic testing for the disease in question.

III. Clinical utility

These serologic tests can be very useful in establishing an etiologic agent in selected cases. It should be stressed that a positive titer for *Borrelia* in a dog with AV block does not necessarily confirm that Lyme disease is the cause of the cardiac arrhythmia. A positive result only confirms previous exposure to the organism. As with all serologic tests, the results must be interpreted in concert with the patient's clinical signs.

IV. Limitations, risks, and costs

A. The limitations are simply those of correct interpretation of serologic testing.

B. No risks are involved.

C. Costs are dependent upon the laboratory.

EXERCISE TESTING

I. Indications

Exercise, or stress, testing may be an appropriate diagnostic technique for patients with clinical signs of collapse, syncope, or exercise intolerance when the diagnosis is not clear after routine evaluation. These techniques may also be useful in the evaluation of patients with known cardiovascular disease, to quantify the degree of disability (i.e., aortic stenosis) or to determine response to therapeutic interventions.

II. Technique

A. In general, the techniques are modified human exercise testing protocols. Standard testing protocols for these techniques have not yet been estab-

lished for veterinary patients. The role of ECG testing following exercise was discussed under the section on special provocative electrocardiographic techniques.
  B. Exercise testing, which is rarely done in cats, typically involves running a dog for a standard time or distance at a given speed. This is most easily accomplished on a treadmill, although alternative testing schemes using stair climbing or walking a specified distance may prove more useful in veterinary patients. A number of variables can be quantified, including the duration or intensity of exercise, heart rate, electrocardiographic findings (such as ST segment changes), blood pressure, venous PO_2, and blood lactate.
III. Clinical utility
  Exercise testing has limited utility at present because of a lack of technique standardization, equipment variability, and lack of clear endpoints. It remains to be determined whether a standard exercise testing protocol will provide information that has therapeutic implications.
IV. Limitations, risks, and costs
  A. Treadmills are usually only available at institutions or universities. Not all patients cooperate during treadmill running or exercise testing, making exercise to near exhaustion impossible. Standardized testing protocols have not been developed and this makes comparisons between institutions difficult.
  B. The potential exists for patient overexertion or the development of severe arrhythmias.
  C. Costs are dependent on facilities and the protocol used.

INVASIVE ELECTROPHYSIOLOGIC STUDIES

  I. Indications
  Invasive electrophysiologic studies (EPS) are indicated in animals with arrhythmias that are refractory to standard antiarrhythmic drug therapies. Invasive electrophysiologic studies can also be used in cases in which it is necessary to specifically map the location or origin of an arrhythmia for surgical or radiofrequency catheter ablation.
  II. Technique
  Multiple catheters are advanced into the heart and intracardiac electrograms are recorded.
  A. For ventricular arrhythmias, premature stimuli are delivered in rapid succession in an attempt to induce sustained ventricular tachycardia or ventricular fibrillation. The ability to induce the arrhythmia is tested again following drug administration.
  B. Invasive electrophysiologic studies can be used to identify and map the location of accessory atrioventricular pathways (i.e., bypass tracts, Wolf-Parkinson-White Syndrome). Electrocautery delivered through the catheter (radiofrequency catheter ablation) or surgery can be used to interrupt the accessory pathway.

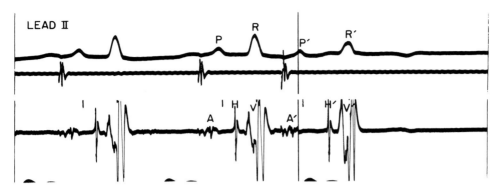

Fig. 5-7. Canine bundle of His electrogram recorded simultaneously with a lead II electrocardiogram (top tracing). Events recorded from the intracardiac electrode catheter: A, atrial deflection; H, His bundle deflection; V, ventricular deflection. His bundle recordings can be useful in determining the origin of aberrant ventricular complexes. The third complex (P′R′) is slightly aberrant because an early premature impulse has not given a portion of the bundle branches enough time to fully recover. The premature impulse is supraventricular because the electrogram shows a prolonged A′-H′ interval. The H′-V′ interval of the premature complex is normal. With ventricular ectopic complexes, the H′ spikes follow, are buried in, or precede V′ by less than the normal H-V interval. The middle tracing is a right atrial electrogram. (From Tilley L: Essentials of Canine and Feline Electrocardiography. 3rd Ed. Lea & Febiger, Philadelphia, 1992, with permission.)

    C. His bundle electrograms can record the site of block within the His bundle and conduction system for advanced forms of atrioventricular block (Fig. 5-7). The information gained from this technique can be used to determine the site of block and the need for pacemaker implantation.

III. Clinical utility

The majority of these techniques, except His bundle electrograms, are only available through collaboration with EPS testing labs at human medical centers. At this time, EPS testing is largely of academic interest in veterinary patients. In a few select cases, permanent cures or therapeutic insights are gained through EPS testing. The most widespread use of this technique in humans is to determine optimal antiarrhythmic drug therapy in a patient who is refractory to conventional therapy.

IV. Limitations, risks, and costs

    A. The limitations are those of cost, training, and limited availability of the equipment required for EPS testing. A debate exists over whether EPS testing for ventricular arrhythmias results in an improved outcome or prolonged survival when compared to drug therapy selected by Holter recording, or simply empirical drug therapy.

    B. The risks are generally those of cardiac catheterization, although the induction of ventricular fibrillation is of greater concern. A defibrillator and personnel familiar with its use *must* be present at the time of testing.

    C. The cost is determined on a case-by-case basis. In most instances, the trained personnel must volunteer their services and equipment time or the costs are excessive.

V. Alternative techniques

Holter monitor recording may provide similar information about response to therapy for ventricular arrhythmias. In veterinary patients, a program of empirical drug therapy and clinical response is used in most cases of ventricular arrhythmia or accessory pathway. Pacemaker implantation is usually adequate therapy for high-grade atrioventricular block, and His bundle electrograms are rarely required.

COMPUTED TOMOGRAPHY AND NUCLEAR MAGNETIC RESONANCE IMAGING

I. Indications

These techniques are useful for noninvasive evaluation of the heart and great vessels. Both techniques permit accurate detection of cardiac masses or thrombi, and are useful in some pericardial disorders and complex congenital defects. Magnetic resonance imaging (MRI) can provide better detail and may be useful in assessing blood flow and in characterizing tissues. There are currently few, if any, cardiovascular disorders in veterinary patients in which these are the techniques of choice.

II. Technique

A. Both MRI and computed tomography (CT) require general anesthesia to immobilize the patient.

B. Computed tomography displays cross sections of cardiac anatomy that are produced by computer reconstruction of information obtained by directing ionizing radiation though multiple angles of the body. MRI provides a similar tomographic view but collects magnetic data following application of a fluctuating radiofrequency impulse. The location of the heart and relationships to local structures is readily appreciated using both techniques.

III. Clinical utility

Computed tomography and MRI are useful in selected patients when, after thoracic radiography and echocardiography, there are still questions regarding the relationship of the heart to surrounding structures.

IV. Limitations, risks, and costs

A. The resolution of most CT scanners available to veterinarians is often inadequate to document small-mass lesions or valvular anatomy. CT scanners are not readily available to most veterinarians, although some human hospitals will permit the use of their equipment for animal imaging. Access to MRI is still very limited and its use is limited largely to research endeavors or selected clinical cases.

B. The risks of both CT and MRI are limited to those of anesthesia.

C. The expense is determined on a case-by-case basis. The costs of CT range from $100 to $500. The cost of MRI is typically unacceptably high unless equipment time and professional personnel are volunteered.

RADIONUCLIDE IMAGING

I. Indications

Radionuclide imaging is a safe and relatively non-invasive technique to evaluate cardiac chamber size, myocardial perfusion, and regional myocardial wall function. The technique provides less detailed information regarding valvular, pericardial, or intracardiac anatomy than echocardiography or cardiac catheterization with angiography. These techniques are particularly useful for non-invasive evaluation of patients with suspected coronary artery abnormalities. Due to the low incidence of coronary artery disease in dogs and cats, these techniques have been used infrequently except in research studies. They do not appear to be superior to the standard diagnostic techniques available for evaluation of animals with cardiovascular disease. The only exception is testing for pulmonary arterial thromboembolism where ventilation and perfusion scans can often confirm the diagnosis.

II. Technique

A radiopharmaceutical is injected intravenously and the radioactivity is then recorded by a radiodetection device, typically a "gamma camera." The resulting image, usually recorded from three projections, is used to help evaluate cardiac function and myocardial perfusion. In some instances, the radioactive component is attached to albumin or red blood cells.

A. Thallium 201 myocardial imaging is most useful for evaluation of myocardial perfusion. A portion of the dose is taken up by the myocardium within the first minute after IV injection. The distribution of thallium to the myocardium is closely related to blood flow. Areas of myocardial infarction or ischemia will demonstrate diminished tracer activity, indicating absent perfusion or altered cell viability. Exercise increases coronary artery blood flow and exercise thallium testing is a very sensitive test for detection of coronary artery disease.

B. Technetium 99m can be used to evaluate cardiac function. The ejection fraction is the most accurate measurement obtained using this technique. Left ventricular end diastolic volume can also be calculated, and from these two measurements, the stroke volume and end systolic volume calculations are available. Regional wall motion abnormalities may also be detected by these techniques.

1. First-pass studies

First-pass radionuclide studies are performed immediately after intravenous injection of a bolus of contrast. The bolus travels through the heart very quickly, allowing for separate imaging of the relative phases of the right and left ventricle.

2. Gated-equilibrium studies

The second type of study done with technetium is a gated-equilibrium study. In the gated-equilibrium study, the images are recorded over several minutes and summed to improve the image quality. The image is simultaneously recorded with an ECG to allow comparison of counts between systole and diastole. The ECG permits the recorded images to be gated to specific times during the cardiac cycle. For example, end diastole is generally accepted to occur at the beginning of the QRS complex. An accurate calculation of end diastolic volume can be made by summing a series of images recorded at the beginning of the QRS complex.

III. Clinical utility

These techniques have limited utility for evaluation of cardiac function in veterinary patients, and their use is typically limited to selected cases or research settings.

IV. Limitations, risks, and costs

A. These techniques are available at very few institutions. The regulations regarding handling and disposal of radiopharmaceuticals must be considered during their use.

B. Patient risk is low, although the technique may require anesthesia.

C. The cost is usually arranged on a case-by-case basis.

V. Alternative techniques

Cardiac catheterization with coronary angiography, although more invasive, is the best alternative for evaluation of coronary arterial anatomy and patency. Echocardiography provides a good alternative for evaluation of myocardial function.

SUGGESTED READINGS

Boucher CA, Kantor HL, Okada RD, Strass HW: Radionuclide imaging and magnetic resonance imaging. p. 1601. In Eagle KA, Haber E, DeSanctis RW et al: The Practice of Cardiology. Little, Brown, Boston, 1989

Guiney TE: Exercise stress testing. p. 1585. In Eagle KA, Haber E, DeSanctis RW et al: The Practice of Cardiology. Little, Brown, Boston, 1989

Kaplan PM: Monitoring. p. 21. In Murtaugh RJ, Kaplan PM (eds): Veterinary Emergency and Critical Care Medicine. Mosby-Year Book, St. Louis, 1992

Keene BW, Kittleson ME, Atkins CE et al: Modified transvenous endomyocardial biopsy technique in dogs. J Am Vet Med Assoc 51(11):1769, 1990

Miller MS, Calvert CA: Special methods for analysing arrhythmias. p. 289. In Tilley LP (ed): Essentials of Canine and Feline Electrocardiography. 3rd Ed. Lea & Febiger, Philadelphia, 1992

Owens JM, Twedt DC: Nonselective angiocardiography in the cat. Vet Clin North Am 7: 309, 1977

Podell M: Use of blood pressure monitors. p. 834. In Kirk RW, Bonagura JD (eds): Current Veterinary Therapy XI. WB Saunders, Philadelphia, 1992

Sisson DD, Daniel GB, Twardock AR: Comparison of left ventricular ejection fractions determined in healthy anesthetized dogs by echocardiography and gated equilibrium radionuclide ventriculography. J Am Vet Med Assoc 50(11):1840, 1989

Suter PF: Special procedures for the diagnosis of thoracic disease. p. 47. In Suter PF (ed): Thoracic Radiography of the Dog and Cat. Peter F. Suter, Wettswil, Switzerland, 1984

6

Acquired Valvular Insufficiency

Clarke E. Atkins

INTRODUCTION

I. Diseases of the heart valves represent an important group of acquired canine cardiac disorders. Valve anatomy and function can be affected directly or indirectly by a variety of diseases, including parasitic disease (heartworms), neoplastic disease (intracardiac tumors), degenerative disease (endocardiosis and cardiomyopathy), traumatic injury, and inflammatory disease (vegetative endocarditis), each of which may produce incompetence.

II. Endocardiosis is the most prevalent and clinically significant of these processes, and most often affects small breeds. The atrioventricular valves are typically involved. Mitral valvular endocardiosis with insufficiency is most commonly encountered, frequently leading to clinically apparent dysfunction and heart failure. The discussion of endocardiosis will center on the left (mitral) atrioventricular valve.

III. As a primary disease this appears to be an infrequent cause of heart failure in the adult cat. Signs and therapy are similar to those of the dog and hence no specific discussion of the cat will be presented here.

IV. Inflammation of the valves is the second most frequently encountered acquired valvular disease in dogs. Vegetative endocarditis of the mitral and aortic valves is most common, and tends to produce devastating consequences.

ACQUIRED ATRIOVENTRICULAR VALVULAR INSUFFICIENCY (MITRAL ENDOCARDIOSIS)

I. Etiology
   A. Valvular endocardiosis (myxomatosis, fibrosis, or chronic valvular disease) is of unknown etiology.
II. Incidence
   A. Males are affected often than females (1.5:1).
   B. Small and toy breeds are predominately affected.
   C. In a survey of canine necropsy specimens, Buchanan (1979) showed that the mitral valve alone was affected in 62 percent, the mitral and the tricuspid valves in 33 percent of cases, and the tricuspid valve alone was af-

fected in only 1 percent of cases. Murmurs of chronic valvular disease are recognized in 10 percent of middle-aged dogs, increasing to approximately one-third in aged dogs.

   D. Florid left-heart or biventricular failure is unusual before the age of 8 to 10 years.

III. Pathophysiology

   A. The mitral valve apparatus is made up of a closely interrelated group of structures, including the mitral valve leaflets; their fibrous point of attachment and fulcrum (the mitral valve annulus); the chordae tendineae, which hold valve leaflets in apposition, preventing eversion; and the left ventricular wall with papillary muscles (Fig. 6-1).

   B. Degeneration begins with subendothelial deposition of mucopolysaccharide, which produces thickening of the valve leaflet. Nodular swellings develop and coalesce, producing plaque-like structures with distortion and valve contracture.

   C. The ultimate result of this degenerative process is a stiff, deformed, and incompetent valve.

   D. Regurgitant volume is small in the early stages of disease, but, as the disease progresses, most of the cardiac output may be ejected into the left atrium. Left atrial pressure rises. The valve annulus and left ventricle dilate, increasing valve dysfunction.

   E. The concomitant drop in forward cardiac output produces certain compensatory mechanisms, such as increased heart rate, fluid retention, and

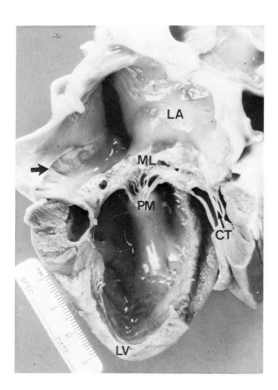

Fig. 6-1. Functional anatomy of the abnormal mitral valve apparatus in a dog that died from severe left-sided heart failure. Mitral valvular regurgitation has resulted in severe left atrial enlargement (LA) and subsequent increase in size of the annulus. Rupture of the left atrial wall *(arrow)* occurs at the site of a jet lesion resulting from regurgitant streams of blood from the left ventricle continuously striking the atrial wall. ML, mitral valve leaflets, grossly thickened and contracted; CT, chordae tendineae; PM, papillary muscle; LV, dilated left ventricular muscle wall.

peripheral vasoconstriction. Initially, these help to maintain cardiac output and blood pressure, but ultimately these processes increase cardiac work, cardiovascular volume, and regurgitant fraction. Thus, a vicious cycle begins.

F. The resultant chronic volume overload is not well tolerated by the left ventricle. In some cases, cardiac output is further reduced by the development of diminished contractility, due in part to left ventricular fibrosis.

G. Heart failure
   1. Falling cardiac output may ultimately produce signs of forward heart failure, such as poor tissue perfusion, exercise intolerance, and syncope.
   2. The rise in left atrial and hence pulmonary venous pressure produces venous congestion and, finally, interstitial and alveolar pulmonary edema.
   3. Prolonged left-heart failure due to mitral regurgitation can uncommonly lead to right-heart failure with systemic venous congestion, hepatosplenomegaly, ascites, and/or hydrothorax, especially when concurrent tricuspid insufficiency exists.

H. Complications
   1. Cardiac arrhythmias
      a) Sinus tachycardia
      b) Supraventricular ectopy, tachycardia
      c) Ventricular ectopy, tachycardia
   2. Rupture of chordae tendineae with decompensation
   3. Tearing of the left atrium with tamponade

IV. Clinical signs
   A. Signs prior to heart failure
   The earliest sign of valvular insufficiency is a midsystolic click and/or an early, low-intensity, mixed-frequency systolic murmur, heard loudest apically at the left fifth intercostal space. As the disease progresses, the murmur becomes longer in duration. The murmur of mitral regurgitation typically antedates by years the onset of clinical signs. Murmur intensity cannot be used to estimate the severity of mitral regurgitation.
   B. Left-heart failure
   1. The phases of heart disease, adapted from the New York Heart Association are presented in Table 6-1. These apply to all heart disease, not just mitral disease.
   2. As left-heart failure ensues, classical signs such as orthopnea, dyspnea, cough, reduced exercise tolerance, syncope, anorexia, and weight loss

TABLE 6-1. FUNCTIONAL CLASSIFICATION OF HEART DISEASE AND FAILURE IN THE DOG

Class I	No clinical manifestation
Class II	Cough or decreased exercise tolerance only with extreme exertion
Class III	Cough, orthopnea, reduced exercise tolerance, ascites, hydrothorax, syncope
Class IV	Signs of class III with the addition of dyspnea at rest

(From Atkins CE: Atrioventricular valvular insufficiency. In Allen DG (ed): Small Animal Medicine. JB Lippincott, Philadelphia, 1991, with permission.)

may be observed. The cough is often worse in the morning and evening hours.

3. Other physical findings
   a) Audible arrhythmias, pulse deficits
   b) Cardiac gallop (S_3 usually)
   c) Respiratory crackles (rales) and dyspnea
   d) Ashen or cyanotic mucous membranes
   e) Prolonged capillary refill time, cold extremities
   f) Weak pulses
   g) Pink froth may be evident in the nostrils and oropharynx terminally

V. Diagnosis
   A. The diagnosis of mitral insufficiency is typically not difficult because of the characteristic murmur, age, and breeds affected. Determining whether the patient is in heart failure and what role cardiac disease plays in the dog's symptomatology may be more challenging. This can be particularly problematic in discerning the role of cardiac disease, if any, in small breed dogs suffering from chronic cough. The cause of the cough may actually be primary respiratory disease with or without concomitant heart disease. Table 6-2 outlines features useful for differentiating whether coughing is due to respiratory disease or due to heart disease.
   B. Another important, but difficult, determination is whether dogs with mitral insufficiency are afflicted with myocardial failure. In other words, is the problem of mitral regurgitation compounded by pump dysfunction? In the majority (80%) of dogs with endocardiosis and heart failure, myocardial dysfunction cannot be documented. Nevertheless, when present,

TABLE 6-2. HISTORICAL AND CLINICAL FINDINGS THAT MAY AID IN DIFFERENTIATION OF COUGH DUE TO MITRAL INSUFFICIENCY FROM COUGH DUE TO CHRONIC RESPIRATORY DISEASE[a]

Heart Failure	Respiratory Disease
Weight loss	Often obese
Cough worse at night; may be accompanied by frothy, pink nasal discharge or sputum	Cough with exercise; may be accompanied by mucopurulent nasal discharge or sputum
Dyspnea variable; often worse at night	Usually not dyspneic
Murmur	With or without murmur
Respiratory crackles or no ALS	Respiratory crackles, wheezes, or no ALS
Sinus tachycardia or other arrhythmias	Normal to slow heart rate with exaggerated sinus arrhythmia
P-mitrale or LVE on ECG	P-pulmonale or RVE on ECG
Pulmonary edema, left atrial enlargement on radiographs	No pulmonary edema, left atrial enlargement mild or absent on radiographs
No airway collapse or bronchial infiltrate on radiographs	Airway collapse or bronchial/parenchymal infiltrate on radiographs
Normal respiratory cytology	Abnormal respiratory cytology
Normal or stress leukogram	Variable inflammatory leukogram
Diuretic responsive	Diuretic unresponsive

Abbreviations: ALS, adventitious lung sounds; ECG, electrocardiogram; LVE, left ventricular enlargement; RVE, right ventricular enlargement.
[a] Each finding need not be present in all cases.
(Adapted from Atkins CE: Atrioventricular valvular insufficiency. In Allen DG (ed): Small Animal Medicine. JB Lippincott, Philadelphia, 1991, with permission.)

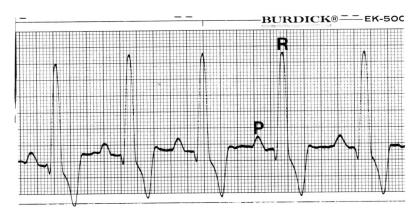

Fig. 6-2. Left ventricle enlargement in a dog with chronic mitral valvular insufficiency. The QRS complexes are wide (0.09-s). The ST segment coving also reflects left-heart enlargement. The P waves are wide (0.06-s), suggesting left atrial enlargement.

it has therapeutic and prognostic relevance. Assessment of myocardial function in the setting of mitral insufficiency is confounded by altered loading conditions, which invalidate commonly used isovolumic (pre-ejection period, Dp/dt) and ejection phase (fractional shortening) indices of myocardial performance.

C. Electrocardiography

    1. The electrocardiographic findings in mitral insufficiency are nonspecific and, unless an arrhythmia is present, are not of great diagnostic utility. In fact, the ECG is frequently normal. The usefulness of the ECG can be enhanced by serial evaluations, and the ECG can be used as an aid in distinguishing cardiac from respiratory causes for chronic cough (Table 6-2).

    2. Common ECG abnormalities

        a) Sinus tachycardia if heart failure is present

        b) Supraventricular and ventricular ectopy and tachycardia

        c) Left atrial enlargement (wide P waves; Fig. 6-2).

        d) Left ventricular enlargement (tall R waves, prolonged QRS duration; Fig. 6-2)

D. Radiography

    1. Thoracic radiography is useful in the diagnosis of cardiomegaly, specific cardiac chamber size, impending (pulmonary venous congestion) or florid heart failure, and the presence of concurrent respiratory disease. In addition, radiographs are helpful in evaluating the efficacy of therapeutic interventions. It must be kept in mind that the radiographic changes associated with mitral insufficiency occur gradually and that serial examinations often amplify the value of this procedure (Figs. 6-3 to 6-7).

    2. Radiographs early in the disease course are unremarkable, but with time and worsening of mitral regurgitation, left-heart enlargement is

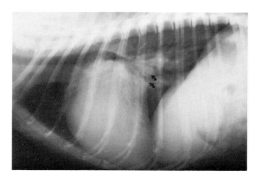

Fig. 6-3. Mitral valvular insufficiency. Lateral projection. The left ventricular border is straightened and there is loss of the caudal waist. There is moderate left atrial dilation *(arrows)*.

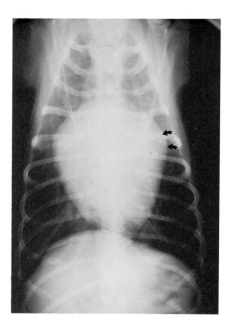

Fig. 6-4. Mitral valvular insufficiency. Dorsoventral projection. The dilated left auricle extends beyond the cardiac border *(arrows)*.

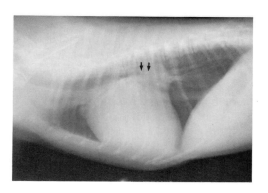

Fig. 6-5. Generalized cardiomegaly. Lateral projection. There is biventricular enlargement and left atrial dilation with elevation and compression of the left mainstem bronchus *(arrows)*.

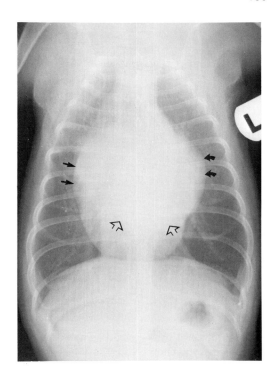

Fig. 6-6. Generalized cardiomegaly. Dorsoventral projection. The marked left atrial dilation is noted by protrusion of the left auricular border beyond the lateral cardiac border *(curved arrows)* and a double density of the enlarged left atrium caudal to the heart base separating the caudal lobar bronchi *(open arrows)*. There is rounding of the right ventricle and bulging of the right atrium *(small arrows)*.

apparent (Figs. 6-3 to 6-6). Left atrial enlargement is an early and relatively consistent sign.

3. As heart failure ensues, the left atrium enlarges further and the hilar pulmonary veins become more radiodense. Together, they produce a left atrial mass, which extends dorsal and caudal to the tracheal carina (Fig. 6-6). Pulmonary venous congestion is indicated by enlargement of the apical pulmonary vein to a size larger than the proximal one-third of the fourth rib or its pulmonary artery (Fig. 6-7).

4. Florid left-heart failure is suspected when hilar interstitial density or diffuse alveolar densities are identified in a dog with mitral insufficiency (Fig. 6-7).

E. Echocardiography

1. In general terms, although the echocardiogram can diagnose myocardial dysfunction (pump or muscle failure), it does not diagnose heart failure. More specifically, without the aid of Doppler studies, it cannot diagnose mitral regurgitation and thus is limited in its ability to diagnose myocardial failure as a completion of mitral regurgitation.

2. Echocardiographic findings of mitral insufficiency
   a) Left atrial and ventricular enlargement (dilatation)
   b) Exuberant left ventricular septal and posterior wall motion is usually noted. A left ventricular shortening fraction that is normal or subnormal, when associated with significant mitral regurgitation, suggests diminished myocardial function.
   c) Thickening of valve leaflets may be recognized.

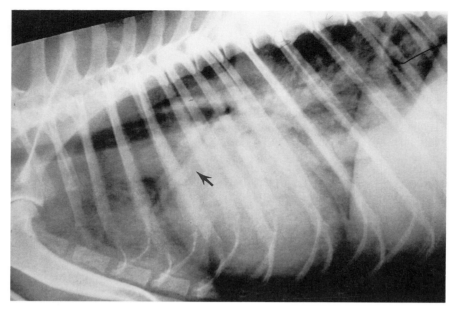

Fig. 6-7. Lateral thoracic radiograph from a dog in florid left-heart failure due to mitral valvular insufficiency. Note the large pulmonary vein *(arrow)* and diffuse alveolar lung density, suggestive of pulmonary edema. (From Atkins CE: Atrioventricular valvular insufficiency. In Allen DG (ed): Small Animal Medicine. JB Lippincott, Philadelphia, 1991, with permission.)

       d) Abnormal valve leaflet motion in the case of ruptured chordae tendineae

       e) Pericardial effusion associated with atrial tears

F. Miscellaneous laboratory tests

    1. When biventricular or right-heart failure is present, the evaluation of thoracic and/or ascitic fluid will help to rule out noncardiac causes for its accumulation. Typically, the fluid associated with heart failure is a modified transudate.

    2. The analysis of arterial blood gas concentrations allows recognition of hypoxemia and metabolic acidosis when present. The respective causes are reduced pulmonary O_2 diffusion and/or ventilation perfusion mismatching and diminished tissue perfusion, the latter being variably associated with lactic acidosis.

    3. Venous blood gas analysis provides similar information about acid-base status, but little information about the ability of the lungs to oxygenate blood. Venous P_{O_2} declines as blood stagnates in the tissues when cardiac output is subnormal. A P_{vO_2} of less than 30 mmHg (normal = 40 mmHg) indicates forward or low output heart failure, and can be used as an adjunct for evaluation of the need for and potential efficacy of vasodilator therapy.

    4. A complete blood count, modified Knott test and/or ELISA antigen

test, serum chemistry and electrolyte panel, and urinalysis should be obtained and evaluated to rule out concurrent disease processes and as a baseline for future evaluations after institution of therapy. Chronic heart failure may modestly raise liver enzymes. Diuretic therapy may result in hypokalemia, hypomagnesemia, metabolic alkalosis, and azotemia.

G. Differential diagnoses
  1. Other causes for murmur
    a) Secondary mitral insufficiency due to hypertrophic or dilated cardiomyopathy
    b) Vegetative endocarditis
    c) Congenital heart disease
    d) Tricuspid insufficiency
    e) Anemia
  2. Signs of left-heart failure (cough, dyspnea)
    a) Primary respiratory disease (Table 6-2) such as bronchitis, airway collapse, pneumonia, neoplasia, and degenerative disease
    b) Pleural diseases with effusion
    c) Anemia
    d) Metabolic acidosis
    e) Other causes of heart failure

VI. Medical Management
  A. The overall therapeutic objective is to enhance both the quality and the duration of life. It should be determined whether failure exists, the nature of its clinical manifestations (forward, backward, or both), whether myocardial failure is present, and whether cardiac rhythm disturbances, respiratory disease, or right-heart failure complicate the clinical picture. A therapeutic approach to the management of mitral insufficiency is detailed in Table 6-3.
  B. Reduction of mitral regurgitation
    1. Surgical correction of valvular dysfunction, although theoretically very appealing, is currently impractical.
    2. Cardiac glycosides and other positive inotropic drugs, diuretics, and vasodilators have the potential to reduce cardiac size and/or afterload, thereby reducing regurgitant fraction.
  C. Positive inotropic therapy: myocardial function is thought to be unaffected in the majority of dogs with symptomatic mitral insufficiency, emphasizing the fact that heart failure can, and often does, exist without concurrent myocardial failure.
    1. The use of cardiac glycosides (digitalis) is controversial. Myocardial failure, and supraventricular arrhythmia, refractoriness to other therapy, and concomitant right or biventricular heart failure are generally accepted indications. Many clinicians feel that digitalis is indicated even without these manifestations because of its ability to reverse baroreceptor dysfunction, known to exist in heart failure.
    2. Other inotropes, such as dobutamine, dopamine, amrinone, and milrinone, are usually not indicated in mitral regurgitation because of the low incidence of myocardial failure. They may be useful in critical, refractory cases, especially when demonstrable myocardial failure exists.

TABLE 6-3. PRINCIPLES OF THERAPY FOR HEART FAILURE DUE TO MITRAL INSUFFICIENCY

Therapeutic Goal	Treatment
Reduce cardiac workload	Exercise restriction Weight loss Cardiovascular volume reduction[a] Vasodilators
Reduce mitral regurgitation	Arterial vasodilators Possibly digitalis Cardiovascular volume reduction
Maintain adequate cardiac output	Vasodilators (arterial or mixed) Digitalis Dobutamine Cardiovascular volume expansion[b]
Reduce venous pressure	Salt restriction Diuretics Vasodilators (venous or mixed)
Improve exercise capacity	Vasodilators (arterial or mixed) Bronchodilators Cough suppressants Treatment of heart failure
Control arrhythmias	Antiarrhythmic drugs Avoidance of hypokalemia Avoidance of digitalis intoxication
Alleviate pleural and abdominal effusion	Diuretics Thoracentesis Abdominal paracentesis Vasodilators (captopril, enalapril) Treatment of heart failure
Avoid complications	Prevention of fluid and electrolyte imbalance Avoidance of drug intoxication Management of extracardiac disorders
Reduce clinical signs	Successful management of heart failure

[a] Using diuretics, salt restriction.
[b] Using fluid therapy.
(Modified with permission from Keene BW, Bonagura JD: Valvular heart disease. p. 311. In: Kirk RW (ed). Current Veterinary Therapy VIII. Philadelphia, WB Saunders, 1983.)
(From Atkins CE: Atrioventricular valvular insufficiency. In Allen DG (ed): Small Animal Medicine. JB Lippincott, Philadelphia, 1991, with permission.)

D. Off-loading therapy
    1. Congestive signs (venous congestion or backward failure) can frequently be reduced or eliminated by the use of off-loading therapies, such as low-salt diet, diuretics, and vasodilators. Of these, cardiac output is enhanced only with arteriolar and mixed vasodilation. Care must be taken because overzealous use of off-loading therapy may reduce filling pressure and cardiac output excessively, thus aggravating signs of forward failure.
    2. Dietary sodium restriction is one of the primary methods for reducing signs of congestive (backward) heart failure. Heavily salted foods should be avoided even prior to onset of signs (Class I). Along with exercise restriction and diuretic therapy, moderate sodium restriction (Kd diet) is instituted at the onset of signs of heart failure (Table 6-4),

TABLE 6-4. SCHEMA BASED ON FUNCTIONAL CLASS OF HEART DISEASE (SEE TABLE 20-2) FOR THERAPY OF HEART FAILURE DUE TO MITRAL INSUFFICIENCY

Treatment	Functional Class		
	II	III	IV
Exercise restriction	Yes	Yes	Yes
Salt restriction	Moderate	Yes	Yes
Diuretics	Yes (late class II)	Yes	Yes
Digitalis	No	Yes[a]	Yes[a]
Vasodilators[b]	No	Yes (late class III)	Yes
Other inotropic drugs	No	No	Yes (late class IV)[c]

[a] Digitalis is indicated when myocardial failure or supraventricular arrhythmias are recognized. Glycosides may also be used to optimize heart rate in the absence of arrhythmias. The use of cardiac glucosides in the treatment of heart failure remains controversial.

[b] The selection of vasodilators depends on the predominance of signs. Each type of vasodilator may be beneficial when congestive signs predominate; when forward failure signs predominate, arterial or mixed vasodilators are preferred. In time, vasodilators, especially angiotensin-converting enzyme inhibitors, will likely be used even earlier in the course of the progression of heart failure.

[c] Dobutamine may be used in critical class IV patients that are unresponsive to other therapy.

(Adapted from Atkins CE: Atrioventricular valvular insufficiency. In Allen DG (ed): Small Animal Medicine. JB Lippincott, Philadelphia, 1991, with permission.)

preferably by feeding the balanced, commercially available low-salt diets. Extreme salt restriction is limited to refractory class IV patients.

3. The diuretics most frequently used include the loop diuretic furosemide, thiazides, and—in cases complicated by hypokalemia—the potassium-sparing diuretics (spironolactone and triamterene). Various combinations of diuretics, for example a thiazide and furosemide, may be used to enhance the efficacy of each, and reduce untoward side effects. Diuretics are used at the lowest dose that alleviates signs of congestion.

4. Vasodilators

   a) Although proven to be effective, the exact role of vasodilators and their method of use have not been clearly defined. Most current recommendations are that they be used when conventional treatments have failed; however, they will clearly be used earlier and earlier in the course of heart failure.

   b) Preload reducing vasodilators (venodilators) reduce signs of congestion but do not improve cardiac output.

      (1) Nitroglycerin paste (used by this author only for short-term emergency use)

      (2) Isosorbide dinitrate

   c) Afterload reducing vasodilators (arteriolar dilators) improve cardiac output, relieve signs of congestion, and may reduce mitral regurgitation, but have a greater tendency to precipitate hypotension than do venodilators.

      (1) Hydralazine (useful for improving cardiac output and reducing mitral regurgitation)

   d) Mixed vasodilators may reduce congestion and enhance cardiac

output. The angiotensin-converting enzyme inhibitors (captopril en-alapril, lisinopril, and benasapril) reduce potassium wasting, are natriuretic, and reduce the negative effects of angiotensin II.
- (1) Prazosin
- (2) Captopril
- (3) Enalapril
- (4) Lisinopril
- (5) Benasapril
- (6) Sodium nitroprusside (IV only; must monitor blood pressure)

D. Miscellaneous therapy
1. Thoracentesis and abdominal paracentesis when right-heart failure complicates left-heart failure.
2. Potassium chloride is infrequently required but its administration may benefit dogs with poor appetites and those requiring high doses of diuretics.
3. Judicious use of fluid therapy (5% dextrose in water, supplemented with potassium, administered at approximately 0.5 mL/lb/h) is indi-cated in some dogs that show poor tissue perfusion and/or dehydration. Monitoring of congestive signs, and possibly central venous pressure, is imperative when fluid therapy is used.
4. Class IV heart failure may dictate the use of cage rest, 40 to 50 percent oxygen by mask, nasal catheter, or oxygen cage, and morphine (for its sedative and potential inotropic and venodilatory benefits).
5. Cough suppressants and bronchodilators, such as aminophylline, the-ophylline, and terbutaline, are usually not used in the treatment of respiratory signs associated with heart failure but may be quite useful in palliation of intractable cough or when primary respiratory disease complicates cardiac disease.
6. Control of supraventricular and ventricular arrhythmias will improve cardiac output by increasing filling time, and by normalizing the se-quence of ventricular depolarization. This is an important adjunct to therapy of mitral insufficiency.

BACTERIAL ENDOCARDITIS

I. General description
A. Infective endocarditis is typically bacterial in origin. It affects the aortic and/or mitral valves most often, and usually spares the tricuspid and pul-monic valves. The mural endocardium may also be involved.
B. Endocarditis may be acute or subacute. Acute endocarditis is caused by highly invasive organisms without the necessity of predisposing anatomic abnormalities. Subacute endocarditis requires predisposing factors.
C. After bacterial colonization of the heart valve, deposition of platelets and fibrin results in the formation of vegetations.
D. Vegetative lesions allow for embolism of other organs. Large vegetations interfere with valve function, producing a volume overload state with eventual heart failure.

II. Incidence and predisposition
    A. Based on postmortem studies, is 1 to 6 percent; rare in cats
    B. Males (70 percent)
    C. Large breeds (>30 kg)
    D. German shepherd dogs
    E. Dogs with congenital heart disease (especially subaortic stenosis and ventricular septal defect)
    F. Septic conditions, indwelling catheters, steroid therapy

III. Etiology
    A. Most cases (>67 percent) are due to one of the following:
        1. *Staphylococcus aureus*
        2. Streptococci
        3. *Escherichia coli*
    B. Other organisms incriminated include *Corynebacterium* species, clostridia, *Enterobacter* species, *Proteus* species, enterococci, *Pseudomonas* species, *Klebsiella* species, *Serratia marcescens*, *Erysipelothrix rhusiopathiae*, and fungi.
    C. Gram positive organisms make up 60 percent of cases; 40 percent are due to Gram negative bacteria.

IV. Clinical signs
    A. Presenting signs can be related to
        1. Sepsis
            a) Fever, anorexia, depression
            b) Hemorrhage (DIC)
            c) Joint and muscle pain
        2. Septic embolism
            a) Dysfunction of organ receiving embolism (e.g., arrhythmias, seizures, renal discomfort, etc.)
            b) Lameness
            c) Sudden death
        3. Cardiac dysfunction
            a) Arrhythmias
            b) Heart failure due to volume overload, with or without myocardial failure (typically dyspnea)
            c) Weakness, exercise intolerance, syncope
    B. Physical findings
        1. Auscultation
            a) Murmur of mitral insufficiency, relative or actual aortic stenosis, and/or aortic insufficiency (with aortic involvement, the murmur may be systolic and diastolic ["to and fro"]; or there may be no audible murmur
            b) A diastolic gallop may be audible if myocardial and/or heart failure is present.
            c) Pulmonary crackles may be heard if left-heart failure is present.
            d) Arrhythmia
        2. Other
            a) Joint and/or muscle pain
            b) Central nervous system dysfunction

        c) Ocular manifestations (retinal hemorrhage or exudate; visual impairment)

        d) Bounding or water-hammer pulse (aortic insufficiency)

V. Diagnosis

  A. The diagnosis can be suspected from the above findings but is usually supported or confirmed by other tests.

  B. Electrocardiography

    1. Left atrial and ventricular enlargement patterns

    2. Ventricular and supraventricular arrhythmias

    3. Atrioventricular conduction disturbances

    4. May be normal

  C. Thoracic radiographs

    1. May be normal

    2. Left ventricular and/or atrial enlargement

    3. Signs of heart failure or pulmonary congestion

  D. Laboratory tests

    1. Findings are variable

    2. Leucocytosis (83 percent)

    3. Monocytosis (84 percent)

    4. Left shift (33 percent)

    5. Normocytic, normochromic anemia (56 percent)

    6. Azotemia (31 percent)

    7. Hypoglycemia (22 percent)

    8. Hematuria, pyuria, or proteinuria (56 percent)

    9. Positive blood culture (72 percent)

  E. Echocardiography

    1. Left atrial and/or ventricular enlargement

    2. Vegetations on aortic and/or mitral valves

    3. Abnormal valve motion; ruptured chordae tendineae

    4. Myocardial dysfunction

VI. Therapeutic approach

  A. The prognosis for vegetative endocarditis is guarded to poor. It is improved if treatment is begun early in the disease, prior to the onset of heart failure. Antibiotic therapy is best based on the results of blood culture. Intravenous therapy, at least initially, is probably preferred and antibiotics should be continued for a minimum of 4 to 6 weeks. Eradication of underlying cause (gingivitis, prostatitis, etc.) should be attempted as well. Corticosteroids are contraindicated.

  B. Infective endocarditis: Potentially useful antibiotics

    1. Gram positive bacteria

      a) Cephalosporins

      b) Aminoglycosides (gentamicin or amikacin)

      c) Chloramphenicol

    2. Gram negative bacteria

      a) Aminoglycosides

      b) Cephalosporins

    3. Anaerobes

      a) Amoxicillin, penicillin

      b) Cephalosporins

       c) Clindamycin
       d) Chloramphenicol
       e) Metronidazole
    4. Negative or no culture
       a) Amikacin or gentamicin plus amoxicillin
       b) Ciprofloxacin plus amoxicillin
C. Heart failure
    1. Diuretics (furosemide)
    2. Digoxin
    3. Enalapril or Benasapril
    4. Salt and exercise restriction
    5. Other vasodilators as needed
D. Other
    1. Arrhythmias
       a) Treat underlying cause
       b) Specific antiarrhythmic drugs
       c) Pacemaker or positive chronotropes for advanced AV block
    2. Analgesics for pain (aspirin, opiates)
    3. Fluids as needed
    4. Symptomatic or specific therapy for accompanying organ dysfunction (e.g., hypoglycemia, seizures, DIC, etc.)
       a) Avoid nephrotoxic antibiotics if renal failure complicates the clinical picture

SUGGESTED READINGS

Atkins CE: Atrioventricular valvular insufficiency. p. 251. In Allen DG (ed): Small Animal Medicine. JB Lippincott, Philadelphia, 1991

Atkins CE: Bacterial endocarditis. p. 299. In Allen DG (ed): Small Animal Medicine. JB Lippincott, Philadelphia, 1991

Buchanan JW: Chronic valvular disease (endocardiosis) in dogs. Adv Vet Sci Comp Med 21:75, 1979

Calvert CA, Greene CE, Hardie EM: Cardiovascular infections in dogs: Epizooitology, clinical manifestations, and prognosis. J Am Vet Med Assoc 187:612, 1985

Harpster NK: The cardiovascular system. p. 820. In Holzworth J (ed): Diseases of the Cat. WB Saunders, Philadelphia, 1987

Keene BW, Rush JE: Therapy of heart failure. p. 939. In Ettinger SJ (ed): Textbook of Veterinary Internal Medicine. 3rd Ed. WB Saunders, Philadelphia, 1989

Opie LH: Drugs for the Heart. 3rd Ed. WB Saunders, Philadelphia, 1991

7

Canine Cardiomyopathy
Clay A. Calvert

INTRODUCTION

Cardiomyopathies are defined as heart muscle diseases of unknown etiology. They exclude primary valvular diseases and congenital heart defects (Table 7-1).

CLASSIFICATION

Based on clinical, hemodynamic, and structural features, the World Health Organization has classified cardiomyopathies as dilated, hypertrophic, or restrictive.

CHARACTERISTICS

 I. Dilated cardiomyopathy (DC)
    Slowly progressive, gradual ventricular dilatation and loss of contractility are the principal features. Diastolic dysfunction also develops when the disease is advanced.
 II. Hypertrophic cardiomyopathy (HC)
    Progressive ventricular hypertrophy and diastolic dysfunction in the absence of cavity dilatation are the cardinal features. Contractility is preserved, although systolic abnormalities may exist.

ETIOLOGIES

By definition, the etiology of cardiomyopathies is unknown. However, hereditary and nutritional components of the etiology are suspected in certain cases.
 I. Primary (idiopathic) cardiomyopathies
    A. Canine dilated cardiomyopathy
       The fact that most dogs with cardiomyopathy are pure bred suggests a hereditary component.
       1. Pure bred dogs are inbred and thus at increased risk for genetic disorders. Familial trends toward cardiomyopathy are common.
       2. Within individual breeds, prevalences of cardiomyopathy vary by geographic location.

145

TABLE 7-1. CLASSIFICATION AND CAUSES OF
CARDIOMYOPATHIES-MYOCARDIAL DISEASE

I. Primary cardiomyopathies
  A. Dilated
  B. Hypertrophic
  C. Restrictive
  D. Intermediate
II. Secondary cardiomyopathies
  A. Metabolic
    1. Endocrine
      a) Hyperthyroidism
      b) Acromegaly
      c) Pheochromocytoma
    2. Nutritional
      a) Taurine deficiency
      b) Carnitine deficiency
    3. Muscular dystrophy
    4. Glycogen storage diseases
  B. Toxic
    1. Doxorubicin
    2. Lead
    3. Cobalt
  C. Inflammatory-Infections
    1. Viral
    2. Microbial
      a) *Toxoplasma* species
      b) *Trypanosoma* species
      c) Bacterial
  D. Infiltrative
    1. Neoplasia
    2. Glycogen storage diseases

    a) Cardiomyopathy is less prevalent in Irish wolfhounds in Ireland than in Irish wolfhounds in England.
    b) Cardiomyopathy in Doberman pinschers appears to be less common in dogs in Europe than in dogs in the United States, Canada, and Australia.
  3. L-carnitine deficiencies have been reported by Keene in boxers and Dobermans.
  4. O'Brien and associates at the University of Guelph have reported cardiac subcellular defects in Doberman pinschers and suggested a hereditary cause.
  5. Most hereditary diseases involve an abnormality in one or more enzymes or biochemical pathways leading to a subcellular defect.
II. Secondary cardiomyopathies (Table 7-1)

PATHOPHYSIOLOGY OF DILATED CARDIOMYOPATHY

I. Idiopathic dilated cardiomyopathy
Dilated cardiomyopathy is a chronic, insidious, slowly progressive disease. The term *dilated* denotes the principal morphologic feature of the later stages of

the disease. Regardless of the proximate cause of cardiomyopathy, there is an initial mild but progressive deterioration of systolic function. As this dysfunction progresses, a stage of compensation begins wherein patients are asymptomatic as a result of various neurohumoral compensatory mechanisms that are activated to maintain resting function; however, maximal function is impaired. Subsequently, a decompensatory stage is entered and is characterized by very high elevations of neuroendocrine factors. Excessive activation of the sympathetic nervous system, alterations in the renin-angiotensin-aldosterone system, and possibly alterations of other humoral factors, such as vasopressin, prostaglandins, and atrial naturitic peptide, characterize the decompensatory stage.

A. Following the initial insult, the compensatory and decompensatory stages are characterized by gradual progressive systolic dysfunction that occurs over a period of years in the adult patient.
   1. Gradual, progressive decrease in ventricular contractility.
   2. Decreased contractility leads to slowly decreasing ejection fraction.
   3. Decreased ejection fraction leads to increased end-systolic volume, limited atrial emptying, and atrial dilatation.
B. In the late decompensatory stage, the large end-systolic ventricular volume and poor contractility lead to relative stasis of blood within the ventricles and atrial, which may lead to intracavitary thrombus formation.
   1. This is common in feline but uncommon in canine DC.
   2. Systemic embolization may result from intracavitary thrombus.
C. Chamber dilatation is associated with inadequate hypertrophy.
   1. Leads to gradually increasing afterload, which eventually becomes extremely high.
   2. Low cardiac output results from intrinsic systolic dysfunction and high afterload.
D. There is an absence of primary valvular pathology.
   1. In some dogs the mitral and/or tricuspid valve margins are focally thickened and fibrotic due to concomitant, unrelated AV valvular endocardiosis.
   2. AV valvular regurgitation is commonly associated with advanced DC.
      a) Dilatation of the AV valve annuli
      b) Papillary muscle dysfunction may contribute
E. Hemodynamic changes are the result of failure of the heart as a pump.
   1. During the compensatory stage, the renin-angiotensin-aldosterone system (RAAS) and sympathetic nervous system become hyperactive.
      a) Increased sodium and water retention contributes to chamber dilation and, hence, the Frank-Starling response.
      b) Endogenous catecholamines (principally plasma norepinephrine and angiotensin II) contribute to increased contractility, heart rate, and vasoconstriction.
   2. As the compensatory stage progresses, reduced stroke volume may be compensated for by tachycardia.
      a) Cardiac output does not increase normally with exercise, which leads to
         (1) Increased left-ventricular end-diastolic pressure (preload)
         (2) Exertional dyspnea

   b) Maximal exercise capacity does not decrease noticeably until the
      ejection fraction is reduced by 30 percent or more.
      (1) Preservation of right ventricular function during exercise
      (2) Frank-Starling principle (increased force of contraction due to
          increased end-diastolic fiber length) maintains stroke volume with
          less myocardial fiber shortening
   3. Ventricular dilatation and compensatory neurohumoral responses, while
      initially beneficial in maintaining cardiac output and blood pressure,
      eventually become detrimental and contribute significantly to cardiac
      decompensation.
      a) Increased afterload causes increased oxygen demand and may con-
         tribute to myocardial degeneration.
      b) Excessive preload leads to pulmonary edema and ascites.
      c) Heart rhythm disturbances and increased heart rate contributed to
         by high levels of norepinephrine and angiotensin II.
F. The microscopic study of the DC heart discloses nonspecific changes.
   1. Variable hypertrophy and atrophy of myocardial cells
   2. Multifocal fibroblast infiltration with collagen deposition
   3. Inflammation is notable by its absence, even in the early stages of the
      disease

INCIDENCE

Dilated cardiomyopathy is the most common type of this disease in dogs. Insidious, slowly progressive enlargement of the ventricles occurs, along with inadequate hypertrophy and gradual impairment of systolic function. The degree of
right-ventricular dysfunction and the frequency-severity of cardiac rhythm disturbances are variable among individuals and breeds.

SIGNALMENT

Cardiomyopathy classically affects middle-aged, large, pure-bred dogs. The Doberman pinscher has the highest disease prevalence. Boxers are commonly affected,
particularly in certain regions of the United States (e.g., the northeast). Some
smaller breeds are affected. Cocker spaniels seem to be predisposed to a DC that
has not been clearly characterized. DC is also seen in English springer spaniels,
bull terriers, and English bulldogs. DC may become evident in puppies or in dogs
over 10 years of age.

HISTORY

I. Occult cardiomyopathy
   A. Following the onset of systolic dysfunction and throughout the compensa-
      tory stage overt signs are absent.
   B. Heart rhythm disturbances: in boxers and Doberman pinschers, heart

rhythm disturbances, primarily ventricular tachyarrhythmias, are inherent from the onset of detectable abnormalities.

1. Syncope due to rapid, sustained ventricular tachycardia is common, particularly in boxers.
2. Sudden, unexpected death is often the first and last indication of occult cardiomyopathy in Doberman pinschers.
3. Arrhythmias may be detected during routine health care maintenance examination or during examination for other problems.
4. Arrhythmias are less frequent in other breeds, making diagnosis during the occult stage more difficult.

II. Symptomatic cardiomyopathy
   A. The decompensatory stage is reached when the normal ejection fraction is reduced by 35 to 50 percent or more. A history of a number of abnormalities related to low cardiac output and elevated preload may be present. During early decompensation, maximal exertion is impaired, but no other overt signs are present. Late in the decompensatory stage nocturnal dyspnea, orthopnea, and exertional coughing develop.
   B. The end-stage of overt decompensation is characterized by signs of CHF at rest, cachexia, and ascites.

PHYSICAL EXAMINATION

I. Occult cardiomyopathy
   A. Early in the disease course there are no obvious abnormalities and physical examination would only be done as a part of an annual examination or for a separate problem. In boxers and Doberman pinschers, a heart rhythm disturbance might be discovered fortuitously. Arrhythmias are less frequent in most other breeds, making occult cardiomyopathy more difficult to detect.
   B. As the early decompensatory stage is reached, the left ventricular ejection fraction has decreased to 35 to 50 percent of normal. Auscultatory abnormalities may be detected.
      1. Systolic heart murmur due to mitral regurgitation
      2. Gallop heart rhythm, due to an abnormal third heart sound, during exertion
      3. Tachyarrhythmias of various types

II. Symptomatic cardiomyopathy
   By the time that overt decompensation occurs, the left-ventricular ejection fraction has often decreased by approximately 60 to 70 percent, leading to a constellation of signs that are variably present.
   A. Coughing, dyspnea, and pulmonary crackles (pulmonary edema) are signs of left-sided CHF.
   B. Evidence of central venous pressure elevation (distended jugular veins and jugular pulses) along with ascites and muffled heart-lung sounds (pleural effusion) are signs associated with right-sided or bilateral CHF.
   C. Weak femoral pulses, pale mucous membranes, prolonged capillary refill time, weakness, and hypothermia are signs of poor cardiac output.

    D. Low intensity systolic heart murmurs usually develop due to dilation and reduced contractility of the AV valve annuli.

    E. Cardiac rhythm disturbances are common.

Diagnosis

It is always desirable to diagnose DC during the occult (preclinical) stage of the disease. This is a difficult proposition since, by definition, by the time that most symptoms appear, the disease is advanced. There is often no particular reason to suspect DC other than breed disposition.

  I. Occult cardiomyopathy

    A. Fortuitous discovery: an abnormality that may be an indication of DC may be discovered during routine annual examination or during examination for a concurrent problem.

      1. Heart rhythm disturbances

      2. A gallop heart rhythm is usually present prior to the emergence of overt heart failure, but is a sign of decompensation.

        a) Usually indicates that overt heart failure is imminent; i.e., days to several months

        b) Accentuated or precipitated by exertion

      3. Systolic heart murmurs may develop prior to the onset of overt congestive heart failure.

        a) If directly related to DC, they indicate advanced disease

        b) May be caused by concomitant disease, such as endocardiosis

    B. History of syncope: syncope due to DC is usually the result of rapid, sustained ventricular tachycardia

      1. Doberman pinschers and boxers

      2. A less frequent sequelum in other breeds

    C. Routine screening: screening of dogs at high risk of DC is not only justified but prudent in certain breeds or circumstances

      1. Doberman pinschers

      2. Familial history of DC

  II. Symptomatic (end-stage) cardiomyopathy

Symptoms of overt or late decompensation, such as exercise intolerance, weakness, lethargy, respiratory abnormalities, muscle wasting, and ascites, are associated with severe systolic dysfunction.

    A. Auscultation

A variety of abnormalities are variably present, including gallop heart rhythm, heart rhythm disturbances, muffled heart and lung sounds due to pleural effusion, and tachycardias of various types.

    B. Thoracic radiographs

Radiography is a useful diagnostic tool, but clinical judgment must be exercised. Dogs with acute, severe left-sided congestive heart failure (pulmonary edema) tolerate little stress.

      1. Generalized globoid cardiomegaly is typical of giant breed DC, but uncommon with Doberman pinscher cardiomyopathy.

      2. Left atrial enlargement is always present in dogs with overt or impend-

ing congestive heart failure and is the most striking cardiac radiographic sign in Doberman pinschers.

3. Lobar vein distention is usually visible in dogs with overt or incipient congestive heart failure
   a) Cranial lobar veins are significantly larger than the corresponding artery and proximal third rib diameter.
   b) Caudal lobar vein is larger than the diameter of the ninth rib at their point of superimposition.

4. Pulmonary edema is the hallmark of left-sided congestive heart failure and is the predominant extracardiac sign of heart failure in Doberman pinschers. Pulmonary edema may coexist with pleural effusion, typically in giant and heavy breeds.

5. Pleural effusion is often associated with pulmonary edema and ascites, and may be mild to severe. Severe effusion obscures much of the cardiac silhouette and embarrasses respiration.

C. Electrocardiography

The static ECG is usually abnormal when heart failure is present or imminent.

1. Cardiac chamber enlargements

2. Low voltage R waves due to global myocardial degeneration are typical in boxers and Doberman pinschers, but can occur in any breed with end-stage DC. When coupled with prolonged QRS duration, the R wave down stroke is slurred.

3. Heart rhythm disturbances are common, but vary by breed.
   a) Atrial fibrillation is present in approximately 60 to 70 percent of giant breed dogs with end-stage DC and may be the factor precipitating cardiac decompensation. Atrial fibrillation is less common in Doberman pinschers and boxers, probably due to their smaller absolute size relative to giant breeds.
   b) Ventricular tachyarrhythmias, while common in all breeds, are most severe in boxers and Doberman pinschers.

D. Cardiac ultrasound

At the time of onset of congestive heart failure, the left-ventricular shortening fraction is decreased by more than 50 percent, and often by 60 to 70 percent. Typical findings include increased left-ventricular end-diastolic dimension, very increased left ventricular end-systolic dimension, decreased septal and posterior wall thicknesses and percent systolic thickening, and increased E-point to septal separation. Right ventricular dilatation varies from mild to severe (Fig. 7-1).

Concomitant Abnormalities

Other abnormalities may be detected as sequelae to DC or as concomitant problems.

I. Hypothyroidism

Hypothyroidism is common in middle- to old-age dogs. It may be present in dogs with DC at any stage, and is probably a concomitant finding of two

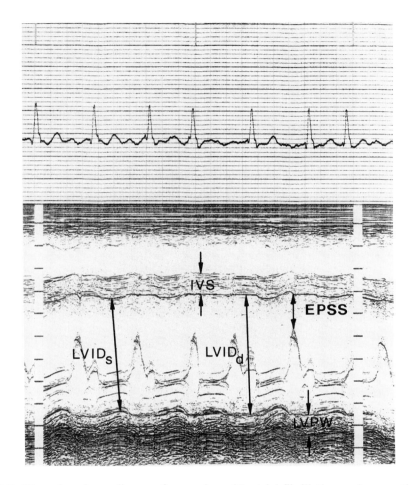

Fig. 7-1. M mode echocardiogram from a dog with atrial fibrillation and congestive heart failure. The left ventricle is dilated and there is severely reduced contractility. IVS, ventricular septum; LVPW, posterior wall; EPSS, E point to septal separation of the anterior mitral valve leaflet, LVID, left-ventricular internal dimension.

common abnormalities. There is no proof of a causal relationship in the vast majority of dogs.

A. Thyroid testing is subject to inaccuracies.

B. Sick euthyroid syndrome is seen in some dogs with acute or protracted congestive heart failure and requires special diagnostic testing (TSH response test or TSH assay).

C. Hypothyroidism may predispose to digoxin toxicity.

II. Azotemia

Azotemia may occur in dogs with end-stage (congestive heart failure) DC and is usually pre-renal as a result of myocardial failure (poor cardiac output). Prerenal or renal azotemia may be aggravated or precipitated by diuretic therapy.

A. Azotemia confounds the use of digoxin since this drug is excreted by the kidneys.
B. Effective therapy usually resolves prerenal azotemia.
   1. Patient feels better and drinks sufficient water to reestablish hydration.
   2. Positive inotropic and afterload reducing therapy may improve renal perfusion.
C. Fluid therapy used cautiously in the face of unstabilized congestive heart failure
   1. May aggravate pulmonary edema
   2. Sodium-containing fluids of greatest concern
      a) Alternate Ringers solution and 5 percent dextrose intravenously (may have to supplement potassium)
      b) Use half-strength Ringers/half-strength (2.5 percent) dextrose intravenously (may have to supplement potassium)
      c) Use Ringers solution subcutaneously
   3. Volume sufficient to provide maintenance and correct dehydration usually aggravates edema
      a) Some clinicians recommend 50 percent of maintenance volume only after pulmonary edema resolved.
      b) Some clinicians recommend full maintenance after pulmonary edema resolved.
      c) Clinical judgment required.
III. Electrolyte abnormalities
   Hyponatremia with or without hyperkalemia may be present at the time of diagnosis, predominantly in association with severe, generalized (bilateral) failure.
   A. Mimics the electrolyte pattern of Addison's disease.
   B. The hyponatremia is dilutional and high normal or high potassium may coexist with hyponatremia. Hyperkalemia may be due to poor renal perfusion, but is not always associated with azotemia.
   C. Usually requires no specific therapy, but resolves with effective therapy for heart failure.

TREATMENT

Treatment of DC entails the use of preload reducers, afterload reducers, positive inotropes, and, in some cases, antiarrhythmic drugs. Specific therapy should be tailored to the patient's needs, which are determined by the stage of disease at the time of diagnosis, the presence or absence of atrial fibrillation, and the severity of ventricular tachyarrhythmias, if present.
I. Occult cardiomyopathy of adult dogs
   The diagnosis of occult cardiomyopathy is difficult, since there are no outward signs suggesting a cardiac problem.
   A. Mild ventricular dysfunction
      During the first year or so after measurable left-ventricular abnormalities can be detected with cardiac ultrasound or Holter recording, dysfunction

is mild. Ultrasound-measured left-ventricular shortening fraction decreases by approximately 10 to 15 percent.
1. Conventional and medical therapy are of no benefit.
2. L-carnitine and taurine may be of benefit in some dogs in which deficiencies have been demonstrated.
3. Arrhythmias, mostly ventricular premature contractions, are present in Doberman pinschers and boxers, but are less likely in most other breeds although exceptions are noted.
    a) Seldom severe in Doberman pinschers during this stage
    b) May be severe in boxers during this stage
    c) Antiarrhythmic therapy indicated in some cases
        (1) Syncope
        (2) Ventricular tachycardia
B. Compensatory stage
During the second year or so after the onset of measurable abnormalities, although patients are asymptomatic, left ventricular dysfunction progresses. Resting cardiac function is adequate but maximal function is impaired. During this stage, the left ventricular shortening fraction decreases to approximately 30 percent below normal.
1. Whether initiating medical therapy during the compensatory stage is beneficial remains unknown.
    a) ACE inhibition and adrenergic blockade is considered inappropriate during this phase in humans.
    b) Digoxin is not indicated
    c) Diuretics are not indicated.
    d) L-carnitine or taurine may be of benefit in some dogs in which deficiencies have been demonstrated.
2. The ventricular tachyarrhythmias of Doberman pinschers and boxers, and occasionally other breeds, may become severe.
    a) Ventricular tachycardia may be detected.
    b) Holter recording is often required for adequate assessment.
    c) Antiarrhythmic therapy may be indicated.
        (1) Procainamide, quinidine, or one of the lidocaine congeners (mexiletine or tocainide)
        (2) Beta-adrenergic blocking drugs (when prescribed, usually in combination with other antiarrhythmic drugs)
C. Early decompensatory stage
Severe ventricular dysfunction (left-ventricular shortening fraction less than 20 percent) subsequently develops. Exercise intolerance develops, but still may not be appreciated in dogs leading sedentary lives.
1. ACE inhibition therapy indicated
2. Digoxin therapy
3. Diuretic therapy
    a) If gallop heart rhythm present
    b) If nocturnal dyspnea occurs
    c) When radiographic evidence of lobar vein distention develops
4. Antiarrhythmic therapy: Arrhythmias are more likely in all patients during this stage, but are most common and most severe in boxers and Dobermans.

a) Ventricular arrhythmias
   (1) See previous section.
   (2) Beta-adrenoreceptor blocking drugs at antiarrhythmic dosages (0.5 to 1.0 mg/kg) should be avoided or used with caution because they exert negative inotropic effects and thus may precipitate overt heart failure.
b) Supraventricular arrhythmias
   (1) Atrial premature contractions are common.
   (2) Atrial fibrillation often develops, particularly in giant breeds, and may precipitate overt congestive heart failure.
       i) May be initially transient
       ii) Digoxin indicated

D. Benefit of medical therapy during the occult stages
If occult cardiomyopathy is detected and appropriate medical therapy prescribed, some benefit is gained.
1. Acute heart failure
   a) Acute, fulminant pulmonary edema may be delayed or rendered less severe when ventricular function becomes critically reduced.
   b) It remains unproven in dogs whether disease progression is altered in a favorable manner.
2. Heart rhythm disturbances
   a) Sudden death due to ventricular tachycardia-fibrillation in a subset of Doberman pinschers and boxers can be delayed but probably not prevented.
   b) Control of severe ventricular tachyarrhythmias can promote more efficient cardiac function and diminish clinical signs such as exercise intolerance and syncope.

II. Late decompensatory stage (overt congestive heart failure)
Unfortunately cardiomyopathy in most affected dogs is not detected until the end-stage of acute congestive heart failure is reached.

A. Acute, immediately life-threatening congestive heart failure
Many, but not all, DC patients are presented with severe, fulminant pulmonary edema, which may be complicated by concomitant right-sided heart failure (pleural effusion and ascites). Aggressive therapy is required to stabilize these patients. Factors suggesting that death is imminent include gray or cyanotic mucous membranes, hypothermia, heart failure fluid coughed or gagged out of mouth or dripping from nose, severe dyspnea and orthopnea, and severe weakness.
1. Oxygen therapy
   a) Intranasal (50 to 100 ml/kg/min)
   b) Oxygen cage or hood administration delivers a higher oxygen concentration.
2. Preload reduction
   a) Nitroglycerin
      (1) Sublingual tablets (0.4 mg): 1 to 2 tablets, initial therapy only
      (2) Paste, 2 percent: ½ to 1 inch TID depending on patient size
      (3) Continued for 1 to 2 days, or occasionally as long as 1 week
   b) Diuretic: Furosemide

(1) 4 to 8 mg/kg IV, SQ or IM
    i) Re-evaluate q4h
    ii) Repeat treatment as indicated
(2) Risk: benefit ratio
    i) Insufficient dose may lead to death
    ii) High-dose therapy produces complications, such as dehydra-
        tion and azotemia
(3) Excessive preload reduction causes decreased cardiac output
    and hypotension.
(4) Taper furosemide dosage over a 1- to 2-day period to mainte-
    nance level

3. Positive inotrope therapy
   a) Rapid-acting, powerful inotropes may be life-saving. However, all
      such drugs may aggravate or precipitate arrhythmias.
      (1) Dobutamine 3 to 5 μg/kg/min constant rate infusion for 24 to 72
          hours.
      (2) Amrinone, 0.75 mg/kg over 3 minutes followed by 5 to 10 μg/kg/
          min
      (3) Milrinone 0.5 to 1.0 mg/kg BID, orally, for several days to several
          weeks [investigational drug]
   b) Digoxin (Lanoxin) is a modest inotrope that requires several days
      or more to exert its effect when given orally. Intravenous administra-
      tion is not recommended.
      (1) Dosage: 0.01 mg/kg daily divided into 2 fractions
      (2) Therapy initiated within 1 to 2 days of start of treatment
      (3) Initiated immediately if atrial fibrillation present
      (4) Combined with rapid-acting inotropes during first few days of
          treatment

4. Afterload reduction: afterload reduction is often deferred initially, since
   systemic arterial pressure is often dangerously low at the time of presentation.
   a) Inodilators such as amrinone and milrinone are usually safe, since
      they increase cardiac output simultaneously with arterial dilatation.
   b) Blood pressure should be stabilized with rapid-acting inotropes prior
      to the administration of afterload reducers
      (1) ACE inhibitors
      (2) Hydralazine

5. Antiarrhythmic therapy: Ventricular tachyarrhythmias may be present
   during acute heart failure (Fig. 7-2). These arrhythmias must be assessed
   and stabilized when appropriate.
   a) Lidocaine
      Of the antiarrhythmic drugs available for IV administration, lido-
      caine has the least detrimental effects on contractility and mainte-
      nance of blood pressure.
      (1) 2 mg/kg, IV bolus (over 30 seconds) for immediately life-threat-
          ening ventricular arrhythmias, such as rapid, wide-complex ven-
          tricular tachycardia and when VPCs are frequent to the point of
          further reducing cardiac output

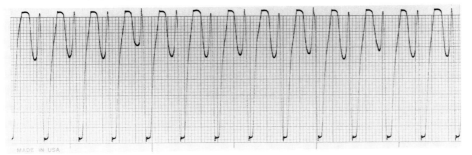

Fig. 7-2. Ventricular tachycardia in a dog with acute CHF.

    (2) Short duration of action (minutes)
    (3) Followed immediately by constant rate infusion of lidocaine at a dosage of 35 to 50 μg/kg
        i) For 24 to 48 hours until maintenance antiarrhythmic therapy established
        ii) Dilute in as low a volume of fluids as practical to avoid aggravating preload
    (4) Takes several half-lives (2 to 3 hours) to establish steady state plasma concentration; increasing infusion rate during that time increases the risk of toxic side effects, such as proarrhythmias and CNS toxicity (seizures and weakness). Individual boluses (2 mg/kg) are recommended to control arrhythmia relapse during the first hours of lidocaine infusion.
  b) Maintenance antiarrhythmic therapy may be required in some dogs, especially Doberman pinschers and boxers.
    (1) Lidocaine congeners exert the least negative effects on contractility and blood pressure: mexiletine (Mexitil) (5 to 10 mg/kg, TID) and tocainide (Tonocard) (15 to 20 mg/kg, TID)
        i) Tocainide should not be administered for longer than 4 consecutive months due to serious adverse effects.
          (*A*) Corneal endothelial dystrophy
          (*B*) Renal complications
        ii) Mexiletine tends to be less efficacious after 4 to 6 months of continued use.
        iii) Mexiletine and especially tocainide are more expensive than procainamide and quinidine.
        iv) Few side effects with mexilitine.
        v) Tocainide often causes anorexia and weakness, and nervousness or anxiety sometimes occurs.
    (2) Procainamide HCl (Procan SR) (15 to 17 mg/kg TID) or quinidine gluconate (Quinaglute) (6 to 10 mg/kg TID)
        i) Greater negative inotropic effect than lidocaine, tocainide, and mexilitine
        ii) Gastrointestinal side effects are common and chronic use leads to subtle appetite decrease and lethargy.

iii) Decreased efficacy after 4 to 6 months of continuous administration in some instances.

iv) Less expensive than the lidocaine cogeners.

B. Acute, not immediately life-threatening congestive heart failure

Many dogs with acute congestive heart failure can be stabilized with less
intensive therapy than described in the previous section. Clinical judgment
is required.

1. Oxygen therapy is always a reasonable treatment for acute heart failure.
2. Preload reduction
   a) Nitroglycerin ointment is safe and can be administered daily for several days. Clinical judgment is required.
   b) Diuretic: furosemide
      (1) 2 to 4 mg/kg orally, SQ, or IM, two to three times daily for one
      to two days
      (2) Dosage tapered during the second day (based on clinical re-
      sponse) to maintenance level
3. Positive inotrope: digoxin
   a) Maintenance dosage: 0.01 mg/kg daily, divided into two fractions
   b) Some clinicians prefer a semi-loading schedule
      (1) 0.01 mg/kg q 12 h or q 8 h for 24 hours followed in 8 to 12 hours
      by the maintenance dosage schedule
      (2) Atrial fibrillation may be an indication for a semi-loading dosage
      schedule
4. Afterload reduction: ACE inhibitors are the only drugs shown by vigorous human and veterinary trials to exert a positive influence on disease
   progression.
   a) Enalapril (Enacard)
      (1) 0.5 mg/kg daily
      (2) 0.5 mg/kg BID if patient unstable after 2 weeks
   b) Hypotension and gastrointestinal disturbances may be encountered.
   c) Defer afterload therapy if pre-existing hypotension is present
5. Antiarrhythmic therapy (see previous section)

C. Maintenance therapy

Maintenance therapy is indicated following treatment of acute heart failure
or as initial treatment in dogs when early, mild pulmonary edema is detected.

1. Preload reduction: furosemide 2 mg/kg BID, orally
2. Positive inotrope: digoxin (See previous section)
3. Afterload reduction: ACE inhibition (See previous section)
4. Antiarrhythmic therapy (See previous section)
5. Maintenance therapy: If heart failure is mild and the initial therapy
   is the maintenance schedule, some clinicians prefer to avoid initiating
   digoxin and an ACE inhibitor simultaneously. Rather, either digoxin or
   an ACE inhibitor is begun and the alternate drug initiated after adverse
   effects, if any, have been evaluated.
   a) Sinus rhythm: either drug may be initiated first
   b) Atrial fibrillation: digoxin should be initiated first

6. Digoxin blood levels should be measured after 7 days of digoxin therapy because the therapeutic index is virtually nonexistent and a large interpatient variability of dose-response exists.
   a) Dosage errors are frequent due to the large size of patients, inaccurate estimate of lean weight, and failure to adjust dosage downward in dogs with ascites.
   b) Recommended therapeutic serum concentrations for DC vary among laboratories but are typically 1 to 2 ng/ml
      (1) Trough (12-hour post-pill) should be 1 to 1.5 ng/ml
      (2) Four-hour post-pill should be 1.5 to 2.0 ng/ml
      (3) May assay at either or both times
   c) Serum concentrations should be evaluated in conjunction with the potential for adverse effects (toxicity), such as gastrointestinal disturbances, trembling, and depression, as well as any clinical response to therapy.
7. Some clinicians advocate the use of blocking drugs in dogs with atrial fibrillation with a rapid ventricular response (> 180/min) following digitalization.
   a) Beta-adrenoreceptor or calcium channel blockers
   b) Low dosages recommended with careful monitoring for hypotension and worsening heart failure
   c) Logic supposes that a slower heart rate will be associated with better ventricular filling, increased contractility, and improved cardiac efficiency.
   d) Holter recording in dogs that are receiving appropriate therapy with appropriate serum digoxin levels indicates that the heart rate in the home environment is slower.
      (1) In hospital or clinic, heart rates influenced by stress-nervousness induced increased adrenergic drive
      (2) Blocking drugs may thus be prescribed inappropriately in some dogs, at least from the standpoint of heart rate control.
8. Beta adrenergic blockade as a treatment for heart failure in humans was first described in 1975. Hemodynamic improvement was first described, and subsequently improved survival was suggested. Initial trials involved small numbers of patients, were nonrandomized, and historical controls were used in one report. Although still a controversial treatment, it is gaining gradual acceptance.
   a) Pathophysiologic basis
      (1) The chronic elevation of endogenous catecholamines associated with heart failure leads to down-regulation of β-1-receptors, which leads to decreased inotropic response to endogenous catecholamines. Beta blockade leads to up-regulation and improved inotropic response during exertion.
      (2) The high plasma norepinephrine levels associated with heart failure may lead to detrimental cardiotoxic consequences associated with excessive intracellular calcium concentrations and dysfunction of contractile proteins.

  b) Controversial aspects
     (1) When to initiate beta-blockade?
     (2) Which drug?
     (3) How much is optimum?
  c) Classification of beta-adrenoreceptor blocking drugs
     (1) First generation: Nonselective blockade (e.g., propranolol)
     (2) Second generation: Selective β-1-blockade (e.g., metoprolol and atenolol)
     (3) Third generation: Selective or nonselective blockade plus unique properties, such as intrinsic sympathomimetic activity via β-2-stimulation or vasodilating capacity via direct action, α-1-blockade, or peripheral β-2-stimulation
  d) Summary of clinical trials in humans
     (1) First-generation drugs not well tolerated due to increased afterload (vasoconstriction) caused by peripheral β-2-blockade
     (2) Some second- and third-generation drugs produced improved hemodynamics, function, and possibly survival. All either had vasodilating effect or did not produce peripheral vasoconstriction.
  e) Species variation: There is considerable variation in the action of these drugs among species. Therefore, extrapolation from human data may not be appropriate.
  f) Principles of therapy
     (1) Start at very low dosages
     (2) Gradual upward titration; one month or longer may be required to reach beneficial levels in humans
     (3) Carefully observe for clinical deterioration and reduce dosage if and when encountered
     (4) No data in dogs

Effect of Medical Therapy on Survival

Medical therapy for DC is generally unsatisfactory once overt or end-stage congestive heart failure develops. Diagnosis during the occult stage allows early intervention, but whether or not disease progression is altered is uncertain and may vary among breeds and individual dogs.

  I. Preload reducers
     Neither diuretics nor nitrates have ever been shown to exert a favorable influence on survival in terms of altering disease progression. Dogs with acute heart failure will die within days without diuretics, and diuretics cannot be withdrawn for extended periods during maintenance therapy. In this context, diuretics prolong survival but disease progression is not altered.
  II. Positive inotropes
     No positive inotrope has ever been shown to exert a favorable influence on disease progression.

A. Rapid acting, powerful inotropes
Drugs such as dobutamine, amrinone, and milrinone are of short-term benefit in that some dogs that would otherwise die during acute heart failure can be stabilized with the assistance of these drugs.
1. Milrinone and vesnarinone have been shown to exert a detrimental effect on survival in humans with end-stage DC when administered chronically.
a) Arrhythmogenic
b) May promote myocardial degeneration
2. Elective replenishment of myocardial norepinephrine concentrations via 48 to 72 hour infusions of dobutamine in patients stabilized from overt CHF.
a) In humans, sustained functional improvement has occurred in some patients. However, survival is not improved and arrhythmia complications can occur.
b) The author has not observed obvious, sustained functional improvement with this treatment in Doberman pinschers and arrhythmias worsened during infusion.
B. Digoxin
Digoxin has not been shown to exert either a favorable or unfavorable influence on survival.
1. Patients most likely to benefit clinically from digoxin exhibit
a) Atrial fibrillation
b) Gallop heart rhythms: audible third-heart sound that implies myocardial failure and is usually due to advanced DC
2. Digoxin withdrawal has recently been demonstrated in humans to result in worsening heart failure in patients also receiving ACE inhibitors and diuretics.
3. Although the therapeutic index of digoxin is poor, digoxin toxicity should not result in serious consequences when appropriate dosages and monitoring are used.
C. Afterload reducers
Direct-acting afterload reducers (arteriolar dilators) have never been convincingly shown to exert a favorable influence on survival.
D. ACE inhibitors
ACE inhibitors are the only group of drugs that have been shown by rigorous, prospective trials to exert a favorable influence on disease progression in humans with severe and moderately severe heart failure and in dogs with severe heart failure.
1. In humans, the effect is exerted through control of heart failure—as opposed to reduction of arrhythmogenic sudden death—by inhibiting detrimental endogenous neurohumoral mechanisms.
2. The author has seen no favorable influence on survival times of Doberman pinschers with end-stage DC.
E. Beta-adrenoreceptor blocking drugs
In humans, uncontrolled or small trials of beta-blockade sometimes demonstrated a favorable influence on survival.

F. Antiarrhythmic therapy
Sudden death due to ventricular tachycardia-fibrillation is a risk, especially in Doberman pinschers and boxers. Antiarrhythmic therapy can prolong survival and short-term (from 3 to 6 months) efficacy is generally good. Efficacy often decreases after 3 to 4 months, and alternate drugs are then required. Antiarrhythmic drugs probably cannot prevent sudden death for an indeterminate time period.

PROGNOSIS

I. Occult cardiomyopathy
When DC is diagnosed in the preclinical (precongestive heart failure stage), survival time depends on how long the disease has existed.
A. DC seems to evolve over a period of several years or more in most adult dogs, and left-ventricular contractility, end-diastolic, and end-systolic dimensions indicate the stage of disease.
B. Sudden death
1. Occurs in approximately 25 percent of Doberman pinschers during the occult stage after shortening fraction has decreased to less than 25 percent
2. Common in boxers
3. Less common in other breeds
II. End-stage cardiomyopathy
Survival times are generally short after the onset of overt congestive heart failure. Many dogs die without ever being stabilized from their first episode of failure. Doberman pinschers probably have the worst prognosis; English springer spaniels can be stabilized from more than one episode of heart failure and often survive over 1 year. In general, a 50 percent, 6-month mortality and 80 to 90 percent 1-year mortality are likely. The average survival time of cardiomyopathic dogs with atrial fibrillation is less than 6 months.

CARDIOMYOPATHY IN DOBERMAN PINSCHERS

Sudden, unexpected deaths and congestive heart failure were first recognized in Doberman pinschers in the early 1950s. The first scientific report of this problem was in 1965 and the first mention of the problem in the veterinary literature was in 1970.

SIGNALMENT

Cardiomyopathy in Doberman pinschers can be diagnosed in puppies and in dogs as old as 14 years. The average age at diagnosis is 7 to 8 years. Approximately 60 to 70 percent of affected dogs are male; there is no obvious correlation with size, coat color, or neutering status.

EVOLUTION OF DISEASE

Cardiomyopathy in Doberman pinschers evolves over a period of 3.5 to 4.0 years, and occasionally longer, after measurable abnormalities can first be detected.

I. Principal characteristics
   A. Heart rhythm disturbances, primarily ventricular tachyarrhythmias, are present throughout the course of the disease. They are initially mild, become progressively more severe, and result in sudden death in 25 percent of affected dogs.
   B. Congestive heart failure is the end-stage of the disease.

II. Initial phase
   A. The earliest detectable abnormalities are disturbances of the heart rhythm.
      1. Ventricular premature contractions
      2. Atrial premature contractions (less frequent)
      3. Usually requires long-term ambulatory ECG (Holter) recording to detect
         a) Less than 100 VPCs/24 hours at the onset
         b) Severe ventricular tachyarrhythmias absent during the first 1 to 1.5 years after the onset of arrhythmia
   B. Ultrasound evidence of left-ventricular dysfunction can be found 1 year after the onset of heart rhythm disturbances. Left ventricular shortening fractions between 25 and 30 percent.
      1. Measurements are equivocal, since the technique has inherent inaccuracies.
      2. Internal dimensions and wall thickness are within normal range for the Doberman pinscher.
      3. Wall thickness of so-called "normal Dobermans" are at the low end or below those parameters of age-, sex-, and weight-matched dogs not prone to cardiomyopathy.

II. Compensatory phase
   A. After 1 to 1.5 years, left ventricular dysfunction progresses so that the ultrasound-measured shortening fraction is less than 25 percent.
      1. Internal dimensions and wall thickness may or may not be within the normal range.
      2. Due to compensatory mechanisms, the shortening fraction decreases more slowly than the progressive increase in left-ventricular end-systolic dimension.
   B. Heart rhythm disturbances gradually worsen
      1. Ventricular tachyarrhythmias are the principal arrhythmia (Fig. 7-3).
      2. Disturbances become life-threatening in approximately 25 percent of affected dogs.
         a) Syncope
         b) Sudden death occurs in approximately 25 percent of affected dogs and occurs during the first or second episode of syncope.
            (1) Left-ventricular shortening fraction has usually progressed to less than 25 percent when syncope/sudden death occurs
            (2) Often is the first evidence of cardiac disease

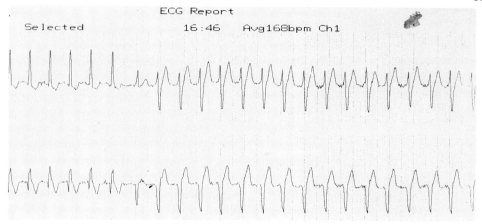

Fig. 7-3. Holter recording demonstrating paroxysmal ventricular tachycardia.

III. Decompensatory stage
  A. Early decompensation
     After 2.5 to 3.0 years from the onset of the earliest detectable abnormalities, the rate of progression of left-ventricular dysfunction accelerates; overt congestive heart failure occurs approximately 1 year later.
     1. Most sudden deaths occur when the left-ventricular shortening fraction is less than 20 percent.
     2. Exercise intolerance is detected in active dogs during the final 6 to 9 months prior to the onset of overt CHF.
     3. Radiographic evidence of left-atrial enlargement is present during the final 9 to 12 months prior to the onset of overt CHF.
     4. Gallop heart rhythms are often detectable during the final 3 months prior to the onset of overt CHF.
     5. Paroxysmal atrial fibrillation develops in a few dogs.
  B. Late decompensatory or end-stage
     Overt CHF seems to occur suddenly and the owners are usually shocked at the apparently sudden deterioration of their dog.
     1. Principal manifestation of acute CHF is pulmonary edema (left-sided CHF) (Fig. 7-4).
     2. Heart rhythm disturbances are present.
        a) Ventricular tachyarrhythmias are potentially life-threatening in approximately 20 to 25 percent of affected dogs.
        b) Atrial fibrillation
           (1) Present at the time of CHF in approximately 25 percent of dogs
           (2) May precipitate overt CHF
     3. Progression after the onset of overt CHF
        a) Survival times are usually short.
        b) Aggressive therapy often provides initial stabilization from pulmonary edema.
        c) A second episode of acute pulmonary edema usually occurs within 3 weeks to 3 months.

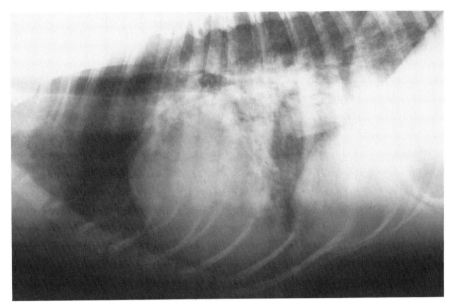

Fig. 7-4. Pulmonary edema in a Doberman pinscher. The dog had a 4 year history of arrhythmias and progressive left-ventricular dysfunction.

    (1) Often preceded by worsening ventricular tachyarrhythmias
    (2) More difficult to stabilize CHF
    (3) If stabilization is achieved, functional impairment is worse
  d) Recovery from a third episode of pulmonary edema is unlikely.
  e) Latent atrial fibrillation heralds the onset of rapid deterioration of clinical status.
  f) Dogs surviving for several months or more after the initial episode of pulmonary edema often develop generalized (bilateral) CHF with ascites.
  g) Approximately 20 to 25 percent die suddenly due to ventricular tachycardia fibrillation, even when pulmonary edema has been resolved.

ETIOLOGY

A hereditary component of cardiomyopathy is strongly supported by the high prevalence of disease in Dobermans, the long history of inbreeding in the breed, and familial trends.
  I. Multiple affected family members, through as many as four consecutive generations, are often observed.
 II. Multiple littermates and nonlittermate full siblings are often affected.
III. Researchers at the University of Guelph have identified subcellular defects in the mitochondria and sarcoplasmic reticulum that may have a genetic basis.

Prognosis

Survival time is dependent on the stage of disease at the time of diagnosis.
  I. Initial stage
     A. Dogs with shortening factors above 25 percent seldom develop CHF in less than 3 to 4 years.
     B. Severe ventricular tachyarrhythmias seldom develop in less than 1 to 1.5 years after the onset of arrhythmia.
 II. Compensatory stage
     A. Barring sudden death, dogs with shortening fractions between 20 and 25 percent tend to develop CHF in 1 to 2 years.
     B. Ventricular tachyarrhythmias become potentially life threatening in at least 25 percent of dogs with shortening fractions below 25 percent.
III. Early decompensatory stage
     A. When the shortening fraction is below 20 percent, CHF usually develops within 1 year.
     B. Approximately 25 percent of affected dogs die suddenly and most of these deaths occur when the shortening fraction is less than 20 percent.
IV. Late decompensatory (end-stage)
     A. The average survival time of dogs presenting with overt CHF with predominant sinus rhythm is approximately 3 months. Dogs presenting with atrial fibrillation and/or bilateral CHF live an average of approximately 1 month, and less than 10 percent of all dogs survive beyond 6 months.
     B. After the onset of overt CHF, approximately 25 percent of dogs die suddenly due to ventricular tachycardia-fibrillation.

CARDIOMYOPATHY IN BOXERS

Cardiomyopathy in boxers is similar to that of Doberman pinschers.
  I. Comparative aspects
     A. Initial stage
        1. Cardiac ultrasound results are commonly within normal parameters in boxers when ventricular tachyarrhythmias are first detected.
           a) Ventricular arrhythmias may be severe during this phase in boxers, whereas they are seldom severe in Dobermans during this phase.
           b) Cardiac ultrasound parameters typically remain within normal limits for more than 1 year after the onset of arrhythmias in boxers, whereas ultrasound evidence of left-ventricular dysfunction usually appears within 1 year after the onset of arrhythmias in Dobermans.
        2. Ventricular premature contractions in boxers almost invariably have a predominant positive polarity in the major leads, whereas the opposite is true in Dobermans.
     B. Syncope/sudden death
        1. Syncope and even sudden death may occur in boxers with left-ventricular shortening factors above 25 percent, where these events in Dobermans

      usually occur in association with a more severe reduction of ejection fraction.
2. Boxers often recover from multiple episodes of syncope over periods of months to years, whereas Dobermans usually die during the first or second episode of syncope that is associated with ventricular tachycardia.
C. Duration of disease
1. In general, most Dobermans will die suddenly or be in CHF by 3.5 to 4 years after the onset of arrhythmia, although a few survive for up to 5 years.
2. The evolution of CM in boxers is generally longer than in Dobermans; left-ventricular weakness and enlargement progress more slowly. The incidence of sudden death is not well documented.

CANINE HYPERTROPHIC CARDIOMYOPATHY

Canine hypertrophic cardiomyopathy (HC) is seldom diagnosed. The occult phase of the disease in adult dogs is associated with few or no symptoms. It is likely that some dogs that die suddenly or that develop left-sided congestive heart failure have HC but the disease is never identified.

INCIDENCE

Hypertrophic cardiomyopathy is uncommonly recognized in dogs, although misdiagnosis or lack of a diagnosis no doubt occurs. During the past 15 years five cases of HC have been diagnosed in the author's practice; over 300 cases of DC have been diagnosed during that time.

SIGNALMENT

Few cases have been documented, and thus dependable data is lacking. Males seem to be affected more often. Symptoms may occur in dogs less than 1 year old or as much as 13 years old. No breed predilection has been convincingly demonstrated, although 4 of 15 reported cases were in German shepherd dogs.

HISTORY

Many affected dogs are asymptomatic. Coughing as a result of left-sided congestive heart failure, ascites, syncope as a result of ventricular tachycardia or advanced heart block, and exercise intolerance may be present.

Physical Examination

Occult HC

Prior to the onset of clinical signs a heart murmur, cardiac rhythm disturbance, or gallop rhythm may be detected. Such patients may be presented for exercise intolerance or syncope, or for routine prophylactic medicine.

Symptomatic HC

Pulmonary crackles due to pulmonary edema, cardiac rhythm disturbances, ascites, jugular pulses, and gallop heart rhythm are variably present in dogs with congestive heart failure or exercise intolerance.

Disease Progression

Assuming that HC is a genetic disease, there is a wide variation in disease progression. Severe hypertrophy may be present prior to 1 year of age in some dogs, while clinical signs in other dogs may not develop until middle to old age. It is possible that variable expression exists so that some dogs may never develop pathology sufficient to cause clinical signs.

Diagnosis

The antemortem diagnosis of HC requires cardiac ultrasound and is unlikely to be made prior to the onset of clinical signs.

  I. Clinical signs
     A. Congestive heart failure is indicated by coughing, dyspnea, pulmonary crackles, gallop heart rhythm, jugular pulses, or ascites.
     B. Heart rhythm disturbances, heart murmurs, syncope, and exercise intolerance may be defected.
 II. Electrocardiography
     The ECG may be normal, but usually indicates heart enlargement, tachyarrhythmias, conduction disturbances, or ST segment abnormalities.
III. Thoracic radiography
     Thoracic radiographs may be normal, may indicate left atrial enlargement or may reveal alveolar pulmonary edema.
 IV. Cardiac ultrasound
     Cardiac ultrasound is the easiest method of diagnosis and evaluation of HC. The abnormalities of canine HC are similar to those seen in cats, although ASH may be more common.

PATHOLOGY

The gross and microscopic appearances of the heart are similar to those of cats and humans. The incidence of ASH is greater than in the cat, but the incidence of myofiber disarray, which is typical in humans with ASH, is detected in the minority of dogs.

TREATMENT

The treatment of canine HC is based on that of humans and cats. Clinical experience is inadequate for conclusions concerning efficacy. Some dogs remain asymptomatic for extended periods even though significant hypertrophy is present.

  I. Blocking drugs
    A. Beta-adrenoreceptor blocking drugs have been used for years in the treatment of HC in humans and cats.
      1. Propranolol 0.5 to 1.0 mg/kg TID
      2. Metoprolol 0.5 to 1.0 mg/kg TID
      3. Atenolol 0.5 mg/kg BID
    B. Calcium channel blocking drugs have been introduced recently and there is less clinical experience with their use.
      1. Diltiazem 0.5 to 1.5 mg/kg TID
      2. Verapamil
        a) Drug of choice in humans
        b) No data in dogs

PROGNOSIS

In general, the prognosis for dogs with HC is uncertain. Asymptomatic dogs can live for over 3 years, albeit with an increased risk of sudden death. The influence of medical therapy on survival is undetermined, but patients with overt heart failure have a poor prognosis.

SUGGESTED READINGS

Atkins CE and Snyder PS: Cardiomyopathy. In Allen DG (ed): Small Animal Medicine. pp. 269–298. JP Lippincott, Philadelphia, 1991

Bonagura JD and Lehmkuhl LB: Cardiomyopathy. In Birchard SJ and Sherding RG (eds): Saunders Manual of Small Animal Practice. pp. 464–480. WB Saunders, Philadelphia, 1994

Calvert CA. Update: Canine dilated cardiomyopathy. In Kirk RW and Bonagura JD (eds): Current Veterinary XI. pp. 773–779. WB Saunders, Philadelphia, 1992

Harpster N. Boxer cardiomyopathy. In Kirk RW (ed): Current Veterinary Therapy VIII. pp. 329–336. WB Saunders, Philadelphia, 1983

Keene BW: Canine cardiomyopathy. In Kirk RW (ed): Current Veterinary X. pp. 240–250. WB Saunders, Philadelphia, 1989

Keene BW: L-carnitine deficiency in canine dilated cardiomyopathy. In Kirk RW and
    Bonagura JD (eds): Current Veterinary Therapy XI. pp. 780–782. WB Saunders, Philadel-
    phia, 1992

O'Brien PJ, O'Grady MR, McCutcheon LJ, et al: Myocardial myoglobin deficiency in
    various animal models of congestive heart failure. J Moll Cell Cardiol 24: 721–730, 1992

O'Grady MR: What's new in the management of dilated cardiomyopathy? p. 795. Proc
    ACVIM, San Diego, CA, 1992

O'Grady MR and Horne R: Occult dilated cardiomyopathy. pp. 232–235. Proc ACVIM,
    San Diego, CA, 1992

8

Feline Cardiomyopathy

Paul D. Pion
Richard D. Kienle

INTRODUCTION

This information applies in general to feline myocardial diseases. Information specific to individual diseases will be addressed in the section *Specific Diseases*, p. 182.

DERIVATION AND DEFINITION

cardio- = heart
mys- = muscle
pathos- = disease

I. The World Health Organization defines a primary (idiopathic) cardiomyopathy as a "primary disease process of heart muscle in absence of a known underlying etiology."
II. A secondary cardiomyopathy is a disease that affects the myocardium secondary to infectious, toxic, metabolic, or other disease processes.

GENERAL COMMENTS

I. Myocardial diseases, the most frequently diagnosed cardiac conditions in cats, were not widely recognized clinical entities until the 1960s.
II. Most cardiomyopathies diagnosed today are of unknown etiology and are currently classified in the literature as representing the hypertrophic or intermediate forms.
III. Dilated cardiomyopathy was, until recently, a common cardiac diagnosis. In 1987, it was determined that many cats presenting with dilated cardiomyopathy were taurine deficient and that supplementation with taurine reversed the myocardial failure. Supplementation of commercial foods with additional taurine has greatly reduced the prevalence of this condition. These findings provide adequate stimulus to continue the search for a cause and cure of other seemingly irreversible and incurable conditions in all species.
IV. Intermediate cardiomyopathy (a classification introduced by Harpster to end the misuse of the term restrictive cardiomyopathy) and restrictive cardiomy-

opathy (an accepted morphologic/pathologic diagnosis in humans that has been misused in the veterinary literature) are poorly defined clinical entities in cats. These diagnoses have been assigned to many feline patients with presumed primary myocardial disease that do not meet the criteria for making a diagnosis of hypertrophic or dilated cardiomyopathy.

V. The introduction of echocardiography (cardiac ultrasound) into speciality veterinary practice in the early 1980s, and more recently into general veterinary practice is the single greatest advance toward more frequent and accurate recognition of myocardial disease.

VI. There is much that we do not understand about the diagnosis, natural history, and treatment of cardiomyopathies.

CLASSIFICATION

I. Primary cardiomyopathies are classified according to their morphologic appearance.
   A. Hypertrophic cardiomyopathy (HCM)
   B. Idiopathic dilated cardiomyopathy (DCM)
   C. Restrictive cardiomyopathy (RCM)
   D. Unclassified (poorly defined) cardio(myo)pathies
   Note: In this chapter, we chose to use the term *unclassified cardio(myo)pathy* as a constant reminder that the only conclusions we can make about these cats' hearts is that they are abnormal. We will avoid use of the term intermediate cardiomyopathy and only briefly discuss restrictive cardiomyopathy because we are unable to make substantiated recommendations regarding diagnosis, treatment, or prognosis.

II. Proven or strongly suspected secondary causes of cardiomyopathy in cats
   A. Nutritional (taurine deficiency)
   B. Metabolic (hyperthyroidism, acromegaly)
   C. Infiltrative (neoplasia, amyloidosis)
   D. Inflammatory (toxins, immune reactions, infectious agents)
   E. Genetic (some hypertrophic cardiomyopathy is strongly suspected; genetic predisposition may also play a role in the development of taurine deficiency–induced myocardial failure)
   F. Toxic (doxorubicin, heavy metals)

III. Within each classification, a wide range of morphologic and clinical presentations are seen.

PATHOPHYSIOLOGY

I. The heart responds to hemodynamic abnormalities in predictable and appropriate ways.
   A. When the ventricle is pumping against an increased pressure load, we speak of a pressure overload. Concentric hypertrophy (thickening of the ventricular walls with minimal or no increase in chamber diameter, and

thus volume) is the means by which the heart responds to a pressure overload.

   B. When the ventricle is pumping an increased volume, we speak of a volume overload. Eccentric hypertrophy (dilatation of the ventricle with minimal or no increase in wall thickness) is the typical response of the heart to a volume overload.

II. Abnormalities in cardiac pump function during systole or diastole can underlie the clinical signs observed.

   A. Systolic dysfunction is present when the ability of the ventricle to eject blood is impaired and may result in signs of low output and possibly congestive heart failure.

   B. Diastolic dysfunction is present when the ability of the ventricle to relax is impaired and may result in signs of congestive heart failure.[*]

III. Ideally, an understanding of the underlying etiology of a disease dictates specific therapy to reverse the condition. However, in most cases treatment of cardiac disease is palliative. Therefore, when tailoring rational therapy for a patient with cardiac disease, the clinical status of the patient is the primary consideration.

   A. Heart disease includes any cardiac abnormality.

   B. Heart failure is a clinical syndrome, not a final diagnosis.

      1. Congestive right-heart failure is present when elevated systemic venous, and therefore capillary pressures resulting from cardiac disease manifest as ascites or peripheral edema.

      2. Congestive left-heart failure is present when elevated pulmonary venous and capillary pressures resulting from cardiac disease manifest as pulmonary edema (and also pleural effusion in cats).[†]

      3. Biventricular congestive heart failure is present when elevated systemic and pulmonary venous and capillary pressures manifest as any combination of the above signs or pleural effusion.[†]

      4. Low-output heart failure or cardiogenic shock is inadequate cardiac output, often a result of myocardial failure.

      5. High-output heart failure is congestive heart failure, left and/or right sided, resulting from excessive flow through a capillary bed.

IV. Chronic congestive heart failure results when compensatory mechanisms (primarily involving the renin-angiotensin-aldosterone system) designed to maintain normal arterial blood pressure and flow increase intravascular volume when cardiac pump function (systolic and/or diastolic) is compromised. Reductions in arterial pressure are detected, stimulating retention of sodium and water, resulting in increased intravascular volume and venous and capillary pressures. Increased capillary hydrostatic pressure leads to an imbalance in Starling forces, resulting in a net fluid efflux from the capillaries into the

---

[*] In order for adequate ventricular filling to occur, ventricular end-diastolic, atrial, venous, and capillary intravascular pressures must be increased.
[†] The pathophysiology of pleural effusion in cats with what appears to be primarily left-heart disease is poorly understood. Some hypothesize that right-heart failure related to pulmonary hypertension (as a result of chronic left atrial hypertension) plays a role. Another possible cause is that the pleural lymphatics in cats may drain into the pulmonary veins in such a way that elevated pulmonary venous pressure may lead to pleural effusion.

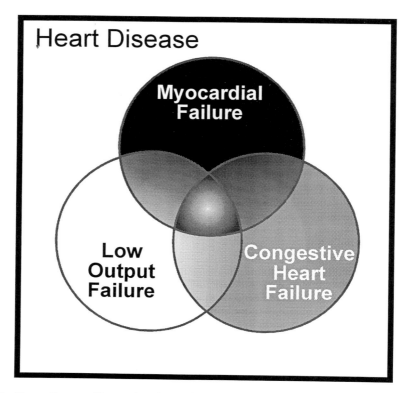

Fig. 8-1. Venn diagram illustrating the various potential combinations of congestive heart (backward) failure, low output (forward) heart failure, and myocardial failure (each represented by a circle) that may be detected in patients with heart disease (the box). As all the circles reside in the box, each represents a form of heart disease and the overlapping portions of the circles illustrate how the conditions may coexist.

interstitial spaces. Edema becomes apparent when interstitial lymphatic clearance mechanisms are overwhelmed.

Myocardial failure is a reduction in myocardial contractility characterized by a reduced shortening fraction and an increased end-systolic dimension on the echocardiogram.

V. It is important to realize that heart failure and myocardial failure represent heart disease and that heart failure, either congestive or low output, may in some cases be a result of myocardial failure. However, heart failure can be, and often is, present in the absence of myocardial failure. Similarly, myocardial failure may be present in association with or in the absence of heart failure. Heart failure may be the result of valvular, systolic, or diastolic dysfunction (Fig. 8-1).

SIGNALMENT AND PRESENTING COMPLAINTS

I. The spectrum of presenting complaints is similar for all forms of myocardial disease and cannot be used to differentiate between them.

II. Most common historical clues in cats with myocardial disease
   A. Dyspnea/tachypnea
   B. Poor general condition, weakness, lethargy, or, rarely, exercise intolerance
   C. Anorexia
   D. Acute posterior paresis or paralysis
   E. Coughing and abdominal distension, common findings in dogs with cardiac disease, are rare findings in cats with cardiac disease.
III. Many present with acute onset of dyspnea, paresis, lethargy, or anorexia. However, many asymptomatic cases are identified after a murmur, gallop sound, or other abnormality is ausculted during a routine physical examination.

PHYSICAL EXAMINATION

I. Early detection of disease should be a primary goal. A thorough physical examination, with careful attention to auscultation, should be performed.
II. Common physical clues suggesting myocardial disease
   A. Systolic murmur (commonly heard along the sternal border); this murmur may relate to either mitral regurgitation or outflow tract obstruction or both.
   B. Gallop sound: at normally rapid heart rates these gallop sounds often represent a summation of the third and fourth sounds.
   C. Arrhythmia
   D. Tachypnea/dyspnea
   E. Muffled or harsh lung sounds
   F. Hypothermia
   G. Jugular pulses/distention
   H. Acute paresis associated with pain in regions that show evidence of reduced peripheral perfusion
III. Systolic murmur, gallop sound, jugular pulses, and arrhythmia are clues that heart disease is present.
IV. Tachypnea/dyspnea, muffled or harsh lung sounds, venous distention, and ascites (though rarely present in adequate amounts to be physically detected) are clues that congestive (backward) heart failure is present.
V. Generalized weakness, lethargy, hypothermia, pale mucous membranes, and weak femoral pulses are clues that low-output (forward) heart failure is present.
VI. Reduced or absent regional peripheral perfusion is a clue that arterial thromboemboli may be present. Thromboembolic events are most common with myocardial disease, but can occur coincident with noncardiac disease (most commonly neoplasia or infection).

ANCILLARY TESTS

Thoracic radiography and electrocardiography may direct or reinforce suspicion that a cardiac disorder is present. Neither electrocardiography nor thoracic radiography is adequate evidence for ruling out, confirming, or classifying feline cardiac disease.

Contrast radiography (with significant risk) or echocardiography (the preferred procedure) is required to confirm (or rule out) and categorize myocardial disease.

  I. Electrocardiography (ECG)
     A. The ECG (normal or abnormal) usually contributes little to the diagnosis.
     B. Left ventricular (LV) (QRS amplitude > 1 mV in lead II) and left atrial (LA) (P wave duration > 0.04 s) enlargement patterns are common.
     C. A shift of the mean electrical axis to the left may be seen. This often has the appearance of a left anterior fascicular block (S wave in leads II, III, and aVF, qR complex in leads I and aVL, MEA −30 to −60 degrees, and a normal QRS duration). However, an actual abnormality of conduction within the left anterior fascicle has not been identified in cats and this pattern may represent an LV enlargement pattern.
     D. Electrocardiography is essential for accurate diagnosis of rhythm and conduction disturbances.
     E. Atrial and/or ventricular arrhythmias are observed in some cases.
 II. Radiography
     A. Radiography is most useful for detecting gross cardiac enlargement and sequelae to cardiac dysfunction (e.g., pulmonary venous congestion, pulmonary edema, enlarged great veins, pleural effusion) (Figs. 8-2 and 8-3).
     B. Restraint for radiographic procedures can be life-threatening to dyspneic cats. Extreme caution should be taken before proceeding with radiography. The authors often delay radiography until after the patient is stabilized (Fig. 8-4).
     C. Diagnostic and potentially therapeutic pleurocentesis should precede radiography in dyspneic cats.
     D. Pulmonary edema may appear as a diffuse, often patchy, interstitial pattern.
     E. Positioning the patient for a ventrodorsal projection or a horizontal beam radiograph taken with the patient held upright (''hanging'') are useful techniques if the cardiac silhouette or mediastinum remain obscured by small amounts of pleural effusion after pleurocentesis.
III. Echocardiography
     A. Echocardiography, including Doppler echocardiography, is essential to determine a functional and anatomic diagnosis noninvasively.
     B. Before assigning a diagnosis of cardiomyopathy based solely upon morphologic/functional appearance, a concerted effort should be made to rule out cardiac and extracardiac diseases that might echocardiographically mimic primary myocardial diseases.
IV. Other diagnostic tests
     A. Results of routine biochemistries, urinalysis, and hemogram usually do not contribute to the diagnosis of myocardial disease. When possible these tests should be performed prior to pharmacologic intervention to establish baseline values for the patient, and to rule out concurrent or secondary metabolic or hematologic disturbances.
     B. In cats with aortic thrombosis, acute renal failure may be observed if the occlusion is at or above the origin of the renal arteries. Stress hyperglyce-

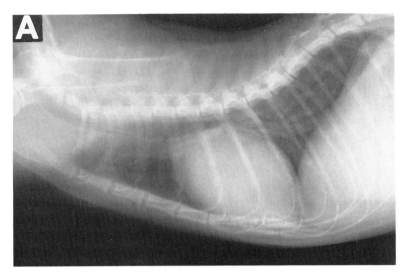

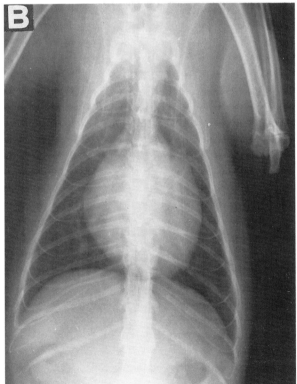

Fig. 8-2. (A) Lateral thoracic radiograph from a cat with dilated cardiomyopathy demonstrating severe generalized cardiomegaly. (B) Dorsoventral thoracic radiograph from the same cat as in Figure A.

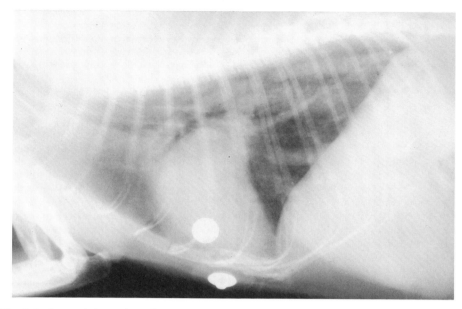

Fig. 8-3. Lateral thoracic radiograph from a cat with hypertrophic cardiomyopathy demonstrating marked left atrial enlargement, pulmonary venous engorgement, and pulmonary edema.

mia, pre-renal azotemia, and leukocytosis are common in cats with arterial thrombosis or forward (low-output) heart failure. Necrosis of muscle tissue can lead to increased concentrations of creatinine phosphokinase, alanine aminotransferase, aspartate aminotransferase, lactic dehydrogenase, and potassium in serum, and taurine in plasma in cats with arterial thrombosis. The concentrations often rise acutely during the early reperfusion period; serum potassium may rise to life-threatening concentrations, requiring therapeutic intervention.

C. Chemical and cytologic evaluation of pleural fluid with respect to protein concentration and cellularity can help determine whether congestive heart failure underlies the production of pleural fluid.

D. Cats with congestive heart failure can develop true chylous effusion. Treating for congestive heart failure resolves this effusion in most cases.

E. Plasma and whole-blood taurine concentrations should be measured in all cats with myocardial failure (see the section *Taurine Deficiency–Induced Myocardial Failure*).

THERAPY

Therapy should be based upon the clinical and functional classification of the disease process in the individual patient and not by following a cookbook approach based solely upon the name of the disease process.

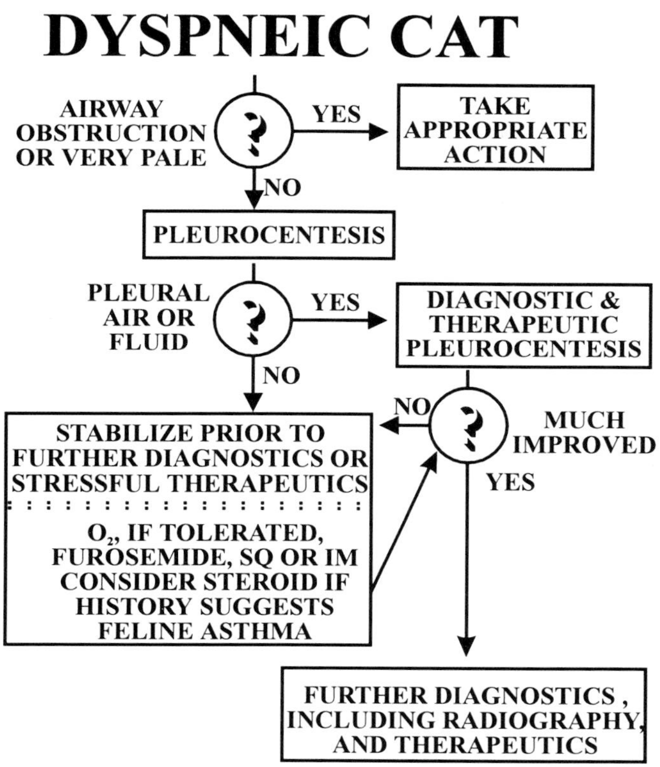

DYSPNEIC CAT

AIRWAY OBSTRUCTION OR VERY PALE — **?** — YES → **TAKE APPROPRIATE ACTION**

NO ↓

PLEUROCENTESIS

PLEURAL AIR OR FLUID — **?** — YES → **DIAGNOSTIC & THERAPEUTIC PLEUROCENTESIS**

NO ↓

STABILIZE PRIOR TO FURTHER DIAGNOSTICS OR STRESSFUL THERAPEUTICS
: : : : : : : : : : : : : : : : : :
O₂, IF TOLERATED, FUROSEMIDE, SQ OR IM CONSIDER STEROID IF HISTORY SUGGESTS FELINE ASTHMA

NO ← **?** → **MUCH IMPROVED**

YES ↓

FURTHER DIAGNOSTICS , INCLUDING RADIOGRAPHY, AND THERAPEUTICS

Fig. 8-4. Algorithm outlining choices and decisions encountered in the management of life-threatening dyspnea in the cat. The most important point illustrated is: do not proceed with stressful diagnostic or therapeutic procedures until the patient is stable. Stressed cats die.

I. With only two exceptions, the indications for and benefits of therapeutic intervention in asymptomatic cats with myocardial disease are controversial. These exceptions are
   A. Myocardial failure secondary to taurine deficiency
   B. Thyrotoxic heart disease
II. Dyspneic cats are easily stressed and may acutely deteriorate and die if stressful diagnostic or therapeutic interventions are initiated too early. An algorithm for management of the dyspneic cat is presented in Figure 8-4.
III. All patients with evidence of significant and life-threatening congestive heart failure (pulmonary edema, pleural effusion) require immediate therapy (i.e., appropriate combinations of pleurocentesis, diuretics, oxygen).
   A. Furosemide is the diuretic of choice. Furosemide may be administered intravenously (1 to 4 mg/kg q1h PRN) or intramuscularly (1 to 4 mg/kg q2h PRN) depending upon the stress level of the cat. Dosing must be dramatically reduced once the respiratory rate begins to decrease. Generally, aggressive diuretic therapy is continued until the respiratory rate is below 40 breaths per minute.

   B. Not all cats respond well to being placed in an oxygen cage. Carefully
      observe the patient after placing it in a closed oxygen cage and opt for
      a quiet, unoxygenated environment if the patient appears more dis-
      tressed in the oxygen cage.
   C. Tranquilization with an agent such as acepromazine may be indicated
      to calm distressed patients.
 IV. Patients with significant pericardial effusion require pericardiocentesis and
     should not receive diuretics prior to pericardiocentesis.
  V. Although the authors do recommend assisting thermoregulation in hypother-
     mic patients with myocardial disease, warming to 97° or 98°F is likely ade-
     quate. Higher temperatures may unnecessarily increase basal metabolic rate
     and demand upon the heart. This recommendation is the authors' opinion
     based upon clinical experience; there is no objective data supporting or
     refuting this recommendation.
 VI. After life-threatening congestive heart failure has been controlled the goal
     of therapy is to prevent further extravascular fluid accumulation with oral
     diuretics and vasodilators.
   A. Lower doses of furosemide (6.25 mg BID to 12.5 mg TID PO) are indi-
      cated for chronic maintenance control of CHF.
   B. Angiotensin-converting enzyme inhibitors (captopril 0.5 to 2.0 mg/kg PO
      q8h or enalapril 0.25 to 0.75 mg/kg PO q12–24h) are also quite effective in
      cats with congestive heart failure.
   C. The use of topical nitroglycerin as a preload reducing agent in acute and
      chronic situations is recommended by some, but evidence of efficacy
      is lacking.
 VII. Antiarrhythmic drugs may be indicated to control significant arrhythmias.
VIII. Inotropic agents may be indicated in patients with myocardial failure and/
      or low-output heart failure.
  IX. The judicious use of intravenous fluids may infrequently be indicated in
      patients with signs of low-output heart failure, primarily in situations where
      the patient has stopped taking in oral fluids, has received excessive diuretic
      treatment, or when concurrent renal dysfunction is present and a concern
      about maintaining adequate renal perfusion exists.
   X. Specific therapies designed to alter the natural history of disease should be
      concurrently instituted and may, in some cases, eliminate the need for drugs
      to control heart failure (see specific conditions).
  XI. All cats with myocardial failure should be supplemented with taurine (see
      the section *Taurine Deficiency–Induced Myocardial Failure*) until proven
      to not be taurine deficient and not taurine responsive.
 XII. Several strategies to prevent an initial thromboembolic event or to avoid
      recurrence of aortic thromboembolism in cats with cardiomyopathy have
      been devised and recommended. None of these strategies has been evalu-
      ated by controlled studies.
   A. Low-dose aspirin (25 mg/kg PO every 2 to 3 days) is the most widely
      used prophylactic measure. Although aspirin is known to exert anti-
      thrombotic effects, there is no objective evidence of its efficacy for the
      prophylaxis of systemic aortic thromboembolism in cats.
   B. Recurrence of thromboembolic events in aspirin-treated cats was as high
      as 75 percent in one study.

C. The failure of aspirin has sparked renewed interest in warfarin as a prophylactic anticoagulant. Preliminary dosage recommendations have been developed (0.05 to 0.5 mg/cat PO q24h), but there is inadequate data to determine if this approach has an acceptable risk-to-benefit ratio. Due to the high risk of complications (bleeding), this alternative should be considered only for indoor cats that can be monitored frequently. Prothrombin time (PT) should be assessed prior to therapy and the aim of therapy should be to maintain a PT approximately 1.5 times baseline, while remaining near the upper limit of normal for the laboratory doing the measurements.

XIII. Treatment of thromboembolic episodes

Left untreated, the outcome of arterial occlusion will depend upon the extent of occlusion and time to spontaneous reperfusion, either via the primary vessel or collateral circulation. Cats may lose the affected leg(s) because of ischemic necrosis, die of toxemia, remain paralyzed from peripheral nerve damage, or regain full or partial function of the leg. Overall, response to presently available conservative or aggressive clinical intervention has been poor.

A. Therapeutic options
1. Surgical removal of emboli
    a) Unreliable results
    b) High anesthetic mortality
2. Catheter embolectomy
    a) Limited experience
    b) Might be effective in conjunction with medical therapies
    c) Risks of anesthesia and acute reperfusion
3. Medical therapies (''benign neglect'')—most are untested and unproven
    a) Anticoagulation with heparin (220 U/kg IV followed 3 hours later by maintenance dose of 66 to 200 U/kg SQ QID) to prevent further thrombosis; adjust dose to maintain the APTT at or slightly above the upper limit of the normal reference range.
    b) Vasodilation with acepromazine (0.2 to 0.4 mg/kg TID, SQ) or hydralazine (0.5 to 0.8 mg/kg PO TID) to promote collateral blood flow
4. Thrombolytic therapy
    a) Streptokinase and urokinase are significantly less expensive than newer fibrinolytic agents (e.g., tissue plasminogen activator), but little clinical experience has been reported.
    b) Tissue plasminogen activator (t-PA): though clinically effective thrombolysis has been documented in the cat, expense, morbidity associated with rapid reperfusion, and inability to prevent recurrence make this option impractical in most cases

PROGNOSIS

I. Inadequate information is available to make broad generalizations regarding prognosis for cats with myocardial diseases.

II. Although echocardiography provides the basis for diagnosis, clinical and radiographic data should be strongly considered for prognostication. Cats with severe myocardial disease and no evidence of heart failure may survive for long periods of time. Conversely, cats with much less severe echocardiographic evidence of disease that present with significant and difficult to control signs of heart failure may survive for very short periods under the best of situations.

III. The long-term prognosis for cats with thromboembolic disease is grave because mortality associated with individual episodes is high and recurrence is common despite prophylaxis.

PATHOLOGY

I. Gross examination of the heart provides useful anatomic information and should be performed when possible to confirm antemortem findings.

II. In most cases histopathologic evaluation adds little useful information and unless readily available at low cost is not recommended unless specific indications are present (see the section *Specific Diseases*).

SPECIFIC DISEASES

PRIMARY CARDIOMYOPATHIES

Feline Hypertrophic Cardiomyopathy

Definition

A disease of the ventricular myocardium (primarily left) characterized by *primary* (inappropriate) *concentric hypertrophy*.

General Comments

I. The etiology is unknown. Autosomal dominant genetic defects have been linked to about 50 percent of the human cases of HCM. Although a genetic basis is suspected in some isolated cat families, the mode of transmission and the genotypic abnormality are currently unknown.

II. Prevalence within the feline population and associated morbidity and mortality are not known.

III. The most commonly diagnosed cardiac condition at this time.

IV. Likely the most commonly overdiagnosed cardiac condition.

V. The degree and distribution of hypertrophy in affected individuals is variable.

VI. The natural history of development of the concentric hypertrophy is unknown.

VII. Left ventricular concentric hypertrophy secondary to other causes (e.g., aortic stenosis, systemic hypertension, acromegaly, hyperthyroidism, etc.) must be ruled out to definitively assign a diagnosis of HCM.

Clinical Classification and Pathophysiology

I. Left ventricular diastolic dysfunction characterized by delayed or incomplete myocardial relaxation and reduced compliance are hypothesized to be the net result of changes in myocardial structure and function occurring in these patients.

II. Systolic anterior motion (SAM) of the anterior mitral valve leaflet may contribute to the development of a late systolic obstruction of flow from the left ventricle and mitral regurgitation. These same factors may be responsible for the systolic murmur auscultated in cats with HCM.

III. The degree to which SAM and mitral insufficiency contribute to the development of left-heart failure in cats with HCM is unknown and deserves further study.

IV. Sudden death may occur in any individual and may be unrelated to disease severity. The incidence of sudden death in cats with HCM is unknown.

Signalment and Presenting Complaints

I. Reported age at diagnosis ranges from 6 months to 16 years (mean age 5 to 7 years).[*]

II. Males are more commonly affected than females.

III. A familial association has been documented in Maine coon cats and is suspected in other breeds.

IV. Presentation is similar to other forms of myocardial disease.

Physical Examination

Similar to other forms of myocardial disease.

Ancillary Tests

I. Electrocardiography: nondiscriminatory between cardiomyopathies

II. Thoracic radiography: nondiscriminatory between cardiomyopathies, though common findings include

   A. Mild to moderate generalized cardiomegaly characterized by a "long" heart with a pointed apex.

   B. Left atrial enlargement, most easily observed on the lateral projection.

---

[*] Although unproven, the authors believe it is likely that the myocardial hypertrophy develops early in life and that clinical signs are not apparent until later in life.

C. Pulmonary edema is more frequently observed than pleural effusion when congestive heart failure is present.

III. Echocardiography

A. Concentric LV hypertrophy (> 6 mm in an average-sized cat) is the hallmark feature; may be symmetric (LV wall = interventricular septum (IVS)) or asymmetric (most commonly IVS > LV wall), global, regional, or localized (Fig. 8-5). Papillary muscle hypertrophy may be the only manifestation of the disease.

B. Several two-dimensional echocardiographic projections should be examined. Determination of wall thickness using standard M-mode echocardiographic projections may overlook or under- or overestimate the degree of hypertrophy present.

C. Left ventricular end-diastolic (LVEDD) or end-systolic (LVESD) dimension may be normal or decreased.

D. An enlarged left atrium indicates increased LV end-diastolic pressure.

E. Occasionally, a thrombus is imaged in the LA or its appendage.

F. Systolic anterior motion of the mitral valve[*] may be identified by two-dimensional or, more commonly by, M-mode examination (Fig. 8-6). SAM may contribute to the presence of dynamic LV outflow tract obstruction.

G. Spectral and color Doppler examination are helpful for identifying rapid or turbulent flow related to mitral regurgitation or LV outflow obstruction.

H. Echocardiograms performed on volume depleted and tachycardic cats may mimic HCM, giving the impression of small chambers (reduced end-diastolic and end-systolic volumes) with significant LV hypertrophy.

IV. Angiography

A. Unnecessary if the diagnosis has been established using echocardiography.

B. Typical findings include LV concentric hypertrophy, small LV cavity, large papillary muscles, LA enlargement, normal transit time, and tortuous pulmonary veins.

Therapy

I. General concepts and the initial management of congestive heart failure are similar to other forms of myocardial disease.

II. Two classes of agents, oral beta blockers and oral calcium channel blockers, have been advocated to improve LV filling and cardiac performance in cats with HCM. Although there is no clear evidence as to which therapy is more beneficial in *symptomatic* individuals, many cardiologists believe patients with documented HCM should receive one or the other as part of their chronic management. Whichever is the initial choice, response to therapy should dictate whether dose adjustment, changing drug class, or discontinuation of therapy is warranted.

---

[*] During ventricular systole the mitral valve should be closed. Systolic anterior motion of the mitral valve is recognized as movement of the anterior mitral valve leaflet toward the ventricular septum during early systole, which returns to normal position just before the onset of diastole.

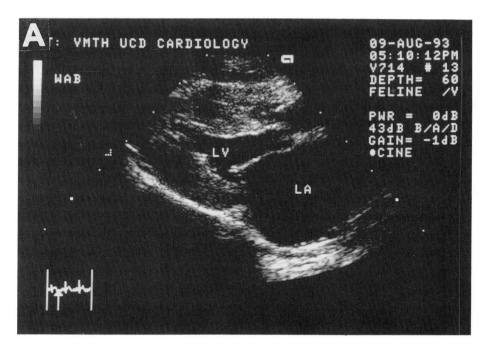

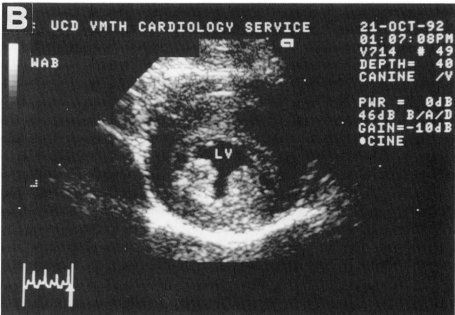

Fig. 8-5. Echocardiograms from a cat with hypertrophic cardiomyopathy. **(A)** Right parasternal, long-axis view, showing concentric hypertrophy of the left ventricle and left atrial dilation; **(B)** Right parasternal, short-axis view, showing the thick interventricular septum and LV wall and a comparatively small LV chamber; **(C)** M-mode echocardiogram at the level of the left ventricle, showing the thickened myocardium and small LV cavity. LV, left ventricle; LA, left atrium. (*Figure continues.*)

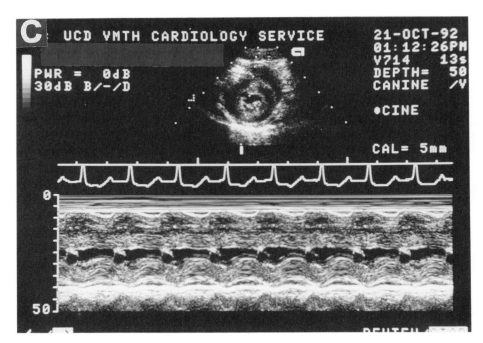

Fig. 8-5. (*Continued*).

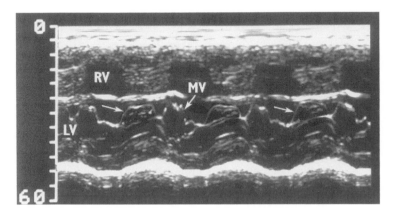

Fig. 8-6. M-mode echocardiogram of the mitral valve from a cat with hypertrophic cardio-myopathy, demonstrating systolic anterior motion (SAM) of the mitral valve. The mitral valve moves toward the interventricular septum in early systole (unlabelled arrows) and returns to normal position shortly before the beginning of diastole. LV, left ventricle; RV, right ventricle; MV, mitral valve. (Courtesy of Mark D. Kittleson, DVM, PhD).

    A. Beta blockade is generally accomplished using propranolol (2.5 to 5.0 mg/cat q8–12h) or atenolol (6.25 to 12.5 mg/cat q12–24 h).

    B. Diltiazem (7.5 mg/cat q8h) is currently the preferred calcium channel blocker.

III. Whether or not *asymptomatic* individuals require or benefit from any of the above therapies is unresolved. The authors recommend treating for 2 to 4 months as a trial. If echocardiographic evidence of hypertrophy is significantly reduced, treatment is continued. If there is no indication of a change in the degree of hypertrophy, there is likely no indication for continuing therapy.

IV. Therapy for the prevention of systemic thromboembolism may be beneficial in some cases.

Prognosis

Prognosis is generally based upon clinical presentation, echocardiographic evidence of elevated intracardiac pressures, and response to therapy. Inadequate data has been published to reach definitive conclusions, therefore, statements on prognosis are largely based upon clinical experience and conjecture. This section reflects the experience of the authors.

I. Asymptomatic cats

    A. Asymptomatic cats with mild to moderate hypertrophy and no left atrial enlargement are believed to have a good long-term prognosis.

    B. Asymptomatic cats with obvious wall thickening and left atrial enlargement are likely at higher risk for developing heart failure. These cats are also believed to be at risk for developing thromboembolic disease.

    C. Asymptomatic cats with severe wall thickening and normal left atrial size are occasionally observed. Although it is tempting to predict that these cats are at greater risk for progressive disease, inadequate data is available.

II. Cats that present in heart failure, in general, have a poor prognosis.

    A. A median survival time after diagnosis of about 3 months is reported.

    B. Cats that present in heart failure and respond favorably to therapy may do well for prolonged periods of time.

III. Cats presenting with aortic thromboembolism, in general, have a poor prognosis.

    A. A median survival, after diagnosis, of about 2 months is reported.

    B. Cats that survive the thromboembolic episode may do well for extended periods. However, these cats are generally at high risk for recurrence of thromboembolism.

IV. Owners should always be warned of the potential for sudden death.

Pathology

I. Postmortem contraction of myocardium tends to falsely increase postmortem-derived estimates of LV wall thickness. Echocardiography provides more accurate estimates of wall thickness in vivo than can be obtained postmortem.

II. In severe cases, the entire LV wall may be impressively thick. Papillary muscle hypertrophy is usually prominent and the LV cavity is usually decreased in size due to encroachment. Both symmetrical and asymmetrical forms of hypertrophy are recognized in cats. The left atrium is often enlarged and occasionally a thrombus is present within it.

III. Cats with milder forms have less dramatic wall thickening and normal or near-normal LV chamber size. The LA may be normal or only mildly enlarged. Occasionally, the disease is manifested only by papillary muscle hypertrophy with normal LV free wall and septal thickness. Considerable variability in the degree and location of the hypertrophy is possible.

IV. Myocyte hypertrophy (a nonpathognomonic finding) is the hallmark of histopathologic examination, with approximately 30 percent of the cases also having myocardial fiber disarray involving at least 5 percent of the septal myocardium.

Feline (Idiopathic) Dilated Cardiomyopathy

Definition

Dilated cardiomyopathy (DCM) is a disease of the ventricular myocardium (predominately left) characterized by *primary* myocardial failure.

General Comments

I. Prior to 1987, DCM was one of the most commonly diagnosed heart diseases in cats.

II. Most cases were probably a secondary cardiomyopathy associated with taurine deficiency.

III. All cats with myocardial failure should be assumed to be taurine deficient until shown to be unresponsive to taurine.

IV. Primary idiopathic DCM is not a common cardiac condition in cats. Because there are no published reports defining differences between cats with myocardial failure associated with taurine deficiency and idiopathic DCM there is very little, if anything, known about idiopathic DCM in cats. There is no reason to expect that clinical findings and results of ancillary tests (other than blood taurine concentration and fundoscopic examination) should be dramatically different between these disorders.

V. Myocardial failure secondary to other causes (e.g., longstanding congenital or acquired left-ventricular volume overload or toxic, ischemic, nutritional, or metabolic problems that may underlie myocardial failure) must be ruled out to definitively assign a diagnosis of idiopathic DCM.

VI. The underlying etiology remains unknown and may represent a common endpoint to many processes.

Pathophysiology

I. The underlying abnormality leading to clinical manifestations in cats with idiopathic DCM is primary systolic myocardial failure.

II. End-systolic LV volume increases due to a reduction in myocardial pump function. As a result, stroke volume and cardiac output decrease.

III. Neurohumoral compensatory mechanisms promote an increase in intravascular volume and end-diastolic pressures that stimulates eccentric hypertrophy.

IV. At these larger LV end-diastolic volumes, the geometry of the ventricle is such that small changes in chamber dimension during systole provide adequate stroke volume and cardiac output.

V. Working at these larger volumes is energetically inefficient for the ventricle.

VI. At any point in this degenerative process that end-diastolic pressures rise too high and/or cardiac output drops too low, the patient may present with signs of congestive heart failure and/or low-output heart failure, respectively.

VII. The factors that contribute to patients going from asymptomatic, well compensated myocardial failure, to a symptomatic, uncompensated state are poorly understood.

VIII. The degree to which alterations in diastolic function contribute to decompensation of patients with DCM is likely larger than previously appreciated.

Signalment and Presenting Complaints

Similar to other forms of myocardial disease.

Physical Examination

Similar to other forms of myocardial disease.

Ancillary Tests

I. Similar to taurine deficiency-induced myocardial failure.

II. Rule out taurine deficiency.

Therapy

I. For acute congestive heart failure see the section on treatment of congestive heart failure in cats.

II. Cats with DCM and signs of low-output heart failure (cardiogenic shock) represent a therapeutic challenge. Suggestions based upon clinical experience with cats with myocardial failure associated with taurine deficiency are presented in the section on this disorder.

Prognosis

I. There are no reports documenting the clinical characteristics of cats with idiopathic DCM that failed to respond to taurine supplementation.
II. There is no evidence that clinical intervention alters the progression of myocardial failure in patients that do not respond to taurine supplementation.
III. The expected survival time for patients is more a function of their clinical condition at the time the diagnosis is made than of the treatment they receive.
   A. Asymptomatic cats diagnosed because a murmur or gallop is identified during a routine physical examination may survive for years with myocardial failure before developing signs of congestive or low-output heart failure.
   B. Cats presenting with signs of congestive or low-output heart failure have a very guarded prognosis. These cats usually either die soon after admission from cardiogenic shock or succumb to refractory congestive heart failure or thromboembolism. Based upon a small number of documented cases, expected survival is 1 to 2 months after diagnosis.

Pathology

I. Although no information is currently available, there is no reason to suspect that findings should be different from taurine-deficient cats with myocardial failure or patients with DCM in other species in which there are no specific or pathognomonic changes found.

Feline Restrictive Cardiomyopathy

Definition

A diverse group of conditions characterized by restriction of diastolic filling.

General Comments

I. Specific clinical and morphologic criteria for diagnosis in the cat have not been clearly defined.
II. Without the use of invasive diagnostic procedures or necropsy examination, it is not possible to distinguish this disorder from infiltrative diseases of the myocardium and unclassified forms of cardio(myo)pathy.
III. Left ventricular pathology predominates in most cases.
IV. Uncommon in the authors' experience. Much of what follows is summarized from the literature and not direct clinical experience.

Pathophysiology

I. Endocardial, subendocardial, or myocardial fibrosis or infiltration impedes ventricular diastolic function resulting in impaired ventricular filling.

II. Left-sided pathology predominates.

III. Systolic function is preserved in most cases.

IV. Papillary muscle fibrosis, distortion of the mitral valve apparatus, and changes in LV geometry may contribute to the development of mitral regurgitation and left-sided congestive heart failure.

V. Similar pathophysiology may result from pericardial fibrosis (restrictive pericarditis) or infiltrative neoplastic and inflammatory diseases of the epicardium or myocardium. Signs referable to biventricular restriction predominate in pericardial disease.

Signalment and Presenting Complaints

I. Signalment is difficult to accurately report since there is little agreement among cardiologists as to which cases fall within this classification.

II. Presenting complaints are similar to other forms of myocardial disease.

Physical Examination

Similar to other forms of cardiomyopathy.

Ancillary Tests

I. Electrocardiography: nondiscriminatory between cardiomyopathies

II. Thoracic radiography: nondiscriminatory between cardiomyopathies. Common findings include
   A. Dramatic left atrial enlargement
   B. Enlarged and tortuous pulmonary veins
   C. When CHF is present, pulmonary edema is more common than pleural effusion

III. Echocardiography
   A. The echocardiographic findings in RCM are quite variable.
   B. Severe LA dilation is a common feature.
   C. Left ventricular internal dimensions are normal or mildly reduced.
   D. Two-dimensional echocardiography may demonstrate loss of normal LV symmetry and distorted or fused papillary muscles. Some authors report increased endocardial echogenicity.
   E. Indices of LV systolic function (e.g., shortening fraction, E-point to septal separation (EPSS), velocity of circumferential fiber shortening) are normal or only mildly depressed.
   F. Mitral regurgitation can be detected with spectral and color-flow Doppler in most affected cats.

IV. Cardiac catheterization and angiography
   A. Expected changes include an increased pulmonary capillary wedge pressure with a prominent a wave, and an elevated LV end diastolic pressure with a characteristic "square root" wave form to the ventricular diastolic pressure tracing.

B. Distortion of the left ventricular chamber with apical obliteration and an irregular endocardial surface has been demonstrated in some cats studied by angiography. Other abnormalities include left atrial enlargement, prominent and tortuous pulmonary veins, mitral regurgitation, and intracardiac thrombi.

Therapy

I. For acute congestive heart failure see the section on treatment of congestive heart failure in cats.
II. No specific therapy is available.
III. Beta blockers and/or calcium channel blockers are not effective for improving diastolic function in RCM. The negative chronotropic, dromotropic, and anti-arrhythmic effects of these drugs may be beneficial in cats with ventricular or supraventricular tachyarrhythmias.

Prognosis

I. As with other forms of cardiomyopathy, prognosis is difficult to predict for individual cases prior to observing the initial response to therapy.
II. A high incidence of serious arrhythmias, systemic thromboembolism, and refractory CHF have been reported by some authors.

Pathology

I. The postmortem changes are unique to this form of cardiomyopathy and may be used to differentiate it from other disorders.
II. Patchy or diffuse endocardial, subendocardial, or myocardial deposition of fibrous tissue is characteristic.
III. Endocardial fibrosis without eosinophilia is the most common form reported in the cat.
IV. Fibrous adhesions between papillary muscles and the myocardium, with distortion and fusion of the chordae tendineae and mitral valve leaflets, may be noted.
V. As with most cardiomyopathies, the LV appears to be most severely affected.
VI. Extreme left atrial and left auricular enlargement are common.
VII. The lesions suggest an inflammatory response; however, causative factors have not been identified.
VIII. A high prevalence of systemic thromboembolism is reported.

Unclassified Feline Cardio(myo)pathies

Definition

Cardio(myo)pathy is a term that the authors' have chosen to apply to a diverse set of cardiac presentations in cats. These are called *unclassified* because the lesions do not conform to expectations for HCM or DCM. The spelling *cardio-*

(myo)pathy denotes that there is no proof that these are in fact primary myocardial diseases.[*]

General Comments

  I. In recent years, an increasing number of cats have been recognized with obviously abnormal hearts that do not fit into any recognized disease classification. Many present in heart failure.
 II. It is not known whether these cases represent a single disease category.
III. It is not known whether these represent congenital or acquired disease.
 IV. It is not known whether these cases are afflicted by a primary myocardial disease or are secondary to or associated with another condition. The information presented here describes the spectrum of lesions that are included in this category at the University of California, Davis.
  V. Although no controlled studies have been performed, taurine deficiency or metabolic abnormalities (e.g., hyperthyroidism) have not been consistent findings in affected cats.

Pathophysiology

 I. Unknown
II. Clinical observations suggest diastolic dysfunction similar to that described for RCM.

Signalment and Presenting Complaints

 I. No known sex, breed, or age predispositions
II. Presenting complaints are believed similar to other forms of myocardial disease

Physical Examination

Similar to other forms of myocardial disease

Ancillary Tests

 I. Electrocardiography: nondiscriminatory between cardiomyopathies

---

[*] In the past, many of these cases have been classified as *restrictive* or *intermediate* forms of cardiomyopathy. The echocardiographic appearance in many cases suggests that the hemodynamics resemble those of restrictive cardiomyopathy; however, few cases have documented characteristic histopathologic lesions. The term intermediate suggests a combination of or transition between states. There is no evidence that this represents a combination of or a transitional state between two forms of cardiomyopathy. In fact, as stated above, there is no evidence that these are cardiomyopathies, and thus we chose a term, cardio(myo)athy, intermediate between cardiomyopathy and cardiopathy.

II. Thoracic radiography: nondiscriminatory between cardiomyopathies. Common findings include
   A. Left or bi-atrial enlargement
   B. When CHF is present, pulmonary edema is more common than pleural effusion
III. Echocardiography
   A. Extremely variable
   B. The most consistent echocardiographic finding is severe dilation of the left atrium (Fig. 8-7). The left ventricle is usually normal-sized or only mildly dilated. Various patterns of mild regional myocardial hypertrophy are observed in the septum or LV free wall of some cats. Enlargement of the right heart is variable, but may be marked in some cases.
   C. Systolic contractile indices may be normal or mildly depressed.
   D. Mitral, and on occasion tricuspid, regurgitation can be detected with spectral and color flow Doppler in most affected cats.
   E. In some cases, a thrombus is observed within the LA (Fig. 8-7B).

Therapy

I. For acute congestive heart failure see the section on treatment of congestive heart failure in cats.
II. Since the underlying etiology and pathophysiology have not been defined, no specific therapy can be recommended for these disorders.

Prognosis

Prognosis is generally based upon clinical presentation, echocardiographic and radiographic evidence of elevated diastolic pressures, and response to therapy.
 I. Asymptomatic cats
   A. Asymptomatic cats with mild left atrial enlargement are believed to have a good long-term prognosis.
   B. Asymptomatic cats with marked left atrial enlargement are likely at higher risk for developing congestive heart failure.
 II. Cats that present in heart failure, in general, have a poor prognosis.
   Cats that present in heart failure and respond favorably to therapy may do well for prolonged periods of time.
III. Cats presenting with aortic thromboembolism, in general, have a poor prognosis.
   A. Cats that survive the thromboembolic episode may do well for extended periods.
   B. However, these cats are generally at high risk for recurrence of thromboembolism.

Pathology

Although pathologic criteria have not been established, severe biatrial enlargement and mild biventricular eccentric hypertrophy appear to be common features in affected individuals.

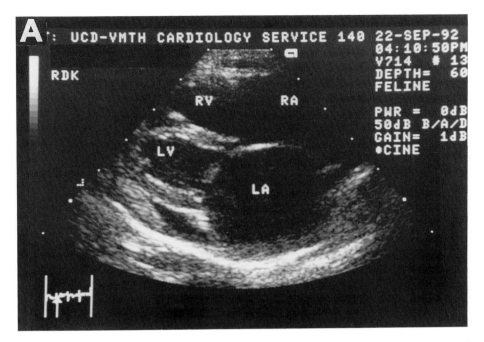

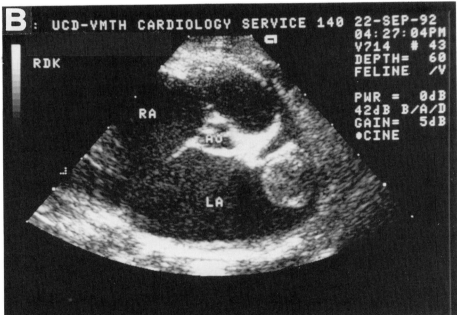

Fig. 8-7. Echocardiograms from a cat with an unclassified form of cardio(myo)pathy. **(A)** Right parasternal, long-axis view. There is marked dilation of both left and right atria and mild dilation of the right ventricle; **(B)** Right parasternal, short-axis view, showing the marked right and left atrial dilation. In addition, a thrombus is visible within the dilated left auricle. (*Figure continues.*)

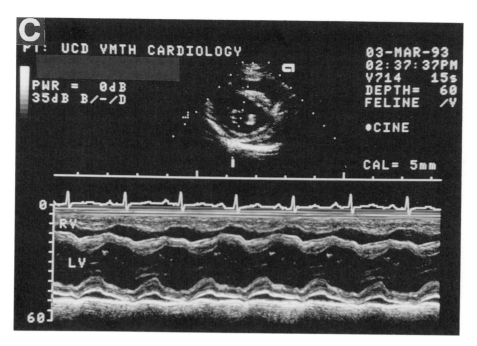

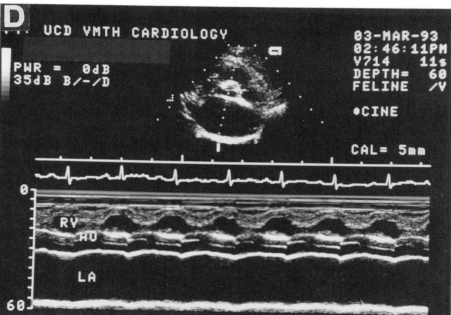

Fig. 8-7. (*Continued*). (**C & D**) M-mode recordings at the ventricular level and aortic level, respectively. The IVS and LV wall thickness are normal. The LV chamber is only mildly dilated and the LV shortening fraction is in the low normal range (30 percent). The left atrium is markedly dilated. LV, left ventricle; LA, left atrium; RV, right ventricle; RA, right atrium; AO, aorta.

Secondary Cardiomyopathies

Nutritional: Taurine Deficiency–Induced Myocardial Failure

Definition

I. Myocardial failure associated with low plasma, whole blood, and tissue taurine concentrations. It is reversible after taurine supplementation.

General Comments

I. In 1987, it was determined that many cats presenting with dilated cardiomyopathy were taurine deficient and that supplementation with taurine reversed the myocardial failure.
II. Therefore, much of the literature referring to idiopathic DCM in cats should be considered to be referring to this condition, not idiopathic DCM.
III. Supplementation of commercial cat foods with additional taurine has greatly reduced the prevalence of this near uniformly fatal condition.
IV. Not all taurine-deficient cats develop myocardial failure. The other factor(s) required for taurine deficiency to lead to the development of myocardial failure are unknown. A genetic predisposition has been proposed.
V. It is reasonable to assume that nutritional taurine deficiency combined with other causes of myocardial failure (e.g., longstanding congenital or acquired left ventricular volume overload or toxic, ischemic, nutritional, endocrine, or metabolic problems) may lead to synergistic complicating effects.
VI. A precise requirement for taurine cannot be determined for all foods because the requirement is dependent upon many factors. No commercial diet should be assumed to be taurine sufficient until the manufacturer has provided feeding trial data documenting that in a trial of at least 6 months, the food maintains normal taurine concentrations in blood and tissue.

Pathophysiology

I. Hemodynamics and pathophysiology are believed similar to idiopathic DCM as previously outlined
II. Taurine deficiency is believed to be nutritionally derived as a result of inadequate amounts of taurine in the diet
III. Taurine is an essential amino acid in the cat; its role in the maintenance of myocardial function remains unknown.

Signalment and Presenting Complaints

Similar to other forms of cardiomyopathy

Physical Examination

I. Similar to other forms of cardiomyopathy
II. Fundoscopic evaluation may reveal the presence of taurine deficiency–induced central retinal degeneration.
   A. Not all taurine-deficient cats with myocardial failure develop central retinal degeneration.
   B. Retinal lesions are permanent. Therefore, documenting retinal degeneration is evidence of taurine deficiency at some time in the cat's life, but is not proof of current taurine deficiency.

Ancillary Tests

I. Electrocardiography: nondiscriminatory between cardiomyopathies
II. Thoracic radiography: nondiscriminatory between cardiomyopathies. Common findings include
   A. Generalized cardiomegaly characterized by a rounded apex
   B. When CHF is present, pleural effusion is more common than pulmonary edema
III. Echocardiography
   A. The primary abnormality is an increase in LVESD (>12 mm) with a reduced shortening fraction (<35 percent). The LVESD is also often enlarged (>18 mm) (Fig. 8-8 and 8-9).
   B. Significant LA enlargement is common.
   C. The EPSS is often increased (>2 mm).
   D. The right ventricle and right atrium are variably affected.
   E. Decreased cardiac output may also lead to a decreased aortic root diameter, with poor aortic root motion.
   F. Mitral regurgitation may be detected with spectral and color-flow Doppler.
   G. In some cases, a thrombus is observed within the body of the left atrium or in the left atrial appendage.
IV. Cardiac catheterization and angiography
   A. Contraindicated if echocardiography is available because of high morbidity and mortality in cats with myocardial failure and heart failure.
   B. Generalized chamber dilatation
   C. Increased transit time of the dye through the circulation in patients with forward heart failure
V. Other
   A. Diet history should be accurately obtained during the initial work-up of any cat with *myocardial failure*. Many owners have managed to formulate diets with inadequate amounts of taurine and need to be educated to prevent recurrence. In addition, it is likely that a small number of cases will continue to be the result of commercial cat foods that contain inadequate amounts of taurine. The veterinary profession, to whom these cats will present for diagnosis and treatment, remains the most effective sentinel for detecting patterns with regard to diet and disease occurrence.
   B. Cats diagnosed with any form of myocardial failure should have plasma

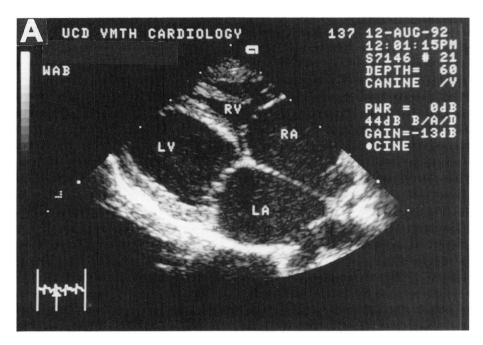

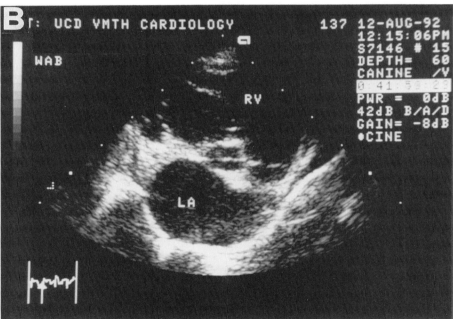

Fig. 8-8. Two dimensional echocardiograms from a cat with myocardial failure associated with taurine deficiency. **(A & B)** Right parasternal, long-axis and short-axis views, respectively, demonstrating marked dilation of all 4 cardiac chambers. LV, left ventricle; LA, left atrium; RV, right ventricle; RA, right atrium.

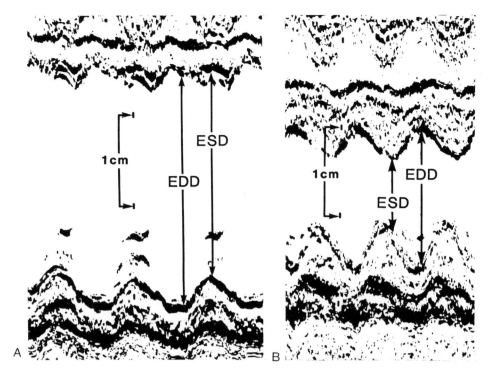

Fig. 8-9. M-mode echocardiograms from a cat with myocardial failure associated with taurine deficiency before **(A)** and after **(B)** taurine supplementation and diet modification. Prior to therapy the LV was markedly dilated and the LV shortening fraction was severely reduced. Those parameters both normalized after taurine supplementation. EDD, left ventricular dimension at end-diastole; ESD, left ventricular dimension at end-systole.

and whole blood taurine concentrations determined from blood samples obtained prior to supplementation.
1. Even a single dose of taurine may make interpretation difficult.
2. Proper sample handling is critical for accurate results. The following guidelines should be used in handling samples for taurine analysis.
    a) Submit both heparinized plasma and heparinized whole blood.[*]
    b) Place the sample on wet ice, or centrifuge the sample and separate the plasma immediately
    c) Make sure the plasma sample contains no clots or hemolysis
    d) Store and ship samples frozen (dry ice or ice packs)
3. Interpretation
    a) Plasma
        (1) Normal—greater than 60 nmol/ml
        (2) At risk—less than 30 nmol/ml
        Note: Plasma taurine concentration is *very* labile; 24 hours of fast-

---

[*] The whole blood analysis is most important.

ing can cause plasma concentrations to fall below 30 nmol/ml.

  b) Whole blood
      (1) Normal—greater than 200 nmol/ml
      (2) At risk—less than 100 nmol/ml
      Note: Whole blood taurine concentration is not as labile. Fasting does not significantly affect values.

Therapy

  I. During the initial phase of therapy proper supportive and symptomatic care for congestive heart failure (as described under general comments on therapy) is *essential* if CHF is present.
 II. The authors *do not* routinely administer digoxin as a part of therapy, but there is no contraindication to doing so.
III. Cats with documented taurine deficiency should be supplemented with 250 mg q12h until echocardiographically determined left ventricular dimensions normalize. This usually occurs within 4 months. Clinical improvement is usually evident within about 2 weeks.
 IV. Diuretics and ACE inhibitors can be discontinued when signs of CHF resolve. The ACE inhibitor should be discontinued first, then the diuretic is tapered over a period of 2 weeks. While withdrawing heart failure medications, the owner should be taught to monitor respiratory rate. Clinical and radiographic evaluation should be repeated 1 week after withdrawing medications to detect any decline in the cat's condition.
  V. The diet should be altered to maintain normal plasma taurine concentrations (>60 nmol/ml).
 VI. Taurine supplementation can be discontinued once echocardiographic values return to within normal limits.
VII. Taurine concentration in plasma and whole blood should be monitored periodically to be certain that the diet fed is maintaining taurine concentrations within acceptable limits. If taurine concentrations are depleted again, many cats will again develop myocardial failure.

Prognosis

  I. Since results of taurine analysis are not immediately known and a recent dietary change may normalize taurine values, all cats with myocardial failure should be supplemented with taurine and given an initially guarded-to-grave prognosis.
 II. In one large study, 30 percent of cats with myocardial failure died within the first week after diagnosis. Hypothermia and thromboembolic disease were associated with a poor prognosis. Taurine supplementation did not provide benefit with regard to survival until 2 weeks after treatment was begun.
III. Cats that survive 1 week and respond to treatment for congestive heart failure can be upgraded to having a fair prognosis.

  IV. Cats that survive 2 weeks and are shown to be taurine deficient can be up-
      graded to a good prognosis.
   V. Most taurine-responsive cats have complete reversal of echocardiographic
      and clinical evidence of myocardial failure after supplementation with taurine
      (Fig. 8-9).
  VI. Cats occasionally may have residual mild myocardial failure (LV shortening
      fraction 25 to 30 percent); however, these cats are generally asymptomatic
      and rarely require any form of therapy other than maintaining normal plasma
      taurine concentrations.

Pathology

No known differences from idiopathic DCM.
   I. Dilatation of the LV and LA
  II. Papillary muscles and trabeculations are less prominent than normal
 III. The RV and RA may also be enlarged
  IV. There are no specific light or electron microscopic lesions

Thyrotoxic Heart Disease

Definition

 I. Cardiac changes resulting from the direct and indirect effects of elevations in
    circulating thyroid hormone (hyperthyroidism).

General Comments

   I. A frequently recognized secondary cardiomyopathy that may be confused
      with primary myocardial diseases in older cats.
  II. Thyrotoxic heart disease does not cause hypertrophic cardiomyopathy.
 III. The prevalence and severity of thyrotoxic heart disease has decreased in
      recent years. This is most likely a result of increased awareness and early
      diagnosis and treatment of hyperthyroidism.

Pathophysiology

   I. The effects of thyroid hormone on the heart are believed to be both direct
      and indirect.
      A. Direct actions
         1. Increased protein synthesis (mitochondrial, ion pump, and contractile
            proteins)
         2. Alteration of myosin subtype ("slow" to "fast" type myosin; V_3 to
            V_1)
         3. Less economical energy conversion from chemical (ATP) to mechani-
            cal force by the myocardium

      4. Increased rate of calcium cycling by the sarcoplasmic reticulum
      5. Up-regulation of cardiac beta receptors
      6. Enhanced rate of spontaneous depolarization by sinoatrial node cells
      7. Shortened action potential duration
  B. Indirect actions
      1. Enhanced metabolic demand by other tissues results in a high-output state. The heart must increase its throughput to meet the increased demands of the peripheral tissues, which are similarly stimulated to a higher metabolic state by the excess circulating thyroid hormone.
      2. Reduced systemic vascular resistance (not the same as hypotension) plays an important role in the overall cardiac status of patients with hyperthyroidism. Afterload is reduced at the same time as preload is increased in the presence of an increased intravascular volume.
      3. In some, hypertension is a predominant finding and leads to
        a) significant concentric hypertrophy of the left ventricle
        b) risk of retinal detachment or hemorrhage

II. The sum of these effects when excess thyroid hormone is present (hyperthyroidism) are a heart that operates at a faster rate (tachycardia), is enlarged (hypertrophied), can contract faster and more powerfully (enhanced contractility), and has a propensity to abnormal electrical depolarizations (arrhythmias).

III. Although these might at first glance sound like beneficial changes (bigger, faster, stronger, more excitable), the thyrotoxic state greatly strains the energy economy of the heart and increases the overall work of the heart. Additionally, the thyrotoxic heart, although hyperkinetic when the patient is at rest, has less "reserve capacity" available for when increased cardiac work is necessary (e.g., exercise). This situation, added to preexisting cardiac disease (e.g., hypertrophic, restrictive, or dilated cardiomyopathy, valvular disease, etc.) can lead to decompensation of a previously well-compensated cardiac disease.

IV. Reduced systemic vascular resistance in the presence of an increased intravascular volume (not documented in cats) associated with significant increases in cardiac output are what define the high-output state of the cardiovascular system in hyperthyroidism. This high-output state can (especially in the presence of underlying primary cardiac pathology) progress to result in clinically apparent signs of congestive heart failure.

V. Despite the reduced systemic vascular resistance that is part of the high-output hyperthyroid state, hypertension rather than hypotension is observed in many hyperthyroid cats (87 percent of 39 cats in one study). Hypertension resolves in most treated cases once a euthyroid state is reached.

Signalment and Presenting Complaints

I. Cats are generally older, with no gender or breed predispositions
II. Most cats present for routine examination or because of signs and symptoms of hyperthyroidism (i.e., polyphagia, PU/PD, weight loss, etc.)
III. Cats occasionally present with CHF and/or low-output heart failure

Physical Examination

  I. Similar to other forms of cardiomyopathy
 II. A thyroid nodule may be palpable

Ancillary Tests

  I. Electrocardiography: nondiscriminatory between cardiomyopathies
 II. Thoracic radiography: nondiscriminatory between cardiomyopathies. Common findings include
     A. Generalized cardiomegaly with or without LA enlargement
     B. When CHF is present, pulmonary edema and pleural effusion are equally likely to be present
III. Echocardiography
     A. Reported echocardiographic changes in cats with hyperthyroidism include
        1. Increased aortic root dimension
        2. Left atrial enlargement
        3. Increased LVEDD and/or LVESD
        4. Mild-to-moderate concentric hypertrophy of the LV free wall and/or septum
        5. An increased (or rarely, decreased) LV shortening fraction
     B. In the authors' experience, the typical echocardiographic changes in cats with hyperthyroidism *without CHF* include hyperkinetic LV wall and septal motion with mild LV dilatation (eccentric hypertrophy) and varying degrees of left atrial enlargement. In general the LV wall and septal thicknesses are not excessive in relation to the chamber dimensions and *do not* resemble the typical changes associated with HCM.
     C. There are reports of cats with myocardial failure, demonstrating marked increases in LVEDD and LVESD, moderate to severe LA enlargement, and a reduction in shortening fraction. The relationship of this presentation to a deficiency of the amino acid taurine is unknown.

Therapy

  I. For acute congestive heart failure see the section on treatment of congestive heart failure in cats.
 II. Signs of CHF may be difficult to control prior to control the hyperthyroid state. Begin with pharmacologic manipulations for both CHF and hyperthyroidism; thyroidectomy or the physical isolation required after radioactive iodine therapy present a high risk to uncompensated animals. Once signs of CHF are well controlled and the hyperthyroid state is attenuated, more specific therapy may be pursued.
III. In cats with asymptomatic thyrotoxicosis, therapy is generally aimed at controlling the hyperthyroid state (i.e., tapazole, thyroidectomy, or radioactive iodine therapy).

IV. Beta-adrenergic blockade is a common recommendation in the literature. However, benefits have not been documented. The authors recommend beta-adrenergic blockade in the following situations
   A. To manage significant supraventricular or ventricular tachyarrhythmias
   B. In noneuthyroid patients undergoing anesthetic procedures

Prognosis

I. Asymptomatic cats can be managed very well without the use of specific cardiovascular therapy prior to appropriate therapy for the hyperthyroid state, and most evidence indicates that the cardiovascular changes are reversible.
II. Most cats with congestive heart failure can be managed successfully if the hyperthyroid state is controlled.

Acromegalic Heart Disease

Definition

Cardiac changes resulting from direct and indirect effects of elevations in circulating growth hormone (hypersomatotropism)

General Comments

I. A syndrome resembling acromegaly in humans has been reported in a group of middle-aged and older cats with growth hormone (GH)–secreting tumors of the pituitary gland.
II. In 14 cases described by Peterson et al, all affected cats had insulin-resistant diabetes mellitus and enlargement of the liver, heart, kidneys, or tongue. Various cardiovascular abnormalities were seen in most of the affected cats.

Pathophysiology

I. The pathogenesis of heart disease in cats with acromegaly is unclear. The importance of a direct trophic effect by excessive growth hormone on the myocardium as opposed to effects resulting from volume expansion, hypertension, or other secondary effects requires further study.
II. The recent finding of increased plasma growth hormone concentration in some cats with HCM suggests a potentially important role for growth hormone in cats with hypertrophic heart disease.

Signalment Presenting Complaints

   I. Cats with acromegaly generally do not present for signs referable to cardiovascular disease.
  II. Presenting complaints commonly include PU/PD and weight loss referable to uncontrolled diabetes.
 III. While no breed predilections have been identified, almost all of the reported cases have occurred in older, neutered male cats.

Physical Examination

   I. Systolic murmurs were noted in 9 of the 14 cats described.
  II. Physical features of acromegaly include prognathia inferior, cranial and abdominal enlargement, organomegaly (especially kidneys and liver), increased body size, and weight gain.
 III. Signs of congestive heart failure may develop late in the course of the disease.

Ancillary Tests

   I. Electrocardiography: abnormalities were not detected in any of the 14 cats reported
  II. Thoracic radiography: nondiscriminatory between forms of myocardial disease
 III. Echocardiography: most reported cats had evidence of septal and LV wall concentric hypertrophy resembling HCM
 IV. Other
    A. The diagnosis of acromegaly is tentatively based on the presence of insulin-resistant diabetes mellitus and/or renal failure in a cat with clinical features of acromegaly.
    B. Documentation of a pituitary mass on CT scan or MRI provide further support.
    C. A definitive diagnosis requires demonstration of increased baseline serum GH concentration.

Therapy

   I. Therapy generally is aimed at controlling the diabetic state and renal failure. If CHF is present, supportive care (diuretics and vasodilators) may also be beneficial.
  II. Successful therapy for feline acromegaly has not been reported. Potential therapeutic modalities include radiation therapy, medical therapy, and hypophysectomy.

Prognosis

   I. The short-term prognosis is good. Pituitary tumors grow slowly and neuro-
      logic signs are uncommon; the diabetes can be relatively well controlled with
      high doses of insulin.
  II. Mild-to-moderate CHF responds fairly well to symptomatic therapy. Six of
      the reported cats developed congestive heart failure. Four of these cats died,
      three of which had concurrent renal failure.
 III. Most cats eventually died or were euthanized due to refractory CHF or renal
      failure. Reported survival ranged from 4 to 24 months after diagnosis.

Pathology

LV hypertrophy is the hallmark pathologic feature. Myocardial histologic lesions
include myofiber hypertrophy, multifocal myocytolysis, interstitial fibrosis, and
intramural arteriosclerosis.

Neoplastic Infiltration of the Heart

   I. Rare in cats
  II. Echocardiography is generally required for nonsurgical detection.
 III. Cardiac tumors reported in cats include
      A. Lymphoma
      B. Chemodectoma
      C. Hemangiosarcoma
      D. Metastatic pulmonary carcinoma
      E. Metastatic mammary gland carcinoma
  IV. Lymphoma is the most common tumor of the feline myocardium. Reported
      cardiac abnormalities in cats with lymphoma include complete heart block,
      pericardial effusion, and congestive heart failure.
   V. Echocardiographic findings in cats with diffuse neoplastic infiltration of the
      myocardium can mimic those of hypertrophic cardiomyopathy.
  VI. Regression of neoplastic infiltration was reported in one cat with lymphoma
      following treatment with combination chemotherapy.

Drugs, Toxins, and Physical Injury

   I. A large number of drugs and toxins are reported to cause myocardial injury
      in domestic animals, but very few are likely to be encountered in clinical
      small animal practice. Of these, doxorubicin has received the most attention
      in cats.
  II. Decreased fractional shortening and increased left ventricular end-systolic
      dimensions were reported in four of six experimental cats given cumulative
      doses of doxorubicin of 170 to 240 mg/m². However, clinical signs of heart
      failure were not observed even after a cumulative dose of 300 mg/m², and no

cat showed ECG abnormalities during the study. As in other species, pathologic studies revealed extensive areas of myocyte vacuolization and myocytolysis. Similar clinical observations have been reported in cats with malignan-
cies treated with doxorubicin. None developed overt heart failure and
arrhythmias were only rarely observed.

III. With the possible exception of heat stroke and hypothermia, physical causes
of myocardial damage are infrequently recognized in cats. Traumatic myocarditis appears to be either uncommon or unrecognized in most cats that experience thoracic trauma.

Infectious Myocarditis

I. Infectious myocarditis is infrequently recognized in cats. Liu et al described
a syndrome of acute nonsuppurative myocarditis in 25 young cats (mean age
2.6 years). Most cats died unexpectedly and necropsy revealed focal or diffuse
infiltration of the endocardium and myocardium with mononuclear cells and
a few neutrophils. A viral etiology was suspected but never identified.

II. A recent report describes a transmissible myocarditis/diaphragmitis in cats.
No organism has been isolated, but transmission between cats by injecting
blood from infected cats is into other cats does reliably reproduce the disease.
All cats developed high fever (103.8° to 105.7°F), were lethargic, and partially
anorexic. CBCs and chemistries were normal in all cats for 6 weeks, except
for an elevation of CPK in three of seven cats. The disease resolved on its
own in these cats. Necropsy revealed pale 1 to 3 mm discrete foci surrounded
by hemorrhage on ventricular myocardium and on the diaphragm. No clinical
signs referable to the cardiovascular system were noticed.

III. The relationship of endomyocarditis to the other cardiomyopathies of cats is
unknown. Other reported causes of myocarditis in cats include toxoplasmosis
and metastatic infection from sepsis or bacterial endocarditis.

SUMMARY

I. Hypertrophic cardiomyopathy is very common and probably represents the
largest percentage of myocardial diseases currently diagnosed in the cat.

II. Presumed myocardial diseases that cannot be classified into one of the primary disorders are increasingly frequent. These lack common features that
allow their classification as a single clinical entity. Little is known about
the etiology, pathophysiology, therapy, and prognosis associated with these
unclassified cardio(myo)pathies.

III. Of the secondary cardiomyopathies discussed, only nutritional (taurine-responsive) dilated cardiomyopathy and thyrotoxic heart disease are encountered with any frequency. Both of these disorders have been well classified
and both respond dramatically to appropriate specific therapy. The other secondary cardiomyopathies occur infrequently and are generally poorly understood. The general approach, diagnosis, and therapy for these disorders are
similar to other feline cardiomyopathies.

IV. The clinician must recognize that associated clinical and diagnostic findings frequently overlap, often making a definitive diagnosis difficult. Echocardiography is the one diagnostic aid that reliably allows differentiation between the different cardiomyopathies encountered in cats. However, even with a thorough ultrasound examination, distinctions are often unclear.

SUGGESTED READINGS

Atkins CE: The role of noncardiac disease in the development and precipitation of heart failure. Vet Clin North Am (Sm Anim Pract) 21:1035, 1991

Fox PR: Feline myocardial disease. p. 435. In Fox PR (ed): Canine and Feline Cardiology. Churchill Livingstone, New York, 1988

Fox PR: Myocardial diseases. p. 1632. In Ettinger SJ (ed): Textbook of Veterinary Internal Medicine. 2nd Ed. WB Saunders, Philadelphia, 1989

Harpster NK: Feline myocardial diseases. p. 380. In Kirk RW (ed): Current Veterinary Therapy IX. WB Saunders, Philadelphia, 1986

Jacobs G, Panciera DL: Cardiovascular complications of feline hyperthyroidism. p. 756. In Kirk RW, Bonagura JD (eds): Kirk's Current Veterinary Therapy XI. WB Saunders, Philadelphia, 1992

Kittleson MD: Management of heart failure: Concepts, therapeutic strategies, and drug pharmacology. p. 171. In Fox PR (ed): Canine and Feline Cardiology. Churchill Livingstone, New York, 1988

Peterson ME, Taylor SR, Greco DS, et al: Acromegaly in 14 cats. J Vet Int Med 4:192–201, 1990

Pion PD, Kittleson MD, Rogers QR: Cardiomyopathy in the cat and its relation to taurine deficiency. p. 251. In Kirk RW (ed): Current Veterinary Therapy X. WB Saunders, Philadelphia, 1989

Pion PD, Kittleson MD: Therapy for feline aortic thromboembolism. p. 295. In Kirk RW (ed): Current Veterinary Therapy X. WB Saunders, Philadelphia, 1989

9

Cor Pulmonale

Dana G. Allen
Andrew Mackin

INTRODUCTION

DEFINITION

I. Cor pulmonale is defined as disease of the right heart (typically, right ventricular hypertrophy and/or dilatation) secondary to pulmonary hypertension associated with either pulmonary vascular or pulmonary parenchymal disease.
II. Although primary cardiovascular diseases, such as left-to-right shunts (patent ductus arteriosus and atrial or ventricular septal defects) and mitral valvular insufficiency, may increase pulmonary vascular resistance and eventually cause secondary pulmonary hypertension with subsequent right ventricular hypertrophy, cor pulmonale specifically refers to right-heart enlargement secondary to primary pulmonary vascular or parenchymal disease.
III. Cor pulmonale may be either acute or chronic. Acute cor pulmonale is defined as acute right-heart disease secondary to pulmonary hypertension, and is usually due to massive pulmonary thromboembolism. Chronic cor pulmonale occurs secondary to chronic pulmonary vascular and parenchymal diseases, such as heartworm infestation and chronic obstructive pulmonary disease.

ETIOLOGY

I. Any disease that affects ventilatory mechanics, alveolar gas exchange or pulmonary vasculature may cause cor pulmonale. Consequently, cor pulmonale may occur secondary to diseases of either pulmonary structures (airway, parenchyma, or vasculature) or the surrounding thoracic cage. Potential causes of cor pulmonale are listed in Table 9-1.
II. Common causes of cor pulmonale in the dog include heartworm (see Ch. 10), pulmonary embolic disorders (other than heartworm), and chronic obstructive pulmonary disease.
III. Pulmonary embolization occurs when thrombi, fat, air, tumor cells or foreign bodies pass through the systemic venous circulation into the right side of the heart, and subsequently lodge within the pulmonary arteries. Pulmonary fat emboli may result from trauma, especially long-bone fractures and contusion of adipose tissue. Air emboli can result from pneumoperitoneum, intravenous

TABLE 9-1. CAUSES OF COR PULMONALE

Pulmonary airway disease
    Chronic obstructive pulmonary disease
        Chronic bronchitis
        Emphysema
        Bronchiectasis
    Airway obstruction
        Tracheal collapse
        Bronchial collapse
Pulmonary parenchymal disease
    Systemic lupus erythematosus
    Systemic mycosis
    Radiation
    Malignant infiltration
    Pulmonary fibrosis
Pulmonary vascular disease
    Heartworm disease
    Pulmonary embolic disease
    High-altitude disease
    Primary pulmonary hypertension
    Compression of pulmonary arteries (neoplasia)
Thoracic cage disease
    Kyphoscoliosis
    Pectus excavatum
    Neuromuscular weakness
    Severe obesity ("Pickwickian syndrome")

infusions, retroperitoneal air injection, and other diagnostic or therapeutic techniques that involve air insufflation. Tumor emboli gain access to the venous circulation from either the primary neoplasm or a metastatic focus. Although embolization of neoplastic cells may eventually result in pulmonary metastatic disease, such emboli are rarely large enough to cause cor pulmonale. Many systemic diseases are associated with pulmonary embolism (Table 9-2).

IV. Chronic obstructive pulmonary disease (COPD) in the dog is frequently associated with chronic bronchitis. Chronic bronchitis in the dog is a common respiratory disease of insidious onset. Potential causes of chronic bronchitis include airway irritation caused by cigarette smoke and other environmental pollutants, allergy airway disease, and respiratory tract infections and parasites.

INCIDENCE

I. The incidence of cor pulmonale in the dog is not well documented. In endemic areas, heartworm disease is probably the most common cause of both acute and chronic cor pulmonale in dogs.

II. The incidence of pulmonary thromboembolism in dogs is unknown, perhaps because minor thromboembolic episodes are presumably undetected.

III. Cor pulmonale is rarely recognized in the cat.

TABLE 9-2. CAUSES OF PULMONARY EMBOLISM

Heartworm disease (embolism of worms and/or thrombus)
Pulmonary thromboembolism
    Hyperadrenocorticism/exogenous glucocorticoids
    Hypothyroidism
    Protein-losing nephropathy
        Amyloidosis
        Glomerulonephritis
    Immune-mediated hemolytic anemia
    Pancreatitis
    Cardiac disease
    Septic processes
    Neoplasia
    Trauma
    Surgical procedures
    Total parenteral nutrition (long-term, large central catheter)
Air embolism
Fat embolism
Neoplastic embolism
Vascular foreign body embolism

(Modified from Rush JE, Atkins CE: Vascular disease. p. 323. In Allen DG (ed): Small Animal Medicine. JB Lippincott, Philadelphia, 1991, with permission.)

PATHOPHYSIOLOGY

I. Both acute and chronic cor pulmonale have in common a disturbance of the pulmonary circulation. Significant reduction in the total cross-sectional pulmonary vascular bed must occur before pulmonary hypertension and subsequent cor pulmonale develop.

    A. Healthy pulmonary vasculature accommodates increased blood volume predominantly by distention and recruitment of underperfused vessels. Distention predominates in dependent areas of the lung where pulmonary venous pressure is greater than alveolar pressure, and recruitment predominates in superior areas of the lung where alveolar pressure is greater than pulmonary venous pressure or where blood vessels are collapsed. Pulmonary arterial pressures initially remain normal despite increased blood volume because as pulmonary blood flow increases, distention and recruitment decrease pulmonary vascular resistance. Pulmonary hypertension occurs when relatively healthy areas of pulmonary vasculature are unable to accommodate augmented blood flow secondary to either increased cardiac output or shunting of blood from more diseased areas of pulmonary vasculature. Persistent pulmonary hypertension induces progressive luminal narrowing of the pulmonary arterial vasculature secondary to structural changes, such as vascular endothelial swelling and myointimal hypertrophy. Pulmonary hypertension becomes self-perpetuating after irreversible medial hypertrophy of the pulmonary arteries develops.

    B. The right ventricle is a low-pressure pump, and is therefore unable to compensate for acute rises in pulmonary arterial pressure. Chronic pulmonary hypertension, on the other hand, initially induces compensatory right ventricular dilatation and hypertrophy. Decreased right-sided cardiac output (and subsequent decreased left-sided cardiac output) promotes sodium and water retention in an attempt to increase blood volume and venous return. The right ventricle is more compliant than the left ventricle, and is able to compensate for increases in blood volume more efficiently than increases in pressure. Eventually, however, the right ventricle can no longer accommodate the combination of spiralling preload and afterload, and right-heart failure develops. Right ventricular end-diastolic pressure, right atrial pressure and central venous pressure increase as the right heart fails.

    C. Overt right-sided congestive heart failure is fortunately an uncommon end result of pulmonary hypertension and cor pulmonale.

II. Pulmonary embolization

    A. The lung is the organ that is most commonly affected by thromboembolic disease in the dog. Thrombi broken free from their original sites of attachment are carried by the systemic venous circulation to the pulmonary arterial vasculature. Thromboembolic disease occludes the pulmonary vascular bed, reducing total pulmonary blood flow and consequently increasing pulmonary vascular resistance. Approximately 25 to 50 percent of the total cross-sectional pulmonary vascular bed must be occluded before pulmonary hypertension develops. Occlusion of over 40 percent of the pulmonary vasculature causes pressure elevations within the right ventricle, right atrium and cranial vena cava. Occlusion of over 60 percent of the vascular bed significantly decreases pulmonary artery blood flow (and consequently cardiac output).

    B. Pulmonary arterial embolism also impairs oxygen exchange (via ventilation-perfusion mismatching) in affected areas of lung. Subsequent local hypoxia causes vasoconstriction of affected pulmonary arterial vasculature. Thromboxane A_2, serotonin, and histamine released from platelets incorporated within thrombi (and possibly histamine released from adjacent pulmonary mast cells) may also contribute to pulmonary arterial vasoconstriction. Thus, pulmonary vasoconstriction secondary to local hypoxia and the release of vasoactive substances exacerbates the pulmonary hypertension initiated by thromboembolic vascular occlusion. Vasoactive substances (such as serotonin and histamine) released during pulmonary thromboembolism may also induce local bronchoconstriction. Bronchoconstriction and subsequent local hypoventilation redirect ventilation to areas of well-perfused lung, thereby encouraging an optimal ventilation-perfusion ratio. Severe pulmonary embolization leads to systemic hypoxemia, widening of the alveolar-arterial oxygen concentration difference, dyspnea and tachypnea secondary to diffuse bronchoconstriction, ventilation-perfusion mismatching, and pleural effusion. Dyspnea and tachypnea may be exacerbated by pleuritic pain and psychological stress.

    C. Thromboembolic occlusion of a large cross-sectional area of the pulmonary vascular bed causes both systemic hypoxemia and marked pulmonary hypertension. Severe pulmonary hypertension may in turn cause cor pulmonale and eventual right-sided heart failure.

    D. Factors predisposing to accelerated thrombogenesis include altered hemodynamics (either turbulence or stasis of blood flow), damage to vascular endothelium, and increased blood coagulability. Pulmonary thromboembolism in dogs with hyperadrenocorticism may result from a hypercoagulable state associated with cortisol excess, hyperlipidemia, hypercholesterolemia, and increased levels of various coagulation factors. Protein-losing nephropathies such as amyloidosis and glomerulonephritis may also cause hypercoagulability secondary to loss of antithrombin III through damaged glomeruli. Antithrombin III in the normal dog attenuates coagulation by neutralizing activated clotting factors.

E. In many cases pulmonary thromboemboli resolve spontaneously. Small emboli typically resolve in approximately 1 to 2 weeks, and larger emboli may take up to 6 weeks to resolve.

F. Heartworm disease causes pulmonary arterial hypertension by both pulmonary vascular obstruction and pulmonary vasoconstriction (see Ch. 10).

III. Chronic obstructive pulmonary disease

A. COPD is defined as chronic airflow obstruction caused by pulmonary diseases such as chronic bronchitis, bronchiectasis, emphysema, and asthma. Chronic bronchitis is characterized by chronic inflammation of pulmonary airways, with subsequent mucus hypersecretion secondary to hypertrophy and hyperplasia of goblet and mucus-secreting cells. Airflow obstruction in chronic bronchitis is due to a combination of bronchoconstriction, excessive mucus production, and edema and inflammation of airway mucosa. Bronchiectasis (irreversible bronchial dilation) and emphysema (enlargement of air spaces and destruction of alveoli) often occur secondarily to chronic respiratory disease. Asthma causes reversible airway obstruction. Although atopic (allergic) asthma typically does not cause chronic cor pulmonale, nonatopic or intrinsic asthma frequently predisposes to chronic bronchitis and subsequent cor pulmonale.

B. Vasoconstriction of small precapillary pulmonary arteries is the main pathophysiologic mechanism for the increased pulmonary vascular resistance seen with chronic respiratory disease. Alveolar hypoxia is usually the most potent stimulus for pulmonary vasoconstriction. Hypoxia-induced local pulmonary vasoconstriction diverts blood flow away from areas of hypoxic lung. Subsequent increased perfusion of well-ventilated lung maintains an optimal ventilation-perfusion ratio. Hypoxia-induced pulmonary vasoconstriction occurs in dogs with COPD, tracheal collapse, major airway obstruction (masses or foreign bodies), lung lobe torsion, and decreased concentrations of inspired oxygen.

C. Hypercapnia (increased Pa_{CO_2}) does not appear to directly affect the pulmonary vascular bed. Local acidosis secondary to the increased hydrogen ion concentrations associated with hypercapnia, however, does induce pulmonary vasoconstriction. Hypoxia and acidosis may synergistically intensify pulmonary vasoconstriction. Local hypoxia, hypercapnia, and subsequent acidosis frequently coexist in respiratory diseases (Fig. 9-1). Reduction or inhibition of local vasodilators (such as endothelial-derived relaxing factor and nitric oxide) and enhancement of local vasoconstrictors (such as endothelial-derived contracting factor) may also contribute to pulmonary vasoconstriction.

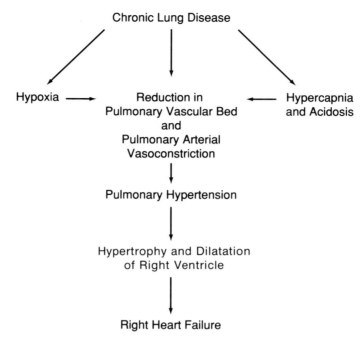

Fig. 9-1. Pathogenesis of cor pulmonale. (Modified from Summer WR: Acute cor pulmonale. p. 285. In Rubin LJ (ed): Pulmonary Heart Disease. Martinus Nijhoff, Boston, 1984, with permission.)

   D. Pulmonary hypertension and subsequent cor pulmonale are the eventual
      sequelae of chronic diffuse pulmonary vasoconstriction.

DIAGNOSIS

HISTORY

Nonspecific clinical signs of pulmonary hypertension and subsequent cor pulmonale include fatigue, exercise intolerance, syncope, dyspnea, and cyanosis. Eventual right ventricular failure may cause obvious ascites.

  I. Pulmonary embolization
      A. Pulmonary embolization may be associated with a variety of clinical signs, including acute unexplained dyspnea, weakness, syncope, cyanosis, and hemoptysis. The clinical presentation depends upon both the degree of occlusion of the pulmonary vasculature and the presence or absence of concurrent pulmonary infarction. Embolization causing only minor occlusion of pulmonary vasculature may be subclinical or induce only subtle transient dyspnea, while major occlusions most commonly induce acute

severe unexplained dyspnea. Hemoptysis associated with pulmonary embolization usually signifies concurrent pulmonary infarction.

B. Pulmonary thromboembolism rarely occurs in isolation. Embolization should be suspected in acutely dyspneic patients with systemic diseases that are known to increase susceptibility to pulmonary thromboembolism (e.g., hyperadrenocorticism, glomerulopathies, pancreatitis, immune-mediated hemolytic anemia, sepsis, and neoplasia) (see Table 9-2).

II. Chronic obstructive pulmonary disease

Diseases causing COPD share a similar clinical presentation, which includes a productive cough, exercise intolerance, dyspnea, cyanosis, and syncope. Chronic bronchitis most commonly affects obese, older dogs. Chronic obstructive pulmonary diseases typically cause exercise intolerance long before precipitating overt cardiac disease.

PHYSICAL EXAMINATION

I. Pulmonary hypertension always precedes the onset of clinical signs characteristic of cor pulmonale. However, since initial pulmonary hypertension is essentially a subclinical disorder, clinical signs associated with increased right atrial pressure and decreased cardiac output tend to predominate.

II. Cardiac auscultation of patients with moderate pulmonary hypertension may reveal increased intensity of the pulmonic valvular component of the second heart sound; auscultation of patients with more advanced pulmonary hypertension may also reveal splitting of the second heart sound, a prominent gallop rhythm, or a right apical systolic regurgitant cardiac murmur due to insufficiency of the tricuspid valve. Pericardial or pleural effusion secondary to severe right-sided congestive heart failure may cause muffling of cardiac sounds.

III. Clinical signs consistent with progressing right-sided congestive heart failure include jugular venous distention, prominent jugular pulses, presence of a positive hepatojugular reflux, hepatomegaly, ascites, and eventual pericardial and pleural effusions. Peripheral edema is rare in dogs with right-sided congestive heart failure, and almost never precedes ascites. Chronic passive pancreatic and gastrointestinal congestion may cause maldigestion and malabsorption, and eventual weight loss.

IV. Pulmonary embolization

A. Patients with severe pulmonary embolization exhibit the characteristic clinical signs of acute cor pulmonale. Severe acute dyspnea is usually the most prominent presenting complaint. Dyspnea is typically unresponsive to oxygen therapy.

B. Physical examination will often also reveal abnormalities consistent with an underlying primary disorder such as hyperadrenocorticism.

V. Chronic obstructive pulmonary disease

A. Patients with severe COPD may exhibit abnormalities consistent with chronic cor pulmonale. However, the clinical signs of the underlying primary respiratory disease (particularly expiratory dyspnea) tend to predominate. Severely affected patients stand with forelegs abducted in an attempt to increase the volume of the thoracic cavity, and extend the head and neck to further facilitate ventilation. Patients with COPD may develop a barrel-shaped thorax as the rib cage expands in an attempt to increase total pulmonary volume. Abdominal musculature may also be used in order to further increase tidal volume.

B. Thoracic auscultation of dogs with COPD frequently reveals increased adventitial lung sounds such as crackles and wheezes. Cyanosis and syncope may occur during episodes of severe respiratory distress.

DIAGNOSTIC TESTING

The minimum data base for a patient with either acute or chronic cor pulmonale should include thoracic radiography, electrocardiography, routine hematology, serum biochemical profile, and, when available, arterial blood gas analysis. Selection of further diagnostic tests is based on results of the initial minimum data base.

Thoracic Radiography

I. Dogs with cor pulmonale frequently exhibit radiographic evidence of right ventricular enlargement, such as increased sternal contact on the lateral projection and prominent bulging of the right ventricular component of the cardiac silhouette on the dorsoventral projection (the so-called "reversed D"). Radiographic signs of right-sided congestive heart failure include persistent enlargement of the caudal vena cava, and pleural or pericardial effusion.

II. Pulmonary embolization should be suspected in patients with moderate to severe dyspnea despite minimal radiographic abnormalities.

A. Radiographic pulmonary vascular abnormalities consistent with embolization include increased diameter of the pulmonary arteries proximal to the thrombus, with attenuation or loss of visualization of more distal lobar arteries and veins.

B. Dorsoventral thoracic radiography may reveal asymmetric vascular diameters, with underperfusion of the obstructed pulmonary vasculature and overperfusion of the unaffected vasculature. Large thrombi may cause prominent local blunting of affected pulmonary arteries.

C. Pulmonary thromboemboli without concurrent hemorrhage or infarction may provide minimal radiographic evidence of pulmonary parenchymal disease. Affected lung lobes may appear relatively hyperlucent as a result of underperfusion and decreased vascular markings. Dorsoventral thoracic radiography of patients with unilateral pulmonary artery thrombosis may reveal asymmetric left- and right-lung field dimensions, as the embolized lung lobes may be smaller due to splinting of the diaphragm. Concurrent pulmonary hemorrhage or infarction may produce focal alveolar infiltrates or atelectasis. Pulmonary infarction may also produce small quantities of pleural effusion.

III. The major (and occasionally the only) radiographic feature of COPD is pulmonary hyperinflation. Pulmonary hyperinflation causes hyperlucency and expansion of lung fields, with associated caudal flattening of the diaphragm.

   A. Chronic bronchitis typically also produces a diffuse increase in bronchointerstitial pulmonary markings.

   B. Bronchiectasis (dilatation of bronchi and bronchioles) may be evident in patients with severe chronic obstructive pulmonary disease.

Electrocardiography

I. The right ventricle must be markedly enlarged before electrocardiographic abnormalities are detectable. Electrocardiographs from patients with documented cor pulmonale are therefore frequently normal. Electrocardiographic abnormalities, when present, usually reflect decreased cardiac output, myocardial hypoxia, and right-sided cardiac enlargement.

II. Decreased cardiac output may lead to compensatory tachycardia, recognized electrocardiographically as sinus tachycardia. Hypoxemia and myocardial hypoxia may cause conduction disturbances and ST segment depression. Right atrial enlargement may increase P wave amplitude (''P pulmonale''), and enable visualization of atrial repolarization as a slight baseline depression following the P wave (the so-called ''Ta'' wave). Electrocardiographic findings (on the frontal plane) consistent with right ventricular enlargement include identifiable S waves in leads I, II, III and aVF, increased S wave depth in leads I and II, and right deviation of the mean electrical axis.

Clinical Pathology

I. Clinical pathologic abnormalities in patients with either acute or chronic cor pulmonale usually reflect underlying disease processes rather than the direct effects of cor pulmonale itself. Prolonged systemic hypoxemia may induce polycythemia for example, and passive hepatic and renal congestion may cause increases in serum alanine aminotransferase, serum alkaline phosphatase, blood urea nitrogen, and serum creatinine.

II. Hematology and biochemistry in patients with pulmonary thromboembolism frequently reveal preliminary evidence of an underlying primary disease, such as hyperadrenocorticism, glomerulopathy, pancreatitis, immune-mediated hemolytic anemia, heartworm disease, sepsis, or neoplasia. Subsequent diagnostic tests that may be indicated in individual patients with pulmonary thromboembolic disease include urinalysis (including urinary cortisol:creatinine ratio), ACTH stimulation or low-dose dexamethasone suppression tests, Coomb's test, blood cultures, and heartworm tests.

III. Hematologic abnormalities occasionally detected in patients with COPD include polycythemia and leukocytosis (neutrophilia and eosinophilia). Further diagnostic tests that may be indicated in individual patients with COPD include fecal parasitology (flotation and Baermann technique) and heartworm tests. Either transtracheal wash or bronchoalveolar lavage should be performed to collect airway secretions for cytology and bacterial and fungal cultures.

Arterial Blood Gas Analysis

I. Arterial blood gas analysis provides supportive evidence for pulmonary thromboembolism. Patients with severe pulmonary thromboembolism are reported to exhibit hypoxemia (decreased Pa_{O_2}) with variable arterial carbon dioxide (Pa_{CO_2}) concentrations. Hypoxemia frequently fails to respond to oxygen supplementation. Patients with mild thromboembolism and coexistent pulmonary hemorrhage or infarction are reported to have normal arterial P_{O_2} with concurrent marked hypocapnia and respiratory alkalosis. Respiratory alkalosis in patients with pulmonary hemorrhage or infarction may be secondary to tachypnea induced by pleuritic pain. Tissue hypoxia with subsequent anaerobic metabolism may cause metabolic acidosis.

II. Patients with COPD are also frequently hypoxemic, and their arterial carbon dioxide concentrations are reported to be variable. Hypoxemia typically responds adequately to oxygen supplementation.

Special Diagnostic Techniques

I. Selective pulmonary angiography (infusion of contrast directly into the pulmonary artery), although relatively invasive, is the procedure of choice for establishing a definitive diagnosis of pulmonary thromboembolism. Nonselective angiography (infusion of contrast via the jugular vein) often achieves adequate opacification of the pulmonary vasculature. Angiographic demonstration of filling defects within the pulmonary arteries confirms the presence of pulmonary thromboembolism. Other angiographic findings consistent with pulmonary thromboembolism include truncation of pulmonary arteries and failure of contrast to completely fill pulmonary vasculature.

II. Cardiac catheterization may be used to confirm pulmonary hypertension (mean pulmonary arterial pressure over 25 mmHg) in dogs with suspected cor pulmonale. Conditions such as pulmonary thromboembolism and canine heartworm may cause profound pulmonary hypertension (mean arterial pressure increased by more than eight times normal baseline values). Patients with cor pulmonale also typically have elevated right ventricular, right atrial, and central venous pressures.

III. The effects of pulmonary hypertension on echocardiographic parameters are not well documented in small animal patients. Echocardiographic findings consistent with pulmonary hypertension in humans include rapid opening slope of the pulmonic valve during early systole, elevation of the ratio of right ventricular pre-ejection period to the right ventricular ejection time, midsystolic semiclosure of the pulmonic valve, and decreased left ventricular internal dimensions. Echocardiographic findings consistent with cor pulmonale include right ventricular hypertrophy, right atrial dilatation and paradoxical motion of the interventricular septum. Visualization of a thrombus within the right atrium provides indirect evidence of pulmonary thromboembolism.

IV. Ventilation-perfusion radionuclide imaging of patients with large pulmonary thromboemboli typically demonstrates normal ventilation of all lung lobes, with concurrent large segmental defects in the perfusion of affected lobes. Results of ventilation-perfusion radionuclide imaging may be inconclusive in patients with multiple smaller thromboemboli.

TREATMENT

I. Diagnosis and specific treatment of the underlying cause of pulmonary hypertension in patients with cor pulmonale is the primary goal of therapy. Concurrent nonspecific supportive therapy (particularly strict cage rest and oxygen supplementation) is recommended in patients with life-threatening cor pulmonale.

II. Overt right-sided congestive heart failure may necessitate such therapy as dietary sodium restriction, diuretics, and digitalis.

III. Pulmonary hypertension may theoretically be alleviated by therapeutic vasodilation of the pulmonary arterial vasculature. Unfortunately, most vasodilators appear to selectively lower systemic vascular resistance to a far greater extent than pulmonary vascular resistance. Production of systemic hypotension with vasodilator therapy is hazardous in patients when compromised cardiac output secondary to pulmonary hypertension is present. Vasodilator therapy should therefore only be considered when conventional therapy (such as oxygen supplementation and bronchodilation) has been shown to be ineffective. Vasodilators such as diltiazem, nifedipine, hydralazine, and prazosin have been demonstrated to improve pulmonary hemodynamics in individual human patients. Systemic blood pressure should be regularly monitored during treatment with vasodilators (Table 9-3).

IV. The only "vasodilator" that consistently reduces pulmonary vascular resis-

TABLE 9-3. DRUGS USED IN THE MANAGEMENT
OF COR PULMONALE IN DOGS

Bronchodilators
  Albuterol (salbutamol) 0.02 to 0.04 mg/kg once to TID; PO
  Aminophylline 10 mg/kg TID; PO, IM, IV
  Oxtriphylline 14 mg/kg TID–QID; PO
  Terbutaline 2.5 to 5 mg TID; PO, SC

Antitussives
  Butorphanol 0.55 mg/kg BID–QID; PO
  Codeine 0.1 to 0.3 mg/kg TID–QID; PO
  Dextromethorphan 2 mg/kg TID–QID; PO
  Hydrocodone 0.22 mg/kg BID–TID; PO

Vasodilators
  Captopril 0.5 to 2 mg/kg BID–TID; PO
  Diltiazem 0.5 to 1 mg/kg TID; PO
  Hydralazine 0.5 to 2 mg/kg BID; PO
  Prazosin 1 mg/15 kg TID; PO

tance without significantly affecting systemic blood pressure is oxygen. Trial oxygen supplementation is therefore recommended in all patients with severe cor pulmonale, even if systemic arterial oxygenation is adequate.

PULMONARY EMBOLIZATION

I. Treatment of pulmonary thromboembolism may be prophylactic or definitive. Prophylactic therapy assumes that the patient's fibrinolytic system will eventually dissolve pre-existing pulmonary thromboemboli. Prophylactic therapy attempts to prevent further thrombus formation and subsequent pulmonary thromboembolization. Definitive therapy for pulmonary thromboembolism, on the other hand, attempts to dissolve or remove the existent thromboemboli.

II. Appropriate prophylactic therapy for dogs with pulmonary thromboembolism is not well established. One currently recommended protocol uses both heparin and warfarin. A loading dose of heparin (100 to 200 U/kg IV) is initiated and is followed within 2 hours by the subcutaneous administration of 200 to 300 U/kg three to four times daily. The goal is to maintain APTT at about 1.5 times baseline values. Heparin is continued for approximately 1 week, at which time warfarin is expected to be fully effective. Oral warfarin therapy (0.1 mg/kg/day PO) is commenced at the time heparin is first given and is titrated to maintain the PT at 1.25 to 2 times baseline values. Chronic oral warfarin therapy is continued for approximately 3 to 6 months (PT is reassessed monthly) unless the primary disease process predisposing the patient to thromboembolism has completely resolved. Iatrogenic hemorrhage is the most frequent complication of combination heparin/warfarin therapy. Concurrent low-dose oral aspirin therapy is considered to be unlikely to prevent recurrence of pulmonary thromboembolism, and is therefore not routinely recommended.

III. Definitive therapy to either dissolve or remove existent pulmonary thromboemboli is infrequently used in veterinary patients. Definitive therapy for pulmonary thromboembolism in humans typically involves either surgical embolectomy or administration of exogenous fibrinolytic agents. Pulmonary embolectomy involves cardiopulmonary bypass techniques to permit open heart surgery, and is associated with high mortality rates (up to 50 percent) in human patients. Fibrinolytic therapy with either urokinase or streptokinase does not improve survival in people with pulmonary thromboembolism, and is complicated by significant iatrogenic hemorrhage. Tissue plasminogen activator is a fibrinolytic agent that may have the potential to enhance medical management of pulmonary thromboembolism. The utility of tissue plasminogen activator has not been clinically evaluated in small animals with pulmonary thromboembolism.

CHRONIC OBSTRUCTIVE PULMONARY DISEASE

I. The principal goal of therapy in patients with cor pulmonale secondary to COPD is to relieve pulmonary hypertension by improving pulmonary gas exchange. Bronchodilators (either beta-agonists such as albuterol and terbutaline, or methylxanthines such as aminophylline and oxtriphylline) are the principal means of nonspecifically improving pulmonary ventilation in patients with COPD. Many dogs with chronic bronchitis will show significant clinical improvement on bronchodilator therapy, although hypoxemia may persist (Table 9-3).

II. Nonspecific management of COPD may include weight control, humidification, coupage, antibiotics, antitussives, and anti-inflammatory agents such as prednisone. Establishment of a definite etiology with subsequent specific therapy is desirable whenever possible.

PROGNOSIS

I. The prognosis for eventual dissolution of pulmonary thromboemboli in a patient surviving the initial embolic event is fair to good provided the original predisposing disease has been effectively treated.

II. The prognosis for resolution of COPD in most dogs is unfortunately guarded. Treatment of COPD is usually only palliative unless a specific etiological agent can be identified and eliminated.

SUGGESTED READINGS

Allen DG: Special techniques. Nonselective angiocardiography. p. 1039. In Allen DG (ed): Small Animal Medicine. JB Lippincott, Philadelphia, 1991

Atkins CE: Vascular disease. p. 323. In Allen DG (ed): Small Animal Medicine. JB Lippincott, Philadelphia, 1991

Brewster RD, Benjamin SA, Thomassen RW: Spontaneous cor pulmonale in laboratory beagles. Lab Anim Sci 33:299, 1983

Burns MG: Pulmonary thromboembolism. p. 257. In Kirk RW (ed): Current Veterinary Therapy VIII. WB Saunders, Philadelphia, 1983

Burns MG, Kelly AB, Hornof WJ, Howerth EW: Pulmonary artery thrombosis in three dogs with hyperadrenocorticism. J Am Vet Med Assoc 178:388, 1981

Cornelissen JM, Wolvekamp WC, Stokhof AA et al: Primary occlusive pulmonary vascular disease in a dog diagnosed by a lung perfusion scintigram. J Am Anim Hosp Assoc 21: 293, 1985

Dennis JS: The pathophysiologic sequelae of pulmonary thromboembolism. Comp Cont Ed Small An Pract 13:1811, 1991

Ettinger SJ, Suter PF. Cor pulmonale. p. 421. In Ettinger SJ, Suter PF (eds): Canine Cardiology. WB Saunders, Philadelphia, 1970

Fox PR: Cor pulmonale. p. 313. In Kirk RW (ed): Current Veterinary Therapy IX. WB Saunders, Philadelphia, 1986

Fluchiger MA, Gomez JA: Radiographic findings in dogs with spontaneous pulmonary thrombosis or embolism. Vet Radiology 25:124, 1984

King RR, Mauderly JL, Hahn FF et al: Pulmonary function studies in a dog with pulmonary thromboembolism associated with Cushing's disease. J Am Anim Hosp Assoc 21:555, 1985

Krotje LJ, McAllister HA, Engwall MJA et al: Chronic obstructive pulmonary disease in a dog. J Am Vet Med Assoc 191:1427, 1987

Kuehn NF, Roudebush P: Chronic bronchitis. p. 397. In Allen DG (ed): Small Animal Medicine. JB Lippincott, Philadelphia, 1991

Lombard CW, Buergelt CD: Echocardiographic and clinical findings in dogs with heartworm-induced cor pulmonale. Comp Cont Ed Small An Pract 12:971, 1983

Maher ER, Rush JE: Cardiovascular changes in the geriatric dog. Comp Cont Ed (Small Anim Pract) 12:921, 1990

McFadden ER, Braunwald E: Cor pulmonale. p. 1597. In Braunwald E (ed): Heart Disease. 3rd Ed. WB Saunders, Philadelphia, 1988

Padrid PA, Hornof WJ, Kurpershoek CJ, Cross CE: Canine chronic bronchitis. A pathophysiologic evaluation of 18 cases. J Am Col Vet Int Med 4:172–180, 1990

Perry LA, Dillon AR, Bowers TL: Pulmonary hypertension. Comp Cont Ed Small An Pract 13:226, 1991

Rawlings CA, Tackett RL: Postadulticide pulmonary hypertension of canine heartworm disease: Successful treatment with oxygen and failure of antihistamines. Am J Vet Res 51:1565, 1990

Spaulding GL: Cor pulmonale. p. 335. In Kirk RW (ed): Current Veterinary Therapy VII. WB Saunders, Philadelphia, 1980

10

Heartworm Disease

Clay A. Calvert

INTRODUCTION

Heartworm infection is distributed widely in the United States. Most veterinarians practice in areas where heartworm disease should be considered in patients with clinical signs referable to the lungs and heart. Even in regions where heartworm infection is not indigenous, such as desert, mountainous, and cold regions, a mobile public may introduce infected animals.

INCIDENCE

Heartworm infection has been reported in all 50 states, but the prevalence is highly variable even within a given locale. If heartworm infection is found in a region, it is unlikely to be eradicated. Infection rates up to 45 percent have been reported within 150 miles of the Gulf and Atlantic coasts from Texas to New Jersey and along the Mississippi River and its tributaries. Most of the remainder of the United States and southern Canada have infection rates up to 5 percent. Heartworm infection occurs throughout much of the temperate world, including Japan and Australia.

I. Epidemiology
   Male dogs are more frequently infected, as are outdoor dogs. Large dogs, probably related to the previous factors, are more commonly infected. Most infected dogs are young to middle aged, reflecting their habitus and inadequate husbandry.
   A. Heartworm infection has spread into the northwestern United States and Colorado.
      1. Hundreds of cases are seen annually in southern Oregon and the Willamette Valley.
      2. Infection rates are very low in Montana, Idaho, Utah, and Washington.
      3. Less than 1 percent of dogs tested in Colorado in 1990 were positive.
         a) Parts of the Western Slope and Arkansas River valley may be endemic.
         b) Infections in the Denver area are limited.
   B. Infection rates have tended to increase in Canada, and a lower proportion of infected dogs have a history compatible with infection obtained elsewhere.

II. Life cycle

Heartworm infection is spread by mosquito species that vary depending on the geographic region. Some mosquito species serve as more effective intermediate hosts and vectors than others.

A. Female mosquitoes serve as the intermediate host and obtain microfilariae (L_1) from infected dogs.

1. Microfilariae develop over a 2-month period and are capable of infecting a dog (third-stage larvae) in 2 to 2.5 weeks.

2. The L_3 enter the host dog via a mosquito bite wound and migrate through the host for approximately 100 days.

3. After 100 days, young adult worms (L_5) enter the vascular system and travel to the pulmonary arteries.

B. Patency occurs approximately 6 months after infection with L_3, and microfilariae numbers increase rapidly over the ensuing 6 months.

C. Disease severity is determined by the number of adult worms and the host-parasite interaction.

1. Dogs that develop a strong immune response to the parasites tend to incur more severe pulmonary pathology.

2. When the infection exceeds one worm per pound, the pulmonary arteries contain many worms and worms are also found in the right ventricle.

D. Transmission of infection is less likely between December and February in the continental United States, even in endemic regions.

PATHOPHYSIOLOGY

Worms in the pulmonary arteries quickly damage the endothelium. Areas of endothelium are sloughed and activated leukocytes and platelets adhere to the subendothelium.

I. Trophic factors

Growth factors may be released by platelets and leukocytes that stimulate migration and multiplication of smooth muscle cells of the tunica media.

A. Smooth muscle proliferation: Villous hypertrophy results from collagen production and invasion of the tunica intima by smooth muscle cells.

1. Villi range in size from a few microns to several millimeters.

2. The villi become covered by an abnormal endothelium that may itself become damaged, leading to complex villus proliferation.

B. Villous hypertrophy occurs in all arteries large enough to accommodate adult worms and regresses following effective treatment.

II. Pulmonary arterial enlargement

Arteries to the caudal and accessory lung lobes are most severely effected.

A. Arteries and arterioles become dilated, sacculated, and tortuous, and lose their normal taperizing arborization.

B. Arterioles whose diameters are less than that of adult worms often are abruptly obstructed.

III. Arterial blood flow
Arterial obstruction results from myointimal proliferation, worms, and thrombosis.
   A. Obstruction of flow leads to collateral recruitment in less involved or noninvolved lung lobes.
   B. Severe infection prevents adequate collateral circulation, which leads to pulmonary hypertension.
IV. Reactive vasoconstriction and hypertension
Regional ischemia produces arterial constriction, further aggravating pulmonary perfusion and hypertension.
 V. Response to dead worms
The pulmonary response to dead worms is an exaggeration of the response to live worms.
   A. Worm fragments are swept into smaller arteries and arterioles, resulting in villous proliferation, thrombosis, and granulomatous inflammation.
   B. Inflammatory reactions: parenchymal lung pathology results from interruption of blood flow, leakage of plasma from damaged small vessels, and inflammation.
VI. Right ventricular afterload
Pulmonary hypertension leads to progressively increasing afterload and right ventricular dilation. Eventually, severe hypertrophy occurs in some patients.
   A. Tends to occur more frequently in dogs with immune-mediated occult infections
   B. Often associated with high worm burdens although chronic infections with residual low worm burdens can also be associated with severe cor pulmonale
   C. The consequences are poor exercise tolerance and right-sided congestive heart failure (ascites)
VII. Occult heartworm disease
Can arise through several methods and accounts for 5 to 67 percent of all infections. In most areas, occult infections are believed to constitute 10 to 40 percent of all infections.
   A. Unisex infections are possible, although not common in highly endemic regions where worm burdens tend to be high.
   B. Immune-mediated occult disease is common.
      1. Antibodies are produced soon after microfilariae appear. They trap microfilariae in the pulmonary capillaries.
      2. Inflammation, consisting predominantly of neutrophils, aids the immune response.
      3. In 10 to 20 percent of immune occult infections the inflammatory response is dominated by eosinophils and an allergic pneumonitis results.
   C. When heartworm testing is performed in the winter and early spring, many infections will be occult because of immature worms.
      1. Patency requires approximately 6 months.
      2. Antigen tests are usually not very sensitive until 7 months after L_3 inoculation.

D. The chronic administration of monthly prophylaxis will reduce or eliminate microfilariae.

HISTORY

Most dogs with heartworm infection have not been receiving prophylaxis. Infected
dogs are often from rural areas and overall husbandry is usually substandard.
Whether or not the owner detects abnormalities depends on the degree of observation by the client, the amount of exercise performed by the dog, the adult worm
burden, and host-parasite interactions.

ASYMPTOMATIC INFECTION

Most dogs tested annually exhibit no signs of infection.

SYMPTOMATIC INFECTION

When infections go undetected for several years or longer coughing and exercise
intolerance may be observed by the owner.

CLINICAL SIGNS

Signs are a reflection of the number of infecting worms, the duration of infection,
and the host response.

THE ASYMPTOMATIC INFECTION

Most dogs have minimal or no signs of infection and detection occurs during
routine testing.

THE SYMPTOMATIC INFECTION

I. Unexplained coughing
   Many dogs are suspected of having heartworm infection because of a mild,
   paroxysmal cough. These dogs frequently have minimal radiographic evidence of heartworm disease.
II. Severe coughing and exercise intolerance
   Heavy worm burdens and occult infections tend to produce severe clinical
   signs. Coughing is frequently exacerbated by exertion. Exercise intolerance
   develops as impaired collateral recruitment and hypertension develop and
   often becomes evident in hunting dogs at the onset of the season. Syncope
   and/or ascites may develop.

III. Hemoptysis

Hemoptysis may be a complication of pulmonary hypertension, thrombosis, and rupture of small blood vessels into the lung parenchyma. It is an indication of severe pulmonary pathology.

IV. Right-sided congestive heart failure

Ascites develops in many dogs with severe pulmonary hypertension. Approximately 70 percent of such infections are occult. Ascites is usually accompanied by cachexia and exertion-associated syncope is common. Dyspnea, coughing, and hemoptysis are common accompanying signs.

PHYSICAL EXAMINATION

Physical examination is unremarkable in most infected dogs. Coughing, tachypnea, dyspnea, splitting of the second heart sound, pulmonary crackles, epistaxis, hemoptysis, cachexia, and ascites are variably detected in symptomatic patients.

AUSCULTATION OF SYMPTOMATIC DOGS

I. Moist pulmonary crackles can be detected when severe pulmonary arterial disease has occurred.
II. Cardiac murmurs are uncommon and associated with severe pulmonary hypertension, often with right-sided congestive heart failure or the caval syndrome.
III. Gallop rhythms indicate right-sided heart failure is present or imminent.
IV. Splitting of the second heart sound may be detected if pulmonary hypertension is severe.

PALPATION

I. Hepatomegaly may be present in association with chronic pulmonary hypertension and should be palpable when heart failure is imminent.
II. Abdominal effusion is balloted in dogs with overt heart failure.
III. Evidence of severe elevation of the central nervous pressure can be obtained by observing or palpating distended jugular veins and jugular pulses.

CLASSIFICATION OF DISEASE SEVERITY

I. Class I dogs are asymptomatic or exhibit only mild clinical signs. Thoracic radiographs may be normal or show slight enlargement of the main pulmonary artery segment and lobar arteries.
   A. Standard treatment is indicated
   B. The prognosis is excellent
II. Class II dogs have moderately severe symptoms, such as frequent coughing and mild-to-moderate exercise intolerance. Thoracic radiographs always indi-

cate enlargement of the lobar arteries but not greater than twice the diameter of the proximal fourth rib (as compared to the cranial lobar arteries) or ninth rib (as compared to the caudal lobar arteries).
A. Standard treatment is indicated
B. The prognosis is good
III. Class III dogs have severe clinical signs, including severe exercise intolerance, syncope, or right-sided congestive heart failure (ascites). Cachexia and poor hair coat are often evident. Thoracic radiograph changes indicate severe enlargement and tortuosity of the lobar arteries. The diameters of the caudal lobar vessels are more than twice that of the ninth ribs at their points of superimposition on the dorsoventral projection.
A. Standard therapy is associated with 40 to 60 percent mortality
B. Alternative treatment protocols are indicated and are associated with 80 percent or greater chance of survival in all but the most severely affected patients.

PROTOCOL FOR DIAGNOSIS

The minimum data base (MDB) can appropriately vary for different patients.

I. Young, asymptomatic patients (Class I)
These patients require only a CBC, BUN, and urine specific gravity.
II. Symptomatic, old, and patients with occult infections
These patients should have a CBC, serum chemistry profile, urinalysis, and thoracic radiographs.
III. Complicated heartworm disease
Patients with renal disease, liver disease, and coagulopathies may require a more extensive data base.

DIAGNOSTIC TECHNIQUES

The diagnosis of heartworm infection is based on the detection of microfilariae and/or circulating adult *Dirofilaria immitis* antigens and is corroborated by clinical and radiographic findings. It is rare that microfilaremic dogs lack adult heartworms. All dogs in endemic regions should be screened annually for heartworm infection. All dogs with clinical signs consistent with infection or unexplained eosinophilia and/or basophilia should be tested for *D immitis* infection. Until recently, the detection of circulating microfilariae of *D immitis* was the basis for the diagnosis of heartworm infection in most instances. With the advent of sensitive and specific immunodiagnostic tests and the use of prophylactic drugs known to eliminate circulating microfilariae the role of microfilarial detection as a screening method has been reduced.

In areas with a cold winter season, testing is performed in the spring, immediately prior to the onset of the transmission season, so as to detect infections acquired late in the previous summer. In year-round warm climates, testing is recommended in March and April. Dogs that test negative in these areas should be retested later in the summer in order to detect infections that occurred in the previous fall and early winter.

DIRECT BLOOD SMEAR

It is customary when performing a microfilariae concentration test to perform a direct blood smear first. If microfilariae of *D immitis* are detected, the more time-consuming concentration test is unnecessary.

I. The direct smear, when negative, should never be considered an indication that heartworm infection is absent.
II. The direct smear is significantly less sensitive than concentration tests.

CONCENTRATION TESTS

Microfilariae are a sign of the presence of mature heartworms and appear approximately 6 to 6.5 months after infection. The modified Knott's test and the filter tests use one milliliter of blood, which has been concentrated prior to examination for the presence of microfilariae.

I. The modified Knott's and filter tests provide comparable diagnostic accuracy.
   A. A concentration test is still employed as the routine screening test by many veterinarians.
   B. A concentration test is indicated in all dogs with positive heartworm-antigen test results.
   C. A concentration test is recommended for all dogs that are to receive prophylaxis for the first time.
   D. A concentration test is essential in all dogs that are going to receive diethyl-carbamazine prophylaxis.
II. If a screening concentration test is negative, an antigen test is indicated in order to assess the possibility of an amicrofilaramic (occult) infection.
III. A concentration test is repeated 3 months following microfilaricide therapy in order to insure that treatment has been complete.

SERODIAGNOSTIC TESTS

There are currently a number of serodiagnostic tests that are widely used for the detection of heartworm infection. These tests are being continually improved and simplified and additional tests will no doubt become available.

I. All of these tests are highly specific; that is, false positive results are rare when the test is performed properly.
   A. Weak-positive test results should be verified by repeating the test, preferably utilizing a different antigen test, and/or by performing corroborative tests such as a microfilarial concentration test or thoracic radiographs.
   B. False-positive tests usually are due to poor technique.

    C. Any positive test result should be followed by a microfilarial concentration test.
  II. The sensitivities of the different tests are good but currently are not all equal. Presumably those tests that are less sensitive will be improved.
 III. A serodiagnostic test may be employed as the routine screening test.
    A. If positive, a microfilariae detection test is indicated.
    B. If negative, no further testing is indicated for 6 to 12 months in adult dogs as long as one is willing to accept a low incidence (less than 5 percent) of falsely negative test results.
  IV. Falsely negative test results can occur.
    A. No worms older than 7 months post-L_3.
    B. If there are less than 3 to 5 adult worms. Some tests detect as few as 1 worm.
    C. If there are no gravid females, since the male worm contributes little or nothing to a positive test result.
    D. There is concern that some of the so-called "stat" tests may be less sensitive.
   V. The serodiagnostic tests are semiquantitative, that is, they indicate an estimated high versus low worm burden.
    A. Rapid, strong reactions indicate a relatively high worm burden.
    B. CITE-HW (Idexx) is marketed as a semiquantitative test.
      1. In the continental United States, most test results indicate a low worm burden.
      2. In the Caribbean and Hawaii, high burden test results are common.
  VI. Serodiagnostic testing is also useful when performed 12 weeks or more following adulticide treatment in order to determine if all adult worms have been killed.

THORACIC RADIOGRAPHY

Radiography is the single diagnostic test that provides the most information relative to disease severity. When heartworm disease is severe, thoracic radiograph abnormalities are virtually pathognomonic (Fig. 10-1).

   I. The dorsoventral projection provides a more sensitive and accurate picture of caudal lobar arterial disease.
  II. Between 80 and 90 percent of dogs with microfilaremic infections have detectable abnormalities.
    A. Inspection for evidence of main pulmonary artery segment enlargement on the ventrodorsal projection is very important.
    B. Assessment for enlargement and tortuosity of the lobar arteries is very important.
      1. The caudal lobar arteries are most severely affected in most dogs.
      2. The diameter of the caudal lobar arteries should not exceed that of the ninth ribs at their points of superimposition.
    C. Excessive emphasis is placed on right-ventricular enlargement, a highly subjective assessment subject to extensive breed variation and requiring excellent patient positioning for accurate evaluation.

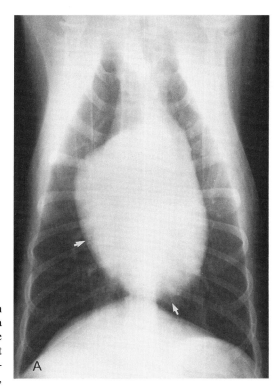

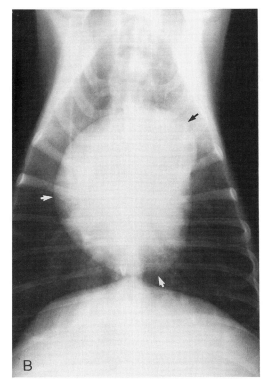

Fig. 10-1. Ventrodorsal radiograph projections of a normal dog **(A)** and a dog with heartworm disease **(B).** There is a main pulmonary artery enlargement *(black arrow)* typical of heartworm infection *(white arrows,* cardiac apex, and right heart). (From Calvert CA, Rawlings CA: Pulmonary manifestations of heartworm disease. Vet Clin North Am 15:991, 1985, with permission.)

III. Severe pulmonary arterial enlargement indicates a high risk of severe post-adulticide therapy thromboembolism.

ELECTROCARDIOGRAPHY

The electrocardiogram is not an integral component of the minimum data base. The ECG of most heartworm-infected dogs is normal.

I. Dogs with severe pulmonary hypertension often have ECG evidence of right-ventricular hypertrophy (RVH).
II. Over 90 percent of heartworm infected dogs with ascites have ECG criteria justifying a diagnosis of RVH.
III. Thoracic radiographs provide more data concerning the severity of infection.
IV. Heart rhythm disturbances are not common, but atrial arrhythmias—including atrial fibrillation—may occur in dogs with severe right atrial enlargement.

ULTRASOUND

Cardiac ultrasound, although not a component of the MDB, is of value in assessing the severity of the heartworm burden and secondary effects on the right ventricle.

THERAPEUTIC APPROACH

ASPIRIN

Aspirin at dosages of 5 to 10 mg/kg once daily results in qualitative platelet dysfunction. This effect can interfere with platelet activation and theoretically with the release of platelet-derived growth factors, which may play a role in myointimal proliferation. Both experimental and clinical studies have suggested a beneficial role in dogs with severe pulmonary pathology.

I. Class I and Class II Infections
   Aspirin is not recommended for routine heartworm infections.
II. Severe pulmonary arterial disease
   Aspirin is reserved for patients with radiographic evidence of severe pulmonary arterial disease.
   A. Moderate to severe clinical signs are usually coexistent.
   B. A dosage of 5 to 10 mg/kg of Bayer or buffered aspirin is prescribed once daily for at least 3 weeks prior to, during, and for 3 to 4 weeks after adulticide therapy.
   C. Aspirin treatment is recommended in conjunction with cage confinement. Therefore, the influence of aspirin on the complications of adulticide therapy or survival cannot be stated (i.e., similar results might be obtained with protracted cage confinement alone).

III. Gastrointestinal bleeding

Gastrointestinal bleeding may occur in association with aspirin administration.

A. Anorexia, vomiting, and melena are signs associated with bleeding into the gastrointestinal tract, but a decreasing hematocrit is a more sensitive indicator of bleeding than melena.

B. Prophylaxis with H_2-blocking antihistamines such as cimetidine, along with protectorants such as sucralfate, may not prevent bleeding.

CORTICOSTEROIDS

Corticosteroids are indicated for the treatment of parenchymal lung complications.

I. Occult heartworm-associated allergic pneumonitis

A. Responds quickly to antiinflammatory dosages of prednisone (1 mg/kg once daily).

B. Adulticide therapy initiated subsequently.

II. Parenchymal complications of pulmonary arterial disease-thromboembolism

A. Anti-inflammatory dosages of corticosteroids are administered for several days up to 1 week in conjunction with cage confinement.

B. Diagnosis based on thoracic radiographs and clinical signs

1. Fever, coughing, dyspnea, hemoptysis, lethargy, and anorexia are variably associated with pulmonary complications.

2. Most often seen 5 to 7 days and 14 to 21 days after adulticide therapy.

III. Routine administration

Routine administration of corticosteroids following adulticide treatment is not recommended, since excessive use of corticosteroids results in decreased pulmonary blood flow, promotes coagulation, and may contribute to thromboembolism.

HEPARIN

Heparin is used for the prevention or treatment of pulmonary thromboembolism.

I. Prevention of thromboembolism

Heparin can be administered in lieu of aspirin, prophylactically, in dogs with severe (Class III) heartworm infection.

A. 75 U/kg, SQ TID initiated 1 week prior to, continued during, and for 3 weeks following adulticide treatment.

B. A similar protocol has been used in Italy by Vezzoni and has resulted in over 90 percent survival.

II. Treatment of thromboembolism

Heparin is the treatment of choice when clinical and radiographic evidence of thromboembolism occurs prior to or following adulticide treatment.

A. 75 U/kg, SQ TID are recommended and generally continued for 5 to 21 days, depending on clinical signs, radiographic findings, the degree of

thrombocytopenia, and the time required for the platelet count to return to normal.
  B. Ancillary therapy is often indicated and includes oxygen, corticosteroids, and cage confinement.

ADULTICIDE THERAPY

Thiacetarsamide is the only approved drug for *D. immitis* treatment. The protocol currently endorsed by the American Heartworm Society has been in effect for over a quarter century.

  I. Protocol
     The adulticide regimen is outlined in Table 10-1. Any deviations from the recommendations of the American Heartworm Society are without justification.
 II. Method of administration
     Thiacetarsamide is stored under refrigeration and administered carefully to avoid extravasation. Discolored and unrefrigerated product should be discarded.
     A. Each injection should be made in a vein as peripherally as feasible.
        1. Do not inject unless proper vein cannulation is 100 percent certain.
        2. Injections often are made using a butterfly needle-catheter and a saline flush to ensure patency.
     B. Indwelling catheters are employed by some clinicians.
        1. Both the catheter tip and thiacetarsamide can contribute to phlebitis and vein rupture.
        2. Multiple injections at the same site lead to phlebitis.
        3. A false sense of security may develop.
     C. Drug extravasation: Pain, heat, and swelling occur within 1 hour of extravasation.
        1. Treatment: DMSO is applied topically for several days.
        2. An Elizabethan collar may help prevent the dog from licking the site.
III. Glucocorticoid hormones
     These drugs have been shown to reduce thiacetarsamide efficacy against female worms and their use during and for 1 to 2 weeks following thiacetarsamide treatment should be avoided if possible.
 IV. Indications to abort therapy
     In most instances it matters little if therapy is given immediately or within

TABLE 10-1. ADULTICIDE TREATMENT REGIMEN

Patient Evaluation	Dosage and Interval
1. Appropriate data base	1. 0.22 ml/kg BID for 2 days
2. Before each dose fraction:	2. Dosage interval (hrs)
a. Physical examination	Maximum: 12
b. Feed and observe appetite	Minimum: 6
c. Check urine for bilirubinuria	

several weeks. For that reason there is little rationale in continuing therapy in the face of acute thiacetarsamide toxicity.

A. Prediction of acute thiacetarsamide toxicity is difficult. Laboratory data usually does not identify dogs at increased risk of acute hepatic toxicity. Liver enzyme activity up to 10-fold increased and BSP retention up to 10 percent have not correlated with increased risk of acute toxicity.

B. Gastrointestinal signs: Persistent vomiting, anorexia, and depression are absolute indications to abort treatment and the risk of this toxicity is greatest after the first injection.

C. Hepatotoxicity: Icterus is an absolute indication to abort treatment.
   1. A proper minimum data base and evaluation should detect pre-existing severe liver disease. Microhepatica should alert the clinician of possible hepatic insufficiency.
   2. Monitoring of liver enzyme activity during treatment is unrewarding, unnecessary, and often not correlated with overt, acute toxicity.
   3. Gross bilirubinuria after one or two injections is an indication to stop treatment.

D. Retreatment: Whenever treatment has been aborted, appropriate supportive therapy is provided prior to discharge.
   1. High carbohydrate, low fat diet is prescribed.
   2. Restriction of activity for 4 weeks is recommended.
   3. "Liver-sparing" drugs containing inositol, choline, and methionine are of no proven value.
   4. Retreatment is scheduled for 4 weeks, is repeated in total, and is rarely associated with acute toxicity.

V. Nonindications to abort therapy
   One or two episodes of vomiting in an otherwise "happy-healthy" appearing dog with a good appetite or occult bilirubinuria are not indications to stop treatment.

VI. Postadulticide complications
   Serious postadulticide complications are usually limited to dogs with moderate-to-severe pulmonary arterial disease as assessed radiographically, are thromboembolic in nature, and occur 1 to 3 weeks postadulticide.

A. Thromboembolic lung disease
   1. Life-threatening severity is characterized by coughing, dyspnea, hemoptysis, tachycardia, and pale mucous membranes.
      a) Confirmed by radiographs.
      b) Biochemical evidence of DIC likely to be present.
      c) Treatment is cage confinement, corticosteroids, oxygen, and possibly heparin [see previous discussion].
   2. Less severe thrombosis is common and characterized by low-grade fever and coughing. Treatment consists of cage confinement and corticosteroids.

B. Azotemia: Renal complications are unusual if renal function is properly assessed prior to treatment. Azotemia is usually prerenal and associated with vomiting and dehydration, and fluid therapy is indicated.

C. DIC: DIC is a sequela to thromboembolic disease and is usually associated with pre-existing, severe pulmonary arterial disease as assessed radiographically.

    1. When present, usually occurs 5 to 21 days postadulticide.

    2. Treatment: Chronic or low-grade DIC is treated with heparin (75 U/ kg SQ TID) for several days to several weeks.

    3. Acute DIC is uncommon, but is usually present when severe pulmonary thrombosis, frank hemorrhage, and death occurs 2 to 3 weeks postadulticide.

  D. Icterus: Icterus and liver failure are uncommon but potentially lethal complications of thiacetarsamide treatment, and can occur within 1 week of treatment.

    1. A thorough MDB with proper assessment may identify dogs with pre-existing severe liver disease.

    2. Otherwise unpredictable

    3. Treatment: Treatment is often unrewarding and involves supportive therapy such as balanced electrolyte fluids, control of gastrointestinal hemorrhage, and treatment for hepatic encephalopathy.

Investigational Adulticide Therapy

Melarsamine dihydrochloride (RM 340), an investigational organoarsenical, has been developed by the Rhône-Merieux Corporation and has undergone extensive laboratory and field testing under controlled conditions.

  I. Efficacy

    The efficacy of RM 340 is excellent. It is very effective against both sexes of adult worms of all ages, as well as developing larvae.

  II. Safety

    The therapeutic index of RM 340 is wider than that of thiacetarsamide. Toxicity necessitating that treatment be aborted is rare.

  III. Advantages over thiacetarsamide

    The three primary advantages are efficacy, safety, and intramuscular administration.

Microfilaracide Therapy Postadulticide

All dogs with circulating microfilariae should receive microfilaricide treatment 4 to 6 weeks postadulticide.

  I. Ivermectin

    Ivermectin is the most effective treatment, although it is not FDA approved for this purpose. Nonetheless, ivermectin has become the "standard of practice" in at least the endemic regions of the United States.

    A. Protocol: Ivermectin is administered as a single, oral dosage in the morn-

TABLE 10-2. IVERMECTIN PROTOCOL

Ivomec: 1:9 dilution with propylene glycol (can be stored) at a dosage of 1 ml/20 kg
Equvalen: 1:9 dilution with water for immediate use at a dosage of 1 ml/20 kg
    1. Administered in morning
    2. Observe patient
    3. Discharge in evening
    4. Microfilariae test in 3 weeks

ing, the patient is observed during the day, and discharged in the evening (Table 10-2).

1. Dosage: 50 μg/kg
2. Side effects
   a) Vomiting and diarrhea possibly accompanied by depression are seen in a few patients.
   b) Evidence of cardiovascular deterioration (tachypnea, tachycardia, weakness, pale mucous membranes) is rare but requires therapy.
      (1) Soluble corticosteroid at shock dosage
      (2) IV electrolyte solution
   c) Mild lethargy and anorexia may be observed in up to 10 percent of dogs 1 to 2 days after treatment.
3. Ivermectin and collies: Ivermectin is safe in collies when prescribed at the recommended dosage.
4. Microfilariae testing: A microfilarial concentration test is indicated at 3 weeks posttreatment.
   a) If positive, ivermectin treatment is repeated.
   b) If negative, a prophylactic drug is prescribed.
   c) Failure to clear microfilariae after two treatments of ivermectin suggests an adulticide failure.
      (1) Place on ivermectin prophylaxis.
      (2) Perform heartworm antigen test 12 weeks post-thiacetarsamide.
         i) If positive, plan to repeat thiacetarsamide treatment in 6 to 12 months.
         ii) If negative, continue prophylaxis.

II. Milbemycin oxime
   The monthly prophylactic drug, milbemycin oxime, is microfilaricidal at the prophylactic dosage.
   A. The manufacturer neither recommends nor supports the use of milbemycin oxime for this purpose.
   B. Acute, usually nonlethal reactions may occur as with ivermectin.

Confirmation of Adulticide Efficacy

Adulticide drugs do not kill every worm in every dog. Young, female adult worms up to 18 months after L_3 inoculation are particularly resistant to thiacetarsamide. Clinical status and pulmonary pathology usually improve even though all worms have not been killed.

  I. Microfilariae concentration testing
     In microfilaremic dogs, a concentration test is indicated 3 weeks after treat-
     ment with ivermectin.
     A. If positive, ivermectin is repeated.
     B. If negative, a prophylactic drug is prescribed.
     C. Failure to clear microfilariae after two treatments of ivermectin suggests
        an adulticide failure.
        1. Place on ivermectin prophylaxis.
        2. Perform antigen test 3 months post-thiacetarsamide.
 II. Antigen testing
     Confirmation of complete or nearly complete adulticide efficacy can be ob-
     tained by antigen testing performed 3 months or more after adulticide therapy.
     This is the only practical method of determination in occult infections. By 12
     weeks postadulticide the strength of reaction is usually markedly decreased.
     A. Weak positive results at 3 months postadulticide are possible because anti-
        genemia occasionally persists. Under these circumstances, the dog should
        be retested after 1 to 2 additional months.
     B. Persistent antigenemia
        1. Retreatment is usually recommended, but deferred for 6 to 12 months
           to allow female worms to age while the dog is maintained on appropriate
           prophylaxis.
        2. Retreatment is not always recommended. This is determined by the
           degree of reduction of antigenemia, the age of the patient, severity of
           the original clinical disease, and the degree of clinical improvement.

SEQUELAE OF HEARTWORM INFECTION

ALLERGIC PNEUMONITIS

This syndrome occurs in 10 to 15 percent of immune-mediated occult infections.
Immune-mediated occult infection results from a state of antibody excess with
entrapment of microfilariae in the lungs. In 10 to 15 percent of these reactions the
cellular infiltrate is dominated by eosinophils producing an allergic pneumonitis.
  I. Clinical signs
     Progressive coughing, crackles, and dyspnea are variably present.
 II. Differential diagnosis
     This syndrome can and has been mistaken for left-sided congestive heart
     failure and blastomycosis.
III. Diagnosis
     The diagnosis is based on several findings
     A. Positive heartworm Ag test
     B. Eosinophilia and/or basophilia are inconsistently present
     C. Thoracic radiographs reveal a diffuse, fine interstitial-alveolar pulmonary
        infiltrate without lymphadenomegaly.
 IV. Treatment
     Prednisone or prednisolone (1 mg/kg daily) or an equivalent dosage of alter-

nate corticosteroid bring about a rapid resolution of clinical signs and pulmonary infiltrates.

V. Adulticide therapy

Thiacetarsamide treatment is recommended as soon as the syndrome has resolved (3 to 5 days).

PREADULTICIDE THROMBOEMBOLIC LUNG DISEASE

Although pulmonary thromboembolism is most commonly encountered post-adulticide, severely affected dogs may present for this complication.

I. Clinical signs

Coughing, dyspnea, and hemoptysis are consistent with pulmonary thrombosis.

II. Physical examination

Labored breathing, epistaxis, hemoptysis, tachycardia, pulmonary crackles, fever, and pale mucous membranes are variably present.

III. Laboratory data

An inflammatory leukogram and thrombocytopenia are often present.

IV. Diagnosis

Thoracic radiography is the most useful diagnostic test.

A. Thoracic radiographs typically reveal severe pulmonary arterial disease, nodular pulmonary infiltrates, and areas of patchy, sometimes indistinct fluid infiltrates.

1. Fluid infiltrates, indicated by alveolar disease, are most likely to be located in the caudal and accessory lobes adjacent to the lobar arteries.

2. Partial consolidation of lung lobes may be present.

B. An inflammatory leukogram with a marked eosinophilia and possibly basophilia is typical.

C. Thrombocytopenia of variable severity is usual.

D. Mild-to-moderate prolongation of the activated clotting time is common.

V. Treatment

A. Cage confinement for 5 to 7 days or until clinical and radiographic resolution of signs has occurred is recommended.

B. Corticosteroids are generally prescribed (e.g., prednisone, 1 mg/kg once daily) but should not be continued beyond the point where clinical and radiographic evidence of resolution has occurred.

1. Treatment of 3 to 7 days is typical.

2. Corticosteroids can reduce pulmonary blood flow if administered long-term, and they also promote coagulation.

C. Heparin (75 U/kg, SQ TID) is also indicated for low-grade disseminated intravascular coagulopathy (DIC) as suggested by the presence of:

1. Severe clinical signs

2. Prolonged activated clotting time

3. Thrombocytopenia

4. Fibrin degradation products (FDPs)

   D. Oxygen therapy provides many benefits, including amelioration of pulmonary arterial constriction.
     1. Cage
     2. Intranasal (50 to 100 ml/kg/min)

DISSEMINATED INTRAVASCULAR COAGULOPATHY

DIC may be a sequela of severe pulmonary arterial disease and thromboembolism. In most instances DIC is low-grade or chronic.

  I. Clinical signs
    DIC is often occult in patients with severe pulmonary disease but the possibility should be investigated when epistaxis, hemoptysis, radiographic evidence of parenchymal lung disease, and thrombocytopenia are detected.
  II. Diagnosis
    The presence of a prolonged ACT and thrombocytopenia should raise the index of suspicion.
    A. A coagulogram should be performed, but may require serum dilution to identify early abnormalities.
    B. FDP assay
  III. Treatment
    Treatment of low-grade or chronic DIC is usually effective.
    A. Cage confinement and supportive therapy, including the judicious use of balanced electrolyte solutions.
    B. Heparin (75 U/kg SQ TID) is recommended for low-grade or chronic DIC.
     1. Therapy continued for several days and occasionally for several weeks
     2. Guided by ACT, platelet count, coagulogram, and clinical signs
  IV. Acute or end-stage DIC is highly fatal and treatment is unrewarding. The disease is suggested by the presence of frank hemorrhage, severe derangements of the coagulogram, plus severe thrombocytopenia.

CAVAL SYNDROME

The caval syndrome is uncommon except in highly endemic areas. Caval syndrome is associated with a heavy inoculation of larvae over a short time span so that a large number of L_5 and adult worms infiltrate the heart and pulmonary arteries. Over 100 or even 200 worms may be present in the pulmonary arteries, heart, and vena cava.

  I. Clinical signs
    Acute cardiovascular collapse, shock, icterus, and hemoglobinuria occur.
  II. Diagnosis
    The diagnosis of caval syndrome is typically a clinical diagnosis made by experienced clinicians in endemic regions.
    A. Age: Most effected dogs are 3 to 5 years of age, but they can be of any age and most are normal prior to the acute onset of the syndrome.

    B. Dyspnea, weakness, pale mucous membranes, icterus, and hemoglobin-uria are typical signs suggesting the diagnosis.

    C. Systolic heart murmur or gallop heart rhythm are usually present.

    D. Radiographs of the chest should not be performed unless necessary due to the adverse effect of stress on survival, but if done reveal right heart and main pulmonary artery enlargement.

    E. ECG evidence of RVH is often present.

    F. Clinical pathology: Evidence of hemolytic anemia, liver disease, and poor cardiac output are typical.

        1. Anemia with hemolytic serum and evidence of regeneration (reticulo-cytosis) are typically present.

        2. Urinalysis reveals hemoglobinuria in most cases.

        3. Increased liver enzyme activity and increased BSP retention are often present.

        4. Prerenal azotemia is common and reflects poor cardiac output.

        5. Microfilaremia is usual.

    G. Cardiac ultrasound provides a definitive diagnosis

III. Treatment

Surgical removal of worms in the manner pioneered by Dr. Ronald F. Jackson is the only effective treatment.

    A. A left-jugular venotomy is performed under local anesthesia. Mild sedation using diazepam or diazepam plus narcotic is used only if necessary.

    B. A specially designed alligator forceps is introduced and passed to the level of the heart.

        1. The jaws of the forceps are opened at the level of the fourth-fifth inter-costal space, advanced slightly, closed, and the forceps withdrawn.

           a) The procedure is repeated until no worms are retrieved on 5 or 6 consecutive passages.

           b) Minimal force is employed during advancement and withdrawal of the forceps since the vena cava and right atrium can be perforated.

           c) When a rigid forceps is employed, the neck often must be extended.

        2. Supportive therapy is provided after surgery.

        3. Arrhythmias may be encountered.

        4. Adulticide therapy is administered approximately 2 weeks later.

IV. Prognosis: In experienced hands, 50 percent or more of the patients can be saved.

SEVERE PULMONARY HYPERTENSION (CLASS III)

Severe pulmonary arterial disease occurs in up to 10 percent of infected dogs in highly endemic regions, and typically occurs in middle-aged dogs without circulating microfilaria.

    I. Clinical signs of severe pulmonary hypertension exist

II. Radiographic evidence of hypertension indicated by severe enlargement of the main pulmonary artery segment and lobar arteries (Fig. 10-2).
   A. The caudal lobar arteries are most severely affected and are large and tortuous.
   B. Secondary parenchymal lung disease may be evident, and results from small vessel damage with leakage of fluid and inflammatory cells into the adjacent lung parenchyma.
      1. Hazy appearance adjacent to arteries
      2. Partial or complete lung consolidation
      3. Occasionally, pleural effusion
III. Anemia-Thrombocytopenia
Fluctuating thrombocytopenia and anemia may persist for over 1 month in dogs with severe pulmonary arterial disease.
   A. Schistocytosis indicates RBC fragmentation by damaged vessels, fibrin, and thrombus.
   B. Regenerative anemia (i.e., reticulocytosis)
IV. Treatment
Standard treatment of dogs with severe pulmonary arterial disease is associated with a 40 to 60 percent mortality, which usually occurs 10 to 21 days after Caparsolate therapy. It is associated with clinical and laboratory data consistent with pulmonary thromboembolism and DIC. There are four alternative management protocols that can decrease mortality to 20 percent or less.
   A. Worm extraction techniques have been developed in Japan by Ishihara and associates in dogs with high worm burdens.
      1. Identification of high worm burden
        a) Ultrasound (Fig. 10-3)
        b) Semiquantitative antigen testing
      2. Technique requires a long, flexible alligator forceps, which is passed repeatedly into the right heart and pulmonary arteries under fluoroscopic guidance to extract worms.
      3. Follow-up adulticide therapy may be required to remove a remaining small worm burden.
      4. Highly effective treatment for dogs with high worm burden when performed by experienced individuals.
   B. A modified RM 340 adulticide regimen has proven highly successful in both European and American field trials.
      1. Investigational drug
      2. Initial treatment uses a reduced drug dosage in order to kill fewer worms and thus reduce the risk of thromboembolism.
      3. Residual worm burden treated with a second course of RM 340 1 month later.
   C. Protracted cage confinement with antiplatelet therapy prior to, during, and for several weeks following Caparsolate therapy.
      1. The patient is placed in strict cage confinement for several weeks prior to, during, and for 3 weeks after adulticide therapy.
      2. Aspirin (5 to 10 mg/kg of Bayer or buffered aspirin once daily) prior to, during, and for 3 weeks after adulticide therapy.

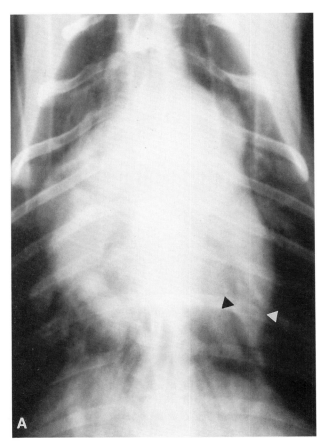

Fig. 10-2. Dorsoventral **(A)** and lateral **(B)** projections of a dog with severe pulmonary artery disease. On the dorsoventral projection the caudal lobar arteries are greatly enlarged *(arrowheads)*. The right cranial lobar *(a)* and caudal lobar arteries *(arrows)* are greatly enlarged on the lateral projection. (From Calvert CA, Rawlings CA: Pulmonary manifestations of heartworm disease. Vet Clin North Am 15:991, 1985, with permission.)

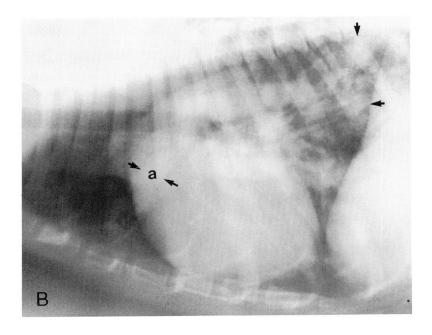

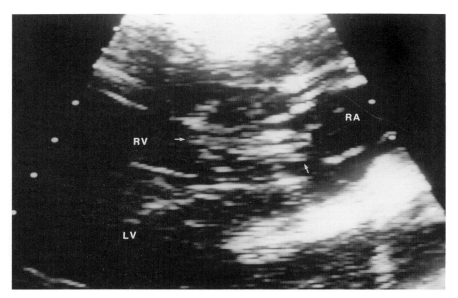

Fig. 10-3. Two-dimensional cardiac ultrasound demonstrating parallel, linear echodensities *(arrows)* representing heartworms in the right atrium and ventricle. The dog had severe pulmonary arterial disease and clinical signs of cor pulmonale. RA, right atrium; RV, right ventricle; LV, left ventricle.

> D. Heparin administration at a dosage of 75 U/kg, SQ TID for 1 week prior to, during, and for 3 weeks following adulticide treatment.
>   1. Should be combined with severe exercise restriction.
>   2. Vezzoni reported better results than with aspirin. Over 90 percent of severely affected dogs survived.
> V. Supportive care for patients receiving aspirin or heparin protocols
>   A. Furosemide and low sodium diet if right-sided heart failure (ascites) present.
>   B. Short-term corticosteroid therapy if parenchymal lung complications due to thromboembolism develop prior to or after adulticide therapy.
>   C. Thrombocytopenia/hemoptysis/overt thromboembolism may occur prior to or after adulticide therapy.
>   1. Patients receiving aspirin should receive heparin (75 U/kg SQ TID) for several days or longer if this complication arises
>   2. Improvement usually occurs within 1 or 2 days of heparin treatment and is often dramatic
>   3. Monitor platelet count and continue until count is normal or near normal.

RENAL DISEASE

Renal disease, when present, is usually characterized as a glomerulopathy and is usually mild.

I. Glomerulopathies
   The diagnosis of glomerulopathies is based on the finding of proteinuria which is best quantitated by a urine protein:creatinine ratio. Moderate-to-severe proteinuria in a dilute urine sample is always a cause for concern.
   A. May be immune-complex disease or amyloidosis.
   B. Hypoalbuminemia may be a sign of severe proteinuria, but may also result from loss into the third space in patients with right-sided CHF (ascites).
   C. Influence on therapy: In general, a mild-to-moderate glomerular disease should not, by itself, influence therapy. However, severe proteinuria may indicate irreversible and progressive glomerular disease.
      1. Nephrotic syndrome: If there is severe proteinuria, ascites, and peripheral edema, heartworm therapy will be unrewarding.
      2. Hypoalbuminemia and proteinuria may indicate that renal disease is irreversible and progressive. Adulticide therapy is administered only if the client is aware, and accepts that the process may be progressive.
      3. Proteinuria with normal serum albumin and BUN-creatinine usually does not progress and heartworm treatment is recommended.
II. Azotemia
   Azotemia may be associated with the nephrotic syndrome, but also may occur in the absence of proteinuria when it is due to interstitial renal disease or prerenal factors.
   A. Influence on therapy
      1. Prerenal azotemia is not, by itself, cause for concern. The cause should be identified and corrected, and adulticide therapy then administered.
      2. Renal azotemia of a mild-to-moderate degree (BUN < 100; creatinine < 3) does not, by itself, exert an adverse influence on heartworm therapy.
         a) Fluid therapy is provided in an attempt to reduce the BUN to less than 50 and the creatinine to less than 2. Fluid therapy is continued during and for several days to 1 week following adulticide therapy.
         b) Appropriate client education is required prior to treatment.

HEPATIC FAILURE

Hepatic failure, outside of that associated with the caval syndrome, is a contraindication to heartworm treatment.

I. Associations
   Hepatic failure, when seen, is usually a sequelae to severe, chronic HWD. Affected dogs usually have severe pulmonary arterial disease, right-sided congestive heart failure, and cachexia.
II. Recognition
   Icterus and renal failure are often present along with biochemical evidence of hepatic failure.
   A. Hypoalbuminemia
   B. Increased BSP retention (in nonicteric dogs), abnormal ammonia tolerance tests, and abnormal bile acids.
   C. Hepatic enzyme activities are increased.
III. Treatment: None

HEARTWORM PROPHYLAXIS

There are a number of highly effective drugs available for the prevention of heartworm infection. Selection of an individual product depends largely on one's preference for daily versus monthly administration, the number of dogs requiring medication, and concomitant intestinal parasite control.

The duration of prophylactic therapy varies by geographic region. In the continental United States, transmission is almost always seasonal. Even in the southeastern United States, little or no transmission occurs in December and January. Preventative medication is begun when the average daily temperature exceeds approximately 55°F. Year-round prophylaxis is not essential in most areas, but is often recommended to reduce the incidence of client failure to reinstitute in the spring.

Preventative medications are recommended for puppies as young as 6 to 8 weeks of age or as soon thereafter as indicated by climate. Adult dogs should be tested for antigens and microfilariae prior to initiation of prophylaxis.

DIETHYLCARBAMAZINE

Diethylcarbamazine (DEC) has stood the test of time and is an excellent product. DEC kills *D immitis* larvae at the L_3-L_4 molt; therefore, it has a short window of opportunity and requires daily administration.

I. Schedule
DEC is recommended year-round in tropical and semi-tropical climates. It is begun with the mosquito season and continued until 2 months after the first frost in temperate zones.
II. Precaution
DEC is never administered without a prior negative microfilarial concentration test.
A. Acute reactions are likely, and may prove fatal, when DEC is initiated in microfilaremic dogs.
1. Non–dose dependent gastrointestinal signs are seen approximately 1 hour after medication is given. Reactions may be mild and self-limiting or may be severe, progressing to shock and death.
2. Reactions recur with each dose
B. Dogs already receiving DEC that are discovered to be microfilaremic may continue on daily DEC.
1. If DEC is withdrawn or for whatever reason is not administered for several days or more, it *can not* be reinstituted.
2. Rather, appropriate workup and treatment is completed prior to restarting a prophylactic drug
C. Antigen positive or antigen unknown dogs without microfilariae may be given DEC
D. If DEC prophylaxis lapses during the transmission season, then macrolide prophylaxis may be substituted. The dog can be retested for microfilariae if the intent is to reinstitute DEC.

III. Formulations
There are a number of tablets, chewable tablets, and liquid forms available.
DEC plus oxybendazole
   1. Controls hookworms and roundworms
   2. Can be associated with hepatoxicity (undetermined, but probably low
      incidence) that is self-limiting after the drug is withdrawn

IVERMECTIN

Ivermectin (Heartgard-30) and ivermectin plus pyrantel pamoate (Heartgard-30
Plus) are highly effective, chewable, monthly, macrolide prophylactics administered at a dosage of approximately 6 to 12 µg/kg. Ivermectin should be initiated
within 1 month of the onset of the transmission season.

   I. Ivermectin and microfilariae
   Ivermectin can be administered to microfilaremic dogs without fear of re-
   action.
   A. Not microfilaricidal at prophylactic dosages
   B. The drug of choice when adulticide therapy failure occurs in microfilare-
      mic dogs and retreatment is to be delayed.
  II. Dogs receiving chronic ivermectin should receive annual heartworm
      screening.
   A. Antigen testing required
   B. Microfilarial testing inaccurate
      1. Chronic (approximately 6 months or longer) therapy eliminates microfi-
         lariae
      2. Common problem with all monthly prophylactic drugs
      3. Requires at least 6 months following withdrawal of drug before microfi-
         laria reappear
 III. Ivermectin plus pyrantel pamoate
   This combination provides monthly prophylaxis as well as control of hook-
   worms and roundworms in a chewable formulation.

MILBEMYCIN OXIME

Milbemycin oxime (Interceptor) is a monthly macrolide prophylactic that also
controls hookworms, roundworms, and whipworms when administered at a dosage of 0.5 to 1.0 mg/kg.

   I. Milbemycin oxime and microfilariae
   This drug is not recommended for microfilaremic dogs since acute, adverse
   reactions are possible.
  II. As with ivermectin, chronic milbemycin oxime use results in reduced microfi-
      larial counts; therefore, antigen testing is required for screening purposes.

III. Milbemycin oxime and collies
This drug is safe for collies when prescribed as recommended.

Moxidectin

Moxidectin is a highly effective and safe macrolide prophylactic drug when administered at a dosage of approximately 3.0 μg/kg. Moxidectin is safe for microfilaremic dogs, is safe for collies when prescribed as recommended, and as with ivermectin and milbemycin oxide, dogs receiving moxidectin require antigen testing
to detect adult worms.

FELINE HEARTWORM DISEASE

The distribution of feline heartworm disease is believed to parallel that of canine
disease, but at a lower rate. Diagnosis of feline heartworm disease is difficult
because of vague clinical signs, lack of circulating microfilariae, and relative lack
of sensitivity of immunodiagnostic tests.

Incidence

The incidence of heartworm disease among privately owned cats varies considerably, though it is less than 10 percent, and averages less than 2 percent. Recent
studies in highly endemic regions have suggested a prevalence in shelter cats of
approximately 3 to 7 percent (approximately 5 to 10 percent of the prevalence in
shelter dogs).

  I. Host resistance
Although most cats are susceptible to *D immitis*, they are relatively resistant
to infection as indicated by a number of factors.
    A. Low adult worm burden
    B. Low survival of transplanted adults as compared to dogs
    C. Low number of inoculated L_3 that reach maturity as compared to dogs
(85 to 90 percent fewer adult worms develop in cats versus dogs when
the same number of larvae are inoculated).
    D. Reduced size of adult worms
    E. Longer period of maturation of adult worms as compared to dogs
    F. Short life span of adult worm in cats compared to dogs
 II. Worm burden
Infected cats seldom harbor more than 6 worms, with 2 to 4 worms being
typical. This low worm burden may be due to several factors.
    A. Increased host resistance
    B. Lower level of exposure to infective mosquitoes
    C. Preference of mosquitoes to feed on dogs
III. Life span

Adult *D immitis* appear to have a life-span in cats of 2 to 3 years. Thus, natural infections may be self limited.

IV. Age-sex distribution

Cats may be infected at any age but the average age at diagnosis is 3 to 6 years. Male cats living outdoors are at greatest risk.

V. Aberrant migration

Larvae tend to migrate to aberrant locations much more often in cats than in dogs. The most common location is the brain, which results in CNS signs.

PATHOPHYSIOLOGY

Although somewhat similar, the pathophysiologic response of the pulmonary arteries of cats to adult *D immitis* is exaggerated compared to that in dogs. The incidence of acute pulmonary and neurologic complications, including sudden death, is higher than in dogs. In contrast, some cats exhibit no signs of infection.

I. Pulmonary endothelial damage and response

The inciting causes and pathologic response to *D immitis* adults is similar to that of dogs (see previous section).

A. The severity of villus proliferation in cats with a typical worm burden is comparable to that seen in dogs with many dead worms.

B. Small- and medium-sized arteries develop myointimal proliferation, but the elastic arteries have a predominance of fibromuscular proliferation.

II. Radiographic changes

Three to five months after L_3 inoculation and within several weeks of transplantation of adult worms, typical radiographic changes can be found.

A. Caudal lobar artery enlargement

B. Diffuse and focal parenchymal lung disease

C. Arteriograms reveal changes similar to those seen in dogs, including decreased perfusion as early as 3 months after L_3 inoculation and severe perfusion defects by 7 months (Fig. 10-4).

III. Obstruction of pulmonary arteries

Obstruction by worms of the caudal lobar arteries is common and comparable to that seen in dogs following adulticide therapy.

A. Obstruction is due to muscular hypertrophy, villus proliferation, vasospasm, worms, and thrombosis.

B. Severe pulmonary hypertension may develop.

CLINICAL MANIFESTATIONS

The clinical signs of heartworm disease in cats may be acute or chronic.

I. Acute signs

Acute signs are associated with pulmonary or CNS disease.

A. Pulmonary signs include coughing, dyspnea, tachypnea, tachycardia, syncope, or sudden death.

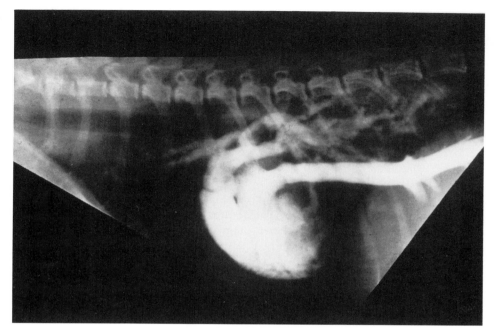

Fig. 10-4. Nonselective angiogram demonstrating enlargement and tortuosity of the caudal lobar pulmonary arteries. Blood flow is decreased in the peripheral regions as indicated by decreased contrast opacity.

    B. CNS signs including seizures, dementia, and blindness are variably seen in cats with worms located in the lateral ventricles.

II. Chronic signs

    Chronic signs are associated with cardiopulmonary and systemic responses.

    A. Cardiopulmonary signs

        1. Congestive heart failure

        2. Relapsing PIE syndrome

    B. Systemic signs

        1. Intermittent vomiting

        2. Unexplained anorexic and lethargy

DIAGNOSIS

The diagnosis of feline heartworm disease is more difficult than in the dog. Thoracic radiography is a useful although difficult to interpret diagnostic aid.

    I. Radiographic changes are similar to those seen in dogs.

    A. The main pulmonary artery segment is not visualized on routine ventro-dorsal or dorsoventral projections.

    B. Enlargement of the caudal lobar arteries is the most diagnostically useful abnormality.

      1. The radiographic picture in normal cats is one of prominent lobar arteries, thus interpretation is made with this in mind.

      2. Blunting and tortuosity may be visible.

  C. Parenchymal lung infiltration viewed on the lateral projection and concentrated in the middle one-third of the caudal lung lobes may be observed.

  D. A PIE syndrome is sometimes observed.

  E. Pleural effusion is seen more commonly than in dogs, is usually associated with CHF, and is a transudate or pseudochylous effusion.

  F. Nonselective arteriography is a useful and practical means of delineating pulmonary arterial pathology, as well as the linear and sometimes coiled filling defects caused by worms. The absence of filling defects and lobar artery abnormalities on a well-performed angiogram weighs heavily against the diagnosis.

II. Electrocardiography

The ECG is often unremarkable.

  A. A right ventricular hypertrophy pattern may be seen with severe, chronic disease and is often associated with CHF (pleural effusion and ascites).

  B. The incidence of heart rhythm disturbances is unknown.

III. Echocardiography

Cardiac ultrasound is a useful diagnostic tool, although worms may not be detected due to their usual low numbers.

  A. A definitive diagnosis is possible if heartworm images are identified in the right atrium, right ventricle, pulmonary artery or vena cava (Fig. 10-5).

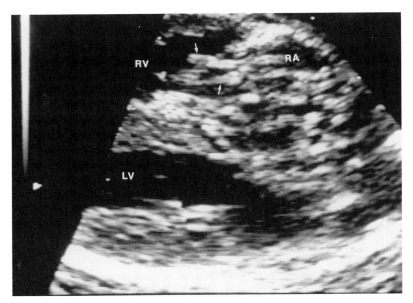

Fig. 10-5. Two-dimensional cardiac ultrasound demonstrating numerous parallel, linear echodensities representing heartworm (arrows) in the right heart of a cat with severe heartworm disease. The cat exhibited dyspnea, weakness, and pleural effusion. LV, left ventricle; RV, right ventricle; RA, right atrium.

    B. Indirect evidence can be obtained if evidence of pulmonary hypertension is seen.
      1. Right ventricular enlargement
      2. Color flow Doppler evidence of abnormally severe pulmonic insufficiency suggestive of pulmonary hypertension
      3. Reduced right ventricular shortening fraction

IV. Clinical pathology

Abnormalities of the CBC and serum chemistry profile are inconsistently observed.

    A. Eosinophilia-basophilia

    These abnormalities are inconsistent and nonspecific, although in combination their presence suggests lung disease.
      1. Experimentally, eosinophilia is routinely present 3 to 7 months after L_3 inoculation.
      2. Within 2 to 3 months of the arrival of worms in the pulmonary arteries, eosinophil counts decrease. Eosinophilia is absent in two-thirds of naturally infected cats at the time of diagnosis.

    B. Hyperglobulinemia

    A polyclonal gammopathy is observed in one-third to one-half of infected cats and is presumably the result of chronic antigenic stimulation.

    C. Other clinical pathology abnormalities are nonspecific and usually absent in early or mild cases.

V. Microfilariae identification

Most cats do not have circulating microfilariae at the time of diagnosis.

    A. Approximately 40 to 50 percent of cats inoculated with L_3 develop microfilaremia.
      1. The time to patency is approximately 7 months.
      2. Microfilaria usually disappear 6 to 8 weeks after their appearance.
      3. Microfilaria, when present, are in low concentrations (usually less than 2 per ml of blood)

    B. Most mosquitoes feeding on cats with low microfilarial concentrations do not become infected, and thus cats are not good intermediate hosts for *D immitis*.

    C. Frequent testing and using larger volumes of blood are usually not rewarding.

VI. Immunodiagnostic testing

ELISA for the detection of adult *D immitis* antigens are specific, somewhat sensitive, and require no special modifications for cats.

    A. False-negative results

    The male *D immitis* contributes little or nothing to a positive antigen test. Thus adequate numbers of female worms, especially gravid worms, are required for reliable test results.
      1. Low numbers of worms
      2. Absence of female worms
      3. Absence of gravid female worms
        Note: Positive results are not likely prior to 7 to 8 months after L_3 inoculation, a fact not restricted to the use of antigen detection in cats.

B. Positive test results

If 3 or more female worms are present at 8 months or more after infection, some tests are more than 70 percent sensitive.
1. False-positive test results do not occur when proper quality control is maintained.
2. The sensitivities of various antigen tests are different. Presumably, those tests that are less sensitive will either be improved or replaced.

C. A very sensitive test is a feline IgG antibody test against heartworm antigens.
1. False-positive test results possible
2. A negative test result weighs heavily against the diagnosis
3. Serodiagnostics Laboratory in St. Louis is the only laboratory currently performing this test.

THERAPY

Whether or not to administer adulticide treatment to cats is controversial. The relatively high incidence of acute, life-threatening pulmonary thrombosis, the uncertain (although probably low) incidence of acute, life-threatening pulmonary drug reactions, and the possibility of self-limitation of infection has clouded this issue.

I. Thiacetarsamide sodium

The only adulticide drug that has received attention is thiacetarsamide sodium.
A. The dosage schedule usually employed (2.2 mg/kg IV BID for 2 days) has not been definitively shown to be the best regimen.
B. The efficacy of thiacetarsamide is controversial: some investigators suggest good efficacy while others question the drug's efficacy.
C. The incidence of drug toxicity is controversial.
1. A high incidence of complications has been observed by some.
a) Lethargy-depression
b) Anorexia-vomiting
c) Respiratory abnormalities
(1) Respiratory failure, pulmonary edema, and death
(2) Respiratory distress or tachypnea of a mild-to-moderate degree
2. Other investigators have observed little or no pulmonary toxicity.
3. Anorexia and vomiting may be encountered after any injection and persistent vomiting and anorexia are an indication to abort therapy.
D. Patient selection
1. The author does not recommend thiacetarsamide treatment for cats with mild or episodic signs that respond to anti-inflammatory dosages of corticosteroids.
a) Episodic dyspnea or coughing
b) Intermittent vomiting
2. Cats with persistent and severe signs should probably be treated. Treated cats should remain hospitalized under close, continuous observation for 2 to 3 weeks after adulticide therapy.

    a) Congestive heart failure
    b) Pulmonary thromboembolism
      (1) Stabilization required prior to treatment
      (2) Cage confinement and corticosteroids, and, if the platelet count is below 100,000/mm^3, heparin

  E. Postadulticide treatment complications
    Acute, life-threatening pulmonary thrombosis is a greater risk in cats than in dogs, occurring in approximately 25 to 40 percent of patients.
    1. Unpredictable and may occur in cats with few worms and minimal pretreatment symptoms.
    2. Occurs from 5 to 21 days after treatment.
    3. Therapy is usually fruitless if symptoms are severe.

II. Worm extraction
  When a high worm burden is identified by cardiac ultrasound, adulticide treatment will probably result in fatal thromboembolism.
  A. Worm extraction after the technique of Ishihara is effective.
    1. Anesthesia required.
    2. Transjugular approach into the vena cava and right heart.
    3. A special flexible alligator forceps is required and the procedure is done with the aid of fluoroscopy.
  B. Response to therapy, in terms of the resolution of clinical signs, is dramatic

III. RM 340
  The investigational adulticide, RM 340, has not been evaluated in cats.

Management of Thromboembolic Lung Disease

  I. Oxygen therapy
    A. Intranasal
    B. Cage
  II. Heparin 75 U/kg, SQ TID for 5 to 21 days
  III. Corticosteroids (antiinflammatory dosages) for several days if there is evidence of parenchymal lung complications.
    A. Radiographic evidence of alveolar lung disease and lobar consolidation
    B. Hemoptysis
    C. Fever
    D. Inflammatory leukogram
  IV. Aspirin is difficult to dose appropriately in cats and has minimal benefits in reducing the severity or incidence of thromboembolic complications. Since platelets in cats are highly activated by heartworm invasion and have a high turnover rate during heartworm infection, more frequent administration at increasing dosages is required to inhibit platelet function. Currently, there is little or no role for aspirin in the treatment of feline heartworm disease.

Microfilaricide Therapy

Since microfilariae are seldom present, treatment is usually not required. Ivermectin may be administered when microfilariae are detected (50 μg/kg). Whether or not such treatment is indicated is questionable since cats are poor reservoir hosts and microfilaria produce little or no pathology.

PROPHYLAXIS

Whether or not to administer heartworm prophylaxis is controversial.

    I. Is heartworm infection a problem in a given area?
    II. Does a particular cat demonstrate a habitus placing it at risk?
    III. A number of prophylactic drugs have been shown to be safe and effective, although none are FDA-approved for this purpose.
        A. Ivermectin (24 μg/kg, orally once monthly)
        B. Milbemycin oxime (0.5 to 0.99 mg/kg, orally, once monthly)

SUGGESTED READINGS

Atkins CE: Heartworm caval syndrome. In Kirk RW (ed): Current Veterinary Therapy XI. WB Saunders, Philadelphia, 1992

Calvert CA, Rawlings CA: Feline heartworm disease. In Sherding RC (ed): The Cat: Diseases and Clinical Management. 2nd Ed. Churchill Livingstone, New York, 1994

Hribernik T: Canine and feline heartworm disease. In Kirk RW (ed): Current Veterinary Therapy XI. WB Saunders, Philadelphia, 1989

Otto GF (ed): Proceedings of the Heartworm Symposium. American Heartworm Society, Washington, DC, 1989

Otto GF (ed): Proceedings of the Heartworm Symposium. American Heartworm Society, Washington, DC, 1992

Rawlings CA: Heartworm Disease in Dogs and Cats. WB Saunders, Philadelphia, 1986

Rawlings CA, Calvert CA: Heartworm disease. In Ettinger SF (ed): Textbook of Veterinary Internal Medicine. WB Saunders, Philadelphia, 1989

Vezzoni A, Genchi C: Reduction of post-adulticide thromboembolism complications with low dose heparin therapy. p. 73. In Otto GF (ed): Proceedings of the Heartworm Symposium. American Heartworm Society, Charleston, SC, 1989

11

Pericardial Disease
Matthew W. Miller

INTRODUCTION

GENERAL

I. It is estimated that clinically significant pericardial disease accounts for only 1 percent of all cardiac disease in the dog and cat.
II. Pericardial disease is, however, an important and frequently overlooked cause of right-heart failure in the dog.
III. Clinically significant pericardial disease is uncommon in the cat.
IV. Pericardial diseases can be categorized as congenital malformations, acquired disease causing pericardial effusion, and acquired disease causing constriction.

ANATOMY AND FUNCTION

I. The pericardial sac is composed of the outer (parietal) and inner (visceral) membranes.
II. The space between these layers is the pericardial sac.
   A. It does not normally communicate with the pleural or peritoneal cavities.
   B. It normally contains a small volume of serous fluid (0.5 to 15 ml).
III. Although not an essential structure, the pericardium functions to limit acute cardiac dilatation, maintain cardiac geometry and ventricular compliance, reduce friction, and provide a barrier to inflammation from contiguous structures.

CONGENITAL DISEASE

GENERAL

I. Peritoneopericardial diaphragmatic hernia (PPDH) is the most common congenital pericardial malformation diagnosed in dogs and cats.
   A. Represents an embryologic malformation of the ventral midline, allowing communication between the pericardial and peritoneal cavities

259

  B. May be associated with other congenital malformations, including sternal deformities (especially in cats), cranial abdominal hernias, and ventricular septal defects
  C. Has been reported in littermates but there is no reported evidence that the lesion is hereditary
II. Pericardial cysts, partial pericardial defects, and complete absence of the pericardial sac represent uncommon congenital pericardial malformations.

PATHOPHYSIOLOGY

  I. Most pericardial defects are clinically silent, however partial defects may allow herniation of part of the heart (usually the atria).
 II. Pericardial cysts usually cause signs as a result of compression of the heart or lungs.
III. With PPDH, the signs are dependent on the nature and amount of abdominal contents that is herniated.
    A. Large amounts of abdominal viscera may cause signs due to compression of the heart or lungs.
    B. Incarceration of abdominal organs, most commonly liver or small bowel, may lead to signs associated with vascular compromise or obstruction.

DIAGNOSIS

  I. Signalment
    A. The age at which clinical signs are first manifest is extremely variable (4 weeks to 15 years) but it is most commonly within the first year of life.
    B. It has been suggested that Weimaraners are predisposed to PPDH.
 II. History
    Most clinical signs are related to the gastrointestinal and respiratory systems.
    A. Vomiting, diarrhea, weight loss, abdominal discomfort
    B. Cough, dyspnea, wheezing
III. Physical examination
    A. Muffled heart sounds on one or both sides
    B. Displaced or attenuated apical cardiac impulse
    C. "Empty" abdomen (PPDH)
    D. Palpable sternal deformity or cranial abdominal hernia
IV. Radiography
    A. Findings are dependent on the size of the defect and the amount and type of abdominal contents that have herniated.
    B. Overlap of the caudal heart border and the diaphragm
    C. Few organs within the abdominal cavity ("empty" abdomen)
    D. Multiple radiographic densities within the cardiac silhouette (omentum, liver, spleen, bowel loops)
    E. Cranial abdominal hernia or sternal deformity
    F. Gastrointestinal barium series may demonstrate bowel loops crossing the diaphragm and within the pericardial sac (more common in dogs than cats)

G. Nonselective angiography can be used to outline the cardiac chamber and giant vessels within the enlarged cardiac silhouette

V. Electrocardiography
   A. Commonly normal
   B. May show decreased complex size if a large amount of abdominal contents has herniated or significant effusion is present. This may only be evident in the chest leads.

VI. Echocardiography
   Will usually allow for definitive diagnosis and identify the nature of the abdominal contents that have herniated. Gas filled bowel loops will interfere with imaging.

THERAPY

I. Surgical closure of the hernia after returning viable organs to their normal location is suggested and usually curative.
II. Surgical removal of pericardial cysts in combination with partial pericardiectomy
III. Most partial pericardial defects are clinically silent; however, partial pericardiectomy is indicated if clinical signs are evident.

PROGNOSIS

If no other significant congenital anomalies or complicating factors are present, the prognosis following surgery is excellent.

PERICARDIAL EFFUSION

GENERAL

I. The term pericardial effusion indicates excessive or abnormal accumulation of pericardial fluid.
II. Diseases resulting in pericardial effusion comprise the majority of clinically significant diseases of the pericardium.
III. Pericardial effusion may develop due to
   A. *Transudation* secondary to CHF, PPDH, cysts, hypoalbuminemia, infections/toxemias or other causes of increased vascular permeability
   B. *Exudation* caused by infective (bacterial, fungal, trypanasomal, or viral) or noninfective pericarditis (uremia)
   C. *Intrapericardial hemorrhage* (with or without secondary pericardial reaction) associated with neoplasia of the heart, heart base, or pericardium (hemangiosarcoma, chemodectoma, ectopic thyroid carcinoma, mesothelioma, and lymphosarcoma), idiopathic pericardial hemorrhage in dogs,

and, less commonly, external trauma or cardiac rupture (usually left atrial rupture secondary to chronic mitral regurgitation)

PATHOPHYSIOLOGY

   I. The hemodynamic effects of pericardial effusion are primarily dependent upon the rate and volume of fluid accumulation and the distensibility or compliance of the pericardium.
  II. Cardiac tamponade refers to the decompensated phase of cardiac compression resulting from an unchecked rise in the intrapericardial fluid pressure.
 III. Cardiac tamponade develops when intrapericardial pressure becomes elevated and compresses the heart. Tamponade is the mechanism by which low cardiac output and congestive heart failure (CHF) develop.
  IV. Important features include: increased (positive) intrapericardial pressure, diastolic collapse of the right atrium (and right ventricle in some cases), reduction of ventricular filling, decreased cardiac output, and arterial hypotension.
   V. Compensatory measures are activated to maintain cardiac output; these include activation of the sympathetic nervous system, vasoconstriction, renal retention of sodium and water, and elevated venous pressures.
  VI. Signs of *right*-heart failure predominate since this thinner chamber is more influenced by high intrapericardial pressures.
 VII. Myocardial systolic function is usually unaffected.

DIAGNOSIS

   I. Signalment
      A. Pericardial effusion is most commonly seen in dogs 5 years old or older.
      B. Pericardial effusion is most commonly observed in large breed dogs and 90 percent or more of the cases are either idiopathic or neoplastic.
      C. German shepherds and golden retrievers are predisposed to both hemangiosarcoma and idiopathic pericardial hemorrhage.
      D. Brachycephalic breeds (Boston terriers, English bulldogs, and boxers) are predisposed to chemodectoma
      E. The most common cause of pericardial effusion in cats is feline infectious peritonitis. Other causes include cardiomyopathy, lymphoma and uremia.
  II. History
      Most historical complaints are associated with congestive heart failure or reduced cardiac output; they include weakness, exercise intolerance, abdominal distension, lethargy, and dyspnea.
 III. Physical examination
      A. The heart sounds may be muffled or seem "distant." Respiratory sounds may be muffled if pleural effusion is present.
      B. Sinus tachycardia is common.
      C. Cardiac murmurs are uncommon unless concurrent valvular or myocardial disease is present.

    D. Clinical signs of elevated systemic venous pressure and right-sided CHF (hepatomegaly/ascites) predominate.

    E. Careful evaluation of the systemic veins is imperative. Overlooking venous distension may lead to an erroneous diagnosis of liver disease or abdominal neoplasia.

    F. Weak arterial pulses

    G. Pulsus paradoxus: an exaggerated decline (>10 mmHg) in arterial pulse pressure during inspiration.

IV. Radiography (Fig. 11-1)

    A. The cardiac silhouette is usually enlarged in cases with significant fluid accumulation.

    B. The cardiac silhouette classically is rounded or globoid, and specific chamber enlargement is not evident. This may not be true when the amount of effusion is small.

    C. The trachea may be elevated, especially if a heart base mass is present.

    D. Other findings may include distention of the caudal vena cava, pulmonary undercirculation, pleural effusion, hepatomegaly, and ascites.

    E. Nonselective angiography will outline the cardiac chambers and great vessels within the enlarged cardiac silhouette; fluoroscopy will demonstrate reduced movement of the cardiac silhouette

V. Electrocardiography (Fig. 11-2)

    A. Arrhythmias other than sinus tachycardia are uncommon

    B. Does not provide a definitive diagnosis, but certain findings should increase suspicion.

        (1) Low amplitude complexes (R < 1 mV in lead II in the dog)

        (2) ST segment elevation (epicardial injury current)

        (3) Electrical alternans

VI. Echocardiography (Fig. 11-3)

    A. Highly sensitive test for detecting pericardial effusion (as little as 15 ml) and pericardial mass lesions.

    B. Echo-free space between the epicardium and pericardium.

    C. Abnormal cardiac motion, often with dramatic side-to-side movement.

    D. Overall cardiac chamber size is usually diminished due to impaired cardiac filling.

    E. Collapse of the right atrium or ventricle indicates markedly increased intrapericardial pressure and is echocardiographic evidence of cardiac tamponade.

    F. Intrapericardial or cardiac mass lesions may be visualized.

    G. If it does not compromise patient care, echocardiography should be performed before pericardiocentesis. The pericardial fluid will greatly enhance the ability to visualize heartbase masses.

THERAPY

I. Pericardiocentesis is the treatment of choice for initial stabilization of dogs and cats with pericardial effusion and cardiac tamponade (Fig. 11-4).

    A. Technique

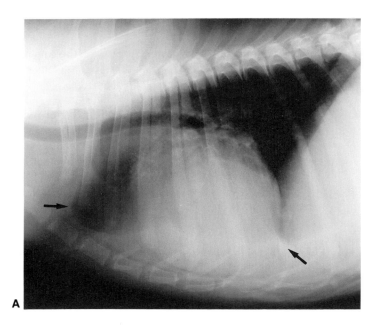

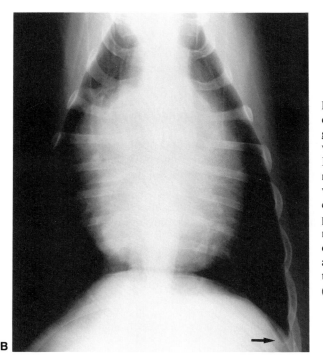

Fig. 11-1. (**A**) Lateral and (**B**) dorsoventral thoracic radiographs obtained from a dog with pericardial effusion. Moderate generalized cardiomegaly is noted on both views without obvious specific chamber enlargement. The pulmonary vasculature is diminished and a small amount of pleural effusion is present as evidenced by mild retraction of the lung margins *(arrows)*.

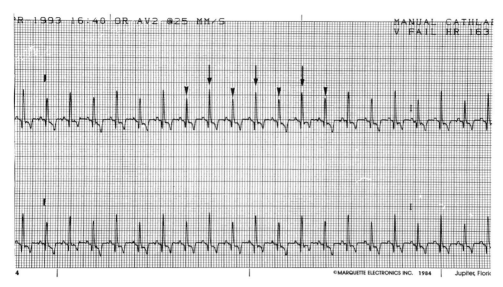

Fig. 11-2. Electrocardiogram from a dog with idiopathic pericardial effusion and signs of cardiac tamponade. Notice how the R waves alternate in amplitude *(arrow* vs. *arrowhead)*. The overall complex size is small and the heart rate is elevated (163 bpm). Lead I, 25 mm/ sec, 2 cm = 1 mV.

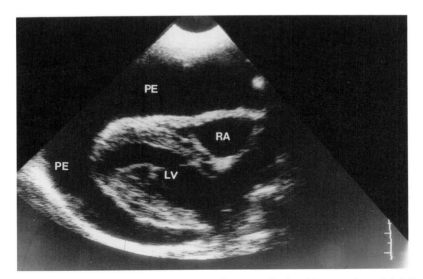

Fig. 11-3. Right parasternal long axis echocardiogram obtained from a dog with idiopathic pericardial effusion. Note the large echo-free space separating the epicardium and pericardium; it represents pericardial effusion (PE). RA, right atrium; LV, left ventricle.

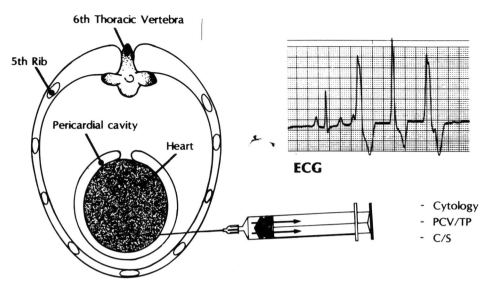

Fig. 11-4. Diagram outlining important aspects of pericardiocentesis, which is most commonly performed between the right fourth and sixth intercostal space. Epicardial contact often results in ventricular premature beats that are upright in lead II and usually self-limiting.

1. Shave and surgically prepare a large area of the right hemithorax (sternum to mid thorax, third to eighth rib).

2. Local anesthesia is usually adequate; however, mild sedation is sometimes necessary. It is important to be sure the pleura has been infiltrated as it seems that penetration of the pleura causes significant discomfort.

3. Place the patient in sternal or lateral recumbency depending on demeanor. Occasionally pericardiocentesis can be accomplished in the standing animal but adequate restraint is essential to prevent cardiac puncture or pulmonary laceration.

4. Electrocardiographic monitoring during the procedure is helpful in that epicardial contact often causes ventricular arrhythmias (Fig. 11-4).

5. The puncture site is usually determined based on the location of the heart on thoracic radiographs. This is most commonly between the fourth and sixth rib spaces at the costochondral junction.

6. Ultrasound guidance is infrequently needed unless the volume of effusion is very small or the effusion is compartmentalized.

7. The size of the needle or catheter used is dependent on the size of the animal. In cats, a 19- or 21-gauge butterfly catheter may be adequate; in large dogs, a 16-gauge over-the-needle catheter (usually with additional side holes) may be needed.

8. The needle or catheter should be attached to a three-way stopcock, extension tubing and a syringe to allow constant negative pressure to be applied during insertion and drainage.

9. Care should be taken to avoid the large vessels that run along the caudal border of the ribs.

10. Once the catheter has been inserted through the skin, negative pressure should be applied.

11. If pleural effusion is present, it will be obtained immediately upon entering the thoracic cavity. It is most commonly a clear to pale-yellow color.

12. As the catheter is advanced and contacts the pericardium, a scratching sensation will be noticed. Minimal advancement will result in penetration of the pericardium.

13. Most pericardial effusions are hemorrhagic and have a "port wine" appearance. Once effusion of this character is obtained, the catheter should be advanced over the needle and the needle removed. The remainder of the drainage should be performed using the catheter.

14. Advancing the needle too far will result in contact with the epicardium. This is often felt as a tapping or more intense scratching sensation and commonly results in ventricular arrhythmias (Fig. 11-4). These arrhythmias are usually self limiting once the needle/catheter is retracted.

15. Pericardial effusion can be differentiated from peripheral blood in that it rarely clots unless it is from very recent hemorrhage, and the PCV is significantly lower than that of peripheral blood.

16. Every attempt should be made to drain the pericardial space as completely as possible.

17. Drainage of the pericardium is often associated with an increase in the complex size on the ECG, a reduction in heart rate, and an improvement in arterial pulse quality.

18. Potential complications include cardiac puncture (with resultant hemorrhage or arrhythmias), coronary artery laceration, lung puncture or laceration, and dissemination of infection or neoplasia throughout the thoracic cavity.

B. Diagnostic evaluations of fluid obtained should include PCV and cytologic evaluation. Bacterial culture and sensitivity should be performed if results of the cytologic evaluation indicate it.

C. Caution should be exercised when evaluating the cellular component of pericardial effusion. Clinically important neoplasia of the heart and pericardium (hemangiosarcoma, chemodectoma) commonly do not exfoliate, resulting in frequent false-negative evaluations. Reactive mesothelial cells within the pericardial sac are commonly overinterpreted as being neoplastic, causing false-positive results.

D. Pericardiocentesis is curative in approximately 50 percent of cases of idiopathic hemorrhagic effusion. If effusion recurs, repeat centesis is indicated.

E. Pericardiocentesis is considered palliative if effusion is neoplastic in origin.

II. Medical management

A. The administration of corticosteroids (prednisone 1 to 2 mg/kg PO in a gradually tapering dose over 10 to 14 days) has been advocated, but controlled studies documenting the efficacy of this therapy are lacking.

B. Since myocardial systolic function is usually not affected, positive inotropic therapy is not indicated.

C. Therapy with diuretics and vasodilators may mildly reduce signs of CHF, but are commonly associated with hypotension and weakness and are not recommended.

III. Pericardiectomy

A. If idiopathic effusion continues following repeated thoracocentesis (>2), subtotal pericardiectomy is recommended and usually curative.

B. Pericardiectomy may provide significant clinical relief in patients with effusion associated with neoplasia. Resection of cardiac mass lesions may be attempted but can be associated with severe complications.

PROGNOSIS

I. Idiopathic pericardial effusion/hemorrhage is usually associated with a good prognosis following pericardiocentesis or pericardiectomy.

II. Hemangiosarcoma is commonly multicentric, poorly responsive to chemotherapy and carries a poor prognosis

III. Chemodectoma is typically a slow growing neoplasm that is late to metastasize. Partial pericardiectomy may provide significant symptomatic improvement for prolonged periods (up to 3 years).

CONSTRICTIVE PERICARDIAL DISEASE

GENERAL

I. Uncommon in the dog and rare in the cat

II. As with pericardial effusion, middle-aged, large breed male dogs seem to be at risk

III. May represent a late sequela of idiopathic pericardial effusion.

PATHOPHYSIOLOGY

I. The major hemodynamic effect is decreased ventricular diastolic compliance, which limits the amount of blood volume that fills the ventricles at any given preload (venous pressure).

II. Thickening of the visceral and or parietal pericardium restricts ventricular filling. In some cases, the visceral and parietal pericardium may fuse and obliterate the pericardial space.

III. In some cases, a small amount of fluid is present within the pericardial sac, resulting in what is referred to as constrictive effusive pericarditis. This form of pericardial disease has characteristics of both constrictive pericardial disease and pericardial effusion.

DIAGNOSIS

  I. History
     Clinical signs and historical complaints are similar to those seen with pericardial effusion. Occasionally there will be a history of a previous diagnosis of pericardial effusion.
 II. Physical examination is similar to that for pericardial effusion.
     A. Venous distention, hepatomegaly, abdominal distention, weak arterial pulses, muffled heart sounds
     B. Pulsus paradoxus not commonly present
III. Radiography
     A. The cardiac silhouette is usually only mildly to moderately enlarged.
     B. Pleural effusion and distension of the caudal vena cava may be noticed, along with ascites and hepatomegaly.
 IV. Electrocardiography
     A. Diminished complex size is present in 75 percent of cases.
     B. Widened P-wave, suggestive of left atrial enlargement, is present in 85 percent of cases.
  V. Echocardiography
     A. The echocardiographic features of constrictive pericardial effusion are less dramatic than those associated with pericardial effusion, and may include a thickened echodense pericardium, diminished cardiac chamber size, paradoxical septal motion, and diastolic flattening of the left ventricular free wall.
     B. In constrictive effusive pericardial disease, the severity of clinical signs relative to the small amount of fluid present should raise suspicion of constrictive disease.

THERAPY

  I. Subtotal pericardiectomy is the therapy of choice.
 II. Pulmonary thromboembolism is reported as a common postoperative complication.
III. If the visceral and parietal pericardium are fused, epicardial stripping may be necessary to relieve ventricular restriction. Pericardial stripping is associated with high morbidity and mortality in humans.
 IV. Supraventricular arrhythmias were common, and especially associated with anesthesia in one study.

PROGNOSIS

The prognosis is good if the epicardium and pericardium are not fused.

SUGGESTED READINGS

Berg RJ, Wingfield W: Pericardial effusion in the dog: A review of 42 cases. J Am Anim Hosp Assoc 20:721, 1984
Bonagura JD: Electrical alternans associatd with pericardial effusion in the dog. J Am Vet Med Assoc 178:574, 1981

Bonagura JD, Pipers FS: Echocardiographic features of pericardial effusion in dogs. J Am
    Vet Med Assoc 179:49, 1981

Gibbs C, Gaskell CJ, Darke PG, Wotton PR: Idiopathic pericardial haemorrhage in dogs:
    A review of fourteen cases. J Small Anim Pract 23:483, 1982

Miller MW, Fossum TW: Pericardial disease. p. 725. In: Kirk RW, Bonagura JD (eds):
    Current Veterinary Therapy XI. WB Saunders, Philadelphia, 1992

Rush JE, Keene BW, Fox PR: Pericardial disease in the cat: A retrospective evaluation
    of 66 cases. J Am Anim Hosp Assoc 26:39, 1990

Thomas WP: Pericardial disorders. p. 1132. In: Ettinger SJ (ed): Textbook of Veterinary
    Internal Medicine. 3rd Ed. WB Saunders, Philadelphia, 1989

Thomas WP, Reed JR, Bauer TG, Breznock EM: Constrictive pericardial disease in the
    dog. J Am Vet Med Assoc 184:546, 1984

Thomas WP, Sisson D, Bauer TG, Reed JR: Detection of cardiac masses in dogs by two-
    dimensional echocardiography. Vet Rad 25:65, 1984

12

Congenital Heart Disease
John-Karl Goodwin

INTRODUCTION

HEREDITARY ASPECTS

I. Congenital heart diseases are the most common type of heart disease in young dogs and cats, and are occasionally diagnosed in adult animals.

II. Congenital heart defects are generally recognized in the young animal and usually represent a hereditary trait or a defect that originated during gestation. A genetic problem often exists for animals with congenital heart disease.

III. Four common forms of congenital heart disease have been shown to be inherited in dogs
   - A. Patent ductus arteriosus in the poodle
   - B. Aortic stenosis in the Newfoundland
   - C. Tetralogy of Fallot in the Keeshond
   - D. Pulmonic stenosis in the beagle

DIAGNOSIS

I. Generally, a congenital heart defect is suspected when a heart murmur is detected in a young dog or cat. Other supporting clinical features may include failure to thrive, exercise intolerance, cyanosis, collapse or seizure, jugular venous distension, electrocardiographic abnormalities and radiographic evidence of cardiac enlargement. A tentative diagnosis is often made based on results of a complete cardiovascular physical examination and routine electrocardiography and radiography (Table 12-1).

II. The specific diagnosis is confirmed in most cases by echocardiography, and rarely by cardiac catheterization. Information obtained echocardiographically is also helpful in determining the severity of the defect, especially if Doppler techniques are used (measurement of blood velocities within the heart).

THERAPY

I. Recent advances allow for the treatment of certain stenotic lesions by balloon valvuloplasty, a technique employing a small balloon located at the end of

TABLE 12-1. DIAGNOSTIC CRITERIA OF COMMON CONGENITAL HEART DEFECTS

Heart Defect	Physical Examination	Electrocardiogram	Thoracic Radiographs	Echocardiography
Innocent (functional murmur)	Murmur usually soft, grade 1/6–3/6, and is early to mid-systolic in timing. It is loudest over the left side, and may change in intensity with positional changes. All else normal.	Normal	Normal	Normal
Patent ductus arteriosus (*left-to-right shunting*)	Continuous machinery-type murmur heard loudest over the left-heart base. The systolic component is usually > grade 3/6. Precordial systolic thrill often present over left heart base. Bounding arterial pulses are typical.	LVH pattern common (tall R-waves, widened QRS) Left atrial enlargement (widened P-waves) pattern common Occasional arrhythmias, especially in long-standing cases	Left-sided cardiomegaly; classically, three "bumps" seen on DV view: main pulmonary artery dilatation, aortic aneurysmal dilatation, and enlarged left atrial appendage Pulmonary hyperperfusion	Dilation of left atrium and left ventricle; often excessive LV fractional shortening. In some cases, visualization of the ductus is possible, especially with Doppler guidance
Patent ductus arteriosus (*right-to-left shunting*)	A soft diastolic murmur of pulmonic insufficiency is frequently present. A split second heart sound may be present. Differential cyanosis.	RVH pattern (rightward shift of the MEA, deep S waves in leads I, II, and III)	Generalized cardiomegaly; prominent main pulmonary artery Pulmonary arteries often enlarged and tortuous	Dilation of right atrium and right ventricle; right ventricular and septal hypertrophy. Contrast studies reveal no intracardiac shunting, yet contrast present in abdominal aorta
Pulmonic stenosis	A prominent (grade 3/6 or greater) systolic ejection murmur over pulmonic valve area	RVH pattern (rightward shift of the MEA, deep S waves in leads I, II, and III)	Right-sided cardiomegaly; prominent main pulmonary artery segment (esp on VD or DV view) Pulmonary arteries often diminuted	Right ventricular dilation and hypertrophy. In most cases, a thickened immobile pulmonic valve is seen. Increased RV ejection velocity (proportional to degree of stenosis)

272

	Auscultation / Physical Examination	Electrocardiography	Radiography	Echocardiography
Subaortic stenosis	Systolic ejection murmur loudest over aortic valve (left base). May radiate cranially to thoracic inlet. Weak and slow rising arterial pulses.	May be normal or indicative of LV enlargement. Ventricular arrhythmias present in severe/long-standing cases	Left-sided cardiomegaly. Prominent ascending aorta due to poststenotic dilatation	Left ventricular hypertrophy is usually prominent. There may be fibrosis (hyperechogenecity) of the myocardium, esp. papillary muscles. A subaortic ridge is often seen. Increased LV outflows velocity, proportional to degree of obstruction.
Ventricular septal defect	Harsh, regurgitant-type systolic murmur heard loudest at right sternal border. Arterial pulses usually normal, may be exaggerated.	May be normal. LVH pattern with large shunts. Partial or complete right bundle branch pattern may be seen	May be normal. Left-sided cardiomegaly usually prominent. There may be enlargement of the right ventricle. Pulmonary hyperperfusion	Echocardiography will usually demonstrate the defect and associated chamber enlargement. Doppler echocardiography will confirm shunting through the defect.
Tetralogy of Fallot	A systolic ejection murmur of pulmonic stenosis is usually present. A split second heart sound may be heard. Evidence of systemic cyanosis.	RVH pattern (rightward shift of the MEA, deep S waves in leads I, II, and III)	Mild-to-moderate right ventricular enlargement; main pulmonary artery segment usually diminished. Pulmonary vasculature diminished	Right ventricular dilatation and hypertrophy. Ventricular septal defect. Overriding and dilated aorta. Obstruction of right ventricular outflow tract. Contrast echo demonstrates right-to-left shunting through the defect
Mitral valve dysplasia	Prominent (>3/6) holosystolic regurgitant murmur over left apex.	Left atrial (widened P-waves) pattern usually present. LVH pattern may be present. Supraventricular arrhythmias (APCs, atrial fibrillation) may be present	Left-sided cardiomegaly with especially prominent left atrium. Enlargement of pulmonary veins	Severely dilated left atrium, with abnormal motion and/or appearance of mitral valve complex. LV dilatation. Doppler confirms moderate-to-severe mitral insufficiency.

Abbreviations: LV, left ventricle; LVH, left ventricular hypertrophy; MEA, mean electrical axis; APC, atrial premature complexes; VD view, ventrodorsal view; DV view, dorsoventral view; RV, right ventricle; RVH, right ventricular hypertrophy.

a cardiac catheter. Surgical correction is the preferred treatment in certain congenital heart defects, such as patent ductus arteriosus.

II. Medical treatment is primarily for the control or prevention of complications such as congestive heart failure, arrhythmias, and endocarditis rather than correction of the defect. Medical therapy is discussed briefly in this chapter.

CANINE

I. The incidence of congenital heart disease in dogs has been reported to be 8 per 1,000 live births. On average, this equates to one case per 15 litters. The actual incidence is likely higher as some defects result in neonatal death and therefore are unreported.

II. The most common congenital heart defects in the dog include patent ductus arteriosus, pulmonic stenosis, subaortic stenosis, ventricular septal defect, and tetralogy of Fallot. Several breed predispositions have been identified (Table 12-2).

TABLE 12-2. CONGENITAL HEART DISEASE: BREED PREDISPOSITIONS

Breed	Disease
Airedale terrier	PS
Beagle	PS
Boxer	AS, ASD
Boykin spaniel	PS
Bull terrier	MD
Chihuahua	PS, PDA,MD
Cocker spaniel	PDA
Collie	PDA
Doberman pinscher	ASD
English bulldog	PS, VSD, TET, MD
English springer spaniel	PDA
Fox Terrier	PS
German shepherd	TD, AS, MD, PDA
German shorthair pointer	AS
Golden retriever	AS, TD
Great Dane	AS, MD, TD
Keeshond	TET
Labrador retriever	TD
Maltese	PDA
Miniature schnauzer	PS
Newfoundland	AS
Pomeranian	PDA
Poodles, Toy and Miniature	PDA
Rottweiler	AS
Samoyed	PS, ASD
Scottish Terrier	PS
Shetland sheepdog	PDA
West Highland white terrier	PS
Weimaraner	TD
Yorkshire terrier	PDA

Abbreviations: AS, aortic stenosis; ASD, atrial septal defect; MD, mitral dysplasia; TD, tricuspid dysplasia; PDA, patent ductus arteriosus; PS, pulmonic stenosis; TET, tetralogy of Fallot; VSD, ventricular septal defect.

III. Less common defects include mitral valve dysplasia, atrial septal defect, tricuspid valve dysplasia, cor triatriatum dexter, and mitral stenosis. Rare defects include persistent truncus arteriosus, tricuspid stenosis, right ventricular hypoplasia, double-outlet right ventricle, and transposition of the great vessels.

FELINE

I. Congenital heart disease is less common in cats than in dogs. In general, the diagnostic and therapeutic approach to congenital heart disease in the cat is the same as that in the dog. No consistent sex or breed predilection has been adequately demonstrated for congenital feline cardiac anomalies, although familial tendencies have been reported.

II. The most common congenital heart defects in the cat include malformation of the mitral valve complex, tricuspid valve dysplasia, ventricular septal defect, aortic stenosis, persistent common atrioventricular canal, endocardial fibroelastosis, patent ductus arteriosus, and tetralogy of Fallot.

III. Less common defects include incomplete sac, persistent truncus arteriosus, pulmonic stenosis, atrial septal defect, tricuspid stenosis, and right ventricular hypoplasia. Vascular ring anomalies are not discussed here, since these defects do not usually produce cardiac disease.

INNOCENT (FUNCTIONAL) MURMUR

Not all young dogs and cats with heart murmurs have congenital heart disease. Such innocent, or functional, murmurs are created by mild turbulence within the heart and great vessels and usually disappear by 6 months of age. The following characteristics of innocent murmurs help differentiate them from pathologic murmurs.

I. Innocent murmurs are systolic in timing, usually occurring early in systole, and are of short duration. They are "soft" (i.e., grade III/VI or less in intensity) and often have a low-pitched, vibrating, or musical quality.

II. Innocent murmurs are usually loudest along the left sternal border and poorly transmitted. Their intensity may vary with changes in position, with the phase of respiration, with exercise, and from day to day.

III. The most important characteristic of the innocent murmur is that it is heard in the absence of any other demonstrable evidence of cardiovascular disease (e.g., lack of clinical signs or radiographic abnormalities).

IV. Loud systolic murmurs (grade IV/VI or greater) and diastolic murmurs are indicative of cardiac disease and should prompt further diagnostics.

SPECIFIC DEFECTS

Patent Ductus Arteriosus

Introduction

In fetal circulation, the ductus arteriosus serves to shunt maternally oxygenated blood into the aorta, thereby bypassing the nonfunctional lungs. Shortly after birth several factors contribute to effect closure of the ductus. Pulmonary vascular resistance drops dramatically, vasodilatory prostaglandin levels decrease, and oxygen tension increases, resulting in a marked increase in pulmonary blood flow and vasoconstriction of the ductus. Following closure by vasoconstriction, the ductus is permanently closed by fibrous contracture, which produces the ligamentum arteriosum. Failure of the ductus to close is termed patent ductus arteriosus (PDA) or persistent ductus arteriosus.

Pathophysiology

The consequences of a PDA depend primarily on the diameter of the ductus and the pulmonary vascular resistance.

  I. When pulmonary vascular resistance is normal, blood will shunt from the aorta (high resistance) into the pulmonary circulation (low resistance). Shunting in this fashion is referred to as left-to-right and represents the most common pattern in PDA. When pulmonary vascular resistance increases and exceeds systemic vascular resistance, blood will shunt from the pulmonary artery into the aorta (so-called right-to-left or reversed PDA).
 II. Blood flow through the ductus is also dependent upon ductal diameter. With a small ductus, the volume of blood shunted is restricted and there may be no hemodynamic effects. In cases with a large ductus and significant shunting, one of two major consequences usually occurs. In most cases, volume overloading of the left atrium and left ventricle results in eventual left-sided failure. Infrequently, the excessive pulmonary blood flow induces dramatic increases in pulmonary vascular resistance and shunt reversal.

Diagnosis

  I. Etiology and breed disposition
     Patent ductus arteriosus occurs in both the dog and cat, with higher frequency in the dog.
     A. Females and the following breeds are predisposed:
        1. Miniature poodle
        2. German shepherd
        3. Collie
        4. Pomeranian

      5. Shetland sheep dog

      6. Toy breeds (e.g., Yorkshire terrier)

   B. The defect has been shown to be hereditary in the miniature poodle, transmitted as a polygenic trait.

II. History and clinical signs

   A. Clinical signs are related to the degree of shunting and may range from none to severe congestive heart failure.

   B. Depending on the degree of heart failure, owners may report signs such as cough, labored breathing, exercise intolerance, and collapse. Reports of seizures and cyanosis are suggestive of a right-to-left shunting PDA.

   C. Cats seldom display signs of cardiac failure until decompensation is advanced.

III. Physical examination

   A. Palpation

      1. Water-hammer, or bounding arterial pulses are usually present in animals with left-to-right shunting PDA. This pulse represents a widened pulse pressure secondary to the loss of diastolic pressure through the ductus, and elevation of systolic blood pressure from the volume-overloaded left ventricle. Usually, the larger the ductus (and therefore the shunt), the more prominent the arterial pulse.

      2. In the majority of cases, a precordial thrill can be palpated over the cranial left-heart base. The left apical impulse is prominent. In cases with right-to-left shunting, there is no precordial thrill and the right apical impulse is more prominent.

   B. General

      1. Cyanosis is an important physical finding in animals with right-to-left shunting PDA. Due to the location of the ductus (distal to the arteries supplying the head and forelimbs), cyanosis is limited to the caudal half of the body. This differential cyanosis is best appreciated by examining caudal mucous membranes, although occasionally cyanosis of the skin caudal to the costal arch can be seen.

      2. Polycythemia (PCV > 60) is usually present in cases with right-to-left shunts.

   C. Auscultation

      1. A continuous-type machinery murmur is a hallmark of left-to-right shunting PDA. The murmur is loudest in mid- to late systole, and gradually decreases in intensity through diastole. In some cases, this characteristic murmur is restricted to the cranial left-heart base, and may be missed if auscultation is limited to the apex. The systolic component of the murmur is usually quite prominent at the cardiac apex.

      2. In cases with a right-to-left shunting PDA, there is no murmur associated with the shunt (in these cases blood *flows* through the shunt rather than "squirting"). A split second heart sound is often present in these cases. Rarely, a diastolic murmur of pulmonic insufficiency is present due to pulmonary hypertension. In cases undergoing reversal of a left-to-right shunting PDA, there is initially a loss of the diastolic component of the continuous murmur followed by a loss of the systolic component.

IV. Electrocardiogram
  A. Electrocardiographic abnormalities are present in most cases of PDA. Evidence of left ventricular and left atrial enlargement include the following.
    1. Tall R waves in lead II (greater than 3.0 mV), III, and aVF.
    2. Deep Q waves are often present in leads II, III, and aVF.
    3. The QRS complexes are increased in duration (>80 ms).
    4. The mean electrical axis may be shifted to the left (<40 degrees).
    5. P-mitrale (widened P-wave) is often present.
  B. Animals with pulmonary hypertension may show evidence of right ventricular hypertrophy: Deep S-waves in leads I, II, III, and aVF; right shift of the mean electrical axis (>100 degrees).
  C. Atrial fibrillation and ventricular arrhythmias may occur in association with congestive heart failure.
V. Thoracic radiographs
  The radiographic signs of patent ductus arteriosus (Figs. 12-1 and 12-2) vary considerably with the volume of blood being shunted, the duration of the problem, and the degree of cardiac decompensation.
  A. Dorsoventral radiographs often reveal three prominences along the left cardiac silhouette.
    1. The aneurysmal bulge of the aortic arch
    2. The enlarged pulmonary outflow tract
    3. The enlarged left atrium
  B. Mild-to-moderate left ventricular and left atrial enlargement is usually present.
  C. Overcirculation of the lung field can often be visualized.
  D. Severe cardiomegaly, pulmonary congestion, and pulmonary edema will be present when there is congestive heart failure.
  E. Right ventricular enlargement and prominent tortuous pulmonary arteries are seen in animals with severe pulmonary hypertension.
VI. Echocardiography
  A. Echocardiographic changes reflect the volume overload state of the left side of the heart and include left atrial dilatation, left ventricular dilata-

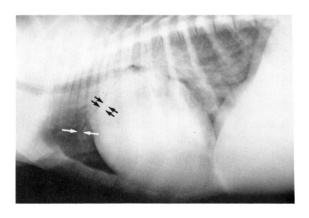

Fig. 12-1. Patent ductus arteriosus (lateral projection). Three month-old poodle. There is generalized heart enlargement, engorgement of the right cranial lobar artery *(white arrows)* and the right cranial lobar vein *(black arrows)*. Vascular engorgement, perivascular congestion and alveolar edema is seen in the caudal lung lobes.

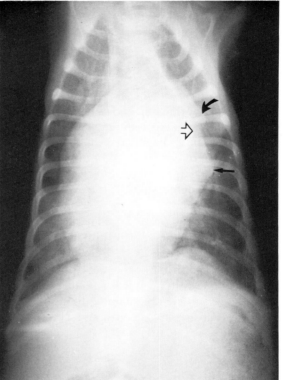

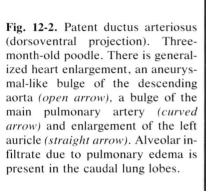

Fig. 12-2. Patent ductus arteriosus (dorsoventral projection). Three-month-old poodle. There is generalized heart enlargement, an aneurysmal-like bulge of the descending aorta *(open arrow)*, a bulge of the main pulmonary artery *(curved arrow)* and enlargement of the left auricle *(straight arrow)*. Alveolar infiltrate due to pulmonary edema is present in the caudal lung lobes.

tion, and normal-to-excessive wall motions (fractional shortening). In some cases the ductus can be visualized.

B. Shunting of blood through the ductus can often be detected by Doppler echocardiography.

C. In cases where pulmonary hypertension with reversed-shunting right ventricular hypertrophy is evident, as well as enlargement of the main pulmonary artery, Doppler echocardiography will reveal pulmonic insufficiency.

D. Contrast echocardiography can be used to confirm the presence of a right-to-left shunting PDA. In this technique, agitated saline is injected into a peripheral vein during echocardiographic examination (first injection) and abdominal aorta imaging (second injection) to detect right-to-left shunting of blood. The absence of intracardiac shunting with the presence of microbubbles within the descending aorta is diagnostic of reversed PDA.

VII. Cardiac catheterization and angiocardiography are rarely needed to confirm the diagnosis of patent ductus arteriosus.

A. Selective angiocardiography

The diagnosis of a left-to-right PDA can be made by injecting contrast media into the ascending aorta. The simultaneous filling of the main pulmonary artery and the aorta is diagnostic for patent ductus arteriosus.

Likewise, a main pulmonary artery contrast injection can be used to confirm the diagnosis of a right-to-left shunt (simultaneous filling of main pulmonary artery and aorta).

B. Nonselective angiocardiography

Nonselective angiocardiography is performed by injecting contrast material through a large diameter venous catheter and taking radiographs in quick succession. Nonselective angiocardiography may be used to support the diagnosis of a right-to-left shunting PDA; however, this technique is of no value in the diagnosis of left-to-right shunts.

VIII. Differential diagnosis

Echocardiography and/or angiocardiographic studies may be used to differentiate patent ductus arteriosus from other congenital cardiac defects. Two cardiac defects that can resemble patent ductus arteriosus are as follows.

A. Aorticopulmonary window

A round or oval communication between the aorta and the main pulmonary artery close to their origin from the heart base. This rare defect usually results in severe pulmonary hypertension.

B. Concurrent aortic stenosis and insufficiency

The systolic murmur of aortic stenosis and the diastolic murmur of aortic insufficiency combine to mimic the machinery murmur of PDA. Echocardiography is usually used to confirm this diagnosis.

Therapy and Prognosis

I. Surgery

As discussed above, several deleterious effects are to be expected in cases with uncorrected PDA. In addition, dogs with long-standing PDA are predisposed to the development of bacterial endocarditis. Therefore, every effort should be made to ligate left-to-right shunting PDA cases.

A. In asymptomatic animals with left-to-right shunting PDA, surgical ligation of the ductus should be performed as soon as possible. Current success rates are 95 percent. Recent studies have shown asymptomatic large dogs and older (>2 years) dogs to have no significant added risk.

B. In cases with mild-to-moderate left-sided heart failure, resolution of pulmonary edema must precede anesthesia and surgery. In cases with severe heart failure, patient stabilization should be attempted; however, these patients are poor anesthetic risks.

C. Correction of patent ductus arteriosus is *contraindicated* when right-to-left shunting is present. Acute right failure and death will occur, as the patent ductus functions as a relief valve for the right ventricle.

II. Medical management

A. In cases deemed unacceptable anesthetic-surgical candidates, medical management of congestive heart failure is indicated (see Ch. 14).

B. There are no drugs currently effective in closing the patent ductus.

PULMONIC STENOSIS

Introduction

Obstruction to the ejection of blood from the right ventricle may occur at the following levels. The latter two types are uncommon.

  I. Valvular (pulmonic valve dysplasia)
 II. Subvalvular
III. Supravalvular

Pathophysiology

  I. The consequences of this defect are in direct proportion to the severity of the obstruction. The major clinical manifestation is right ventricular failure secondary to pressure overload.
 II. Hemodynamically, valvular pulmonic stenosis results in a pressure gradient across the stenotic valve because of resistance to right ventricular outflow. The severity of the lesion is directly related to this pressure gradient. Right ventricular hypertrophy is almost always present; the degree varies with the amount of stenosis.
III. Turbulence associated with the increase in velocity of blood across the stenotic valve is the cause of the poststenotic dilatation in the main pulmonary artery segment.

Diagnosis

  I. Etiology and breed disposition
     Pulmonic stenosis occurs in both the dog and cat
     A. The defect is more common in the following breeds.
        1. English bulldog
        2. Fox terrier
        3. Miniature schnauzer
        4. Chihuahua
        5. Samoyed
        6. Beagle
     B. A polygenic inheritance has been identified in the beagle.
 II. History and clinical signs
     A. Animals with mild or moderate pulmonic stenosis are usually asymptomatic. Many animals may live apparently normal lives with mild degrees of pulmonic stenosis.
     B. Symptomatic animals with pulmonic stenosis have clinical signs of dyspnea and fatigue secondary to low cardiac output. Exercise-induced syncope may occur, because of the limitation in cardiac output imposed by the stenotic valve.
     C. Decompensation and signs of right-heart failure occur when right ven-

tricular output is decreased because of a fall in the contractile state of the right ventricular myocardium.

III. Physical examination
  A. Palpation
     Animals with moderate-to-severe pulmonic stenosis have easily palpable right ventricular impulses. A precordial thrill is usually present at the left lower third or fourth intercostal space. Jugular venous distension and pulsations may be present.
  B. Auscultation
     A systolic crescendo-decrescendo murmur is heard best at the left lower third or fourth intercostal space. If the murmur is severe, it may radiate over the cranial thorax and be audible at the thoracic inlet. A split second heart sound due to delayed closure of the pulmonic valve may also be present.

IV. Electrocardiogram
  A. Signs of right ventricular hypertrophy are present in almost all cases. There are deep S waves present in leads I, II, and III, and a right shift of the mean electrical axis in the frontal plane (>120 degrees).
  B. Arrhythmias are uncommon.

V. Thoracic radiographs
   The primary radiographic features (Figs. 12-3 and 12-4) include the following.
  A. Right ventricular enlargement and right atrial enlargement.
  B. Enlargement of the main pulmonary segment.
  C. Decreased pulmonary vascularity; pulmonary arteries are smaller than normal.

VI. Echocardiography
   Echocardiography has proven to be highly sensitive in the diagnosis and determination of severity of pulmonic stenosis. Characteristic findings include the following.
  A. Right ventricular dilatation and hypertrophy of the right ventricular wall and interventricular septum. Due to increased pressures within the right ventricle the septum is typically flattened.
  B. The right ventricular outflow tract is often dilated and in cases of valvular stenosis the pulmonic valve cusps are thickened and immobile. A poststenotic dilatation of the main pulmonary artery is usually evident.

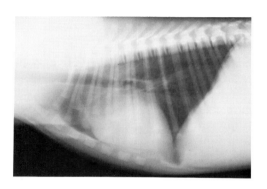

Fig. 12-3. Pulmonic stenosis (lateral projection). Two-month-old mixed breed. There is increased sternal contact of the right heart, due to right-heart enlargement, and normal to slightly diminished pulmonary vasculature.

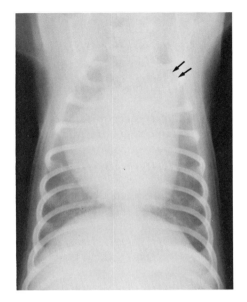

Fig. 12-4. Pulmonic stenosis (dorsoventral projection). Two-month-old mixed breed. There is marked right-heart enlargement and prominence of the main pulmonary artery *(arrows)*.

C. Doppler echocardiography provides a very sensitive and noninvasive method of determining the severity of the stenosis. The velocity of blood (ms) through the stenosis, measured by Doppler echocardiography, provides a very reliable measure of the pressure gradient of the stenosis. The pressure gradient (in mmHg) can be readily derived with the equation

$$4 \times (\text{maximum velocity})^2$$

VII. Other diagnostic techniques

Cardiac catheterization may be used to confirm the diagnosis of pulmonic stenosis, although this procedure is usually unnecessary since the advent of echocardiography. Cardiac catheterization and angiography are occasionally used when multiple cardiac defects are suspected.

VIII. Differential diagnosis

A. Atrial septal defect: The volume overload placed on the right ventricle by a left-to-right shunting atrial septal defect may result in a systolic ejection murmur over the pulmonic valve. Such murmurs are usually softer than those associated with pulmonic stenosis.

B. Innocent or physiological murmurs: These murmurs are usually much softer than typical pulmonic stenosis murmurs and do not typically persist beyond 6 months of age.

Therapy and Prognosis

The need for treatment and the prognosis are dependent upon the severity of the defect as determined by Doppler echocardiography or cardiac catheterization. Cases with mild stenosis (<30 mmHg; ejection velocity <2.7 m/s) do not require treatment and have a favorable prognosis. Those with severe stenosis (>70 mmHg;

ejection velocity >4.2 m/s) are candidates for surgery or balloon valvuloplasty, and have a poor prognosis if uncorrected. Intermediate cases should be followed to monitor for progression of the stenosis.

   I. Surgery
     A. The method of surgical correction depends on the type of stenosis present and its severity.
     B. Supraventricular PS may be palliated by circumventing the stenosis with a conduit.
     C. Repair of valvular or discrete subvalvular PS can be accomplished by pulmonary arterotomy (using inflow occlusion). The patch graft technique is effective in young animals with valvular PS. The bistoury technique or the modified Brock's procedure have also been used effectively.
  II. Balloon Valvuloplasty
     A. Balloon valvuloplasty, an alternative to surgical correction, has recently been introduced in veterinary medicine. In this procedure a special cardiac catheter is guided through the stenotic valve and a balloon situated at the end of the catheter is inflated, effectively enlarging the valve diameter. A number of veterinary institutions have balloon valvuloplasty capabilities.
     B. Generally, balloon valvuloplasty results in a significant (40 to 60 percent) decrease in the pressure gradient. Long-term effects have not been reported at this time in the veterinary literature, but it appears this technique is a viable option to surgical intervention.
 III. Medical management
    Signs of right-sided congestive heart failure should be treated as described in Chapter 14.

AORTIC STENOSIS

Introduction

   I. Anatomy
     A. Aortic stenosis is a narrowing or reduction of the left ventricular outflow tract dimensions at the subvalvular (fibrous ring or muscular), valvular, or supravalvular level.
     B. The subvalvular form (subaortic stenosis) is the most common form in the dog. In this defect, a fibrous band or ring located just below the aortic semilunar valves impedes left ventricular emptying.
     C. The supravalvular type is the most common form in the cat.
  II. Pathophysiology
     A. Stenosis of the left ventricular outflow tract forces a pressure overload on the left ventricle. The left ventricle responds to this chronic pressure overload by undergoing hypertrophy.
     B. As blood is forced through the stenotic area, its velocity increases, resulting in turbulent flow, a systolic ejection murmur, and a poststenotic dilatation of the aorta. The velocity of blood through the lesion is directly proportional to the degree of stenosis.

   C. Left ventricular hypertrophy places a higher oxygen demand on the heart. Myocardial hypertrophy, decreased capillary density, and increased wall tension all contribute to produce myocardial hypoxia.

   D. These cases are prone to sudden death, presumably from fatal ventricular arrhythmias induced by hypoxia. Infrequently, left-sided heart failure develops. These cases also are prone to the development of infective endocarditis.

Diagnosis

  I. Etiology and breed predisposition
    A. A polygenic inheritance has been identified in the Newfoundland.
    B. Other common breeds include the following:
      1. Golden retriever
      2. Rottweiler
      3. German shepherd
      4. Boxer
  II. History and clinical signs
    A. In mild-to-moderately affected cases, there are often no clinical signs, and the suspicion of aortic stenosis is made when a murmur is detected during routine examination.
    B. In severe cases, owners may report failure to thrive, exercise intolerance, collapse, and labored breathing. In some cases, the first clinical sign is sudden death.
 III. Physical examination
    A. Palpation
      Animals with aortic stenosis have easily palpable left ventricular impulses and those with severe stenosis usually have a palpable precordial thrill over the aortic valve area. Femoral pulses are often weak.
    B. Auscultation
      Aortic stenosis is manifested by a systolic ejection-type murmur heard best over the left fourth intercostal space at the level of the costochondral junction (aortic valve area). Frequently, the murmur radiates up the carotid artery and can be auscultated in the mid-cervical area. Occasionally, the murmur may be loudest in the right third or fourth intercostal space midway up the thorax. Rarely, a concurrent diastolic murmur of aortic insufficiency may be present.
 IV. Electrocardiogram
    A. The ECG may be normal.
    B. There may be evidence of left ventricular hypertrophy (tall R waves in lead II [greater than 3.0 mV], III, and aVF).
    C. Ventricular or supraventricular arrhythmias are occasionally detected.
  V. Thoracic radiographs
    A. Radiographic changes tend to parallel severity of the stenosis. Character-

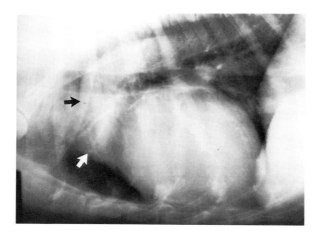

Fig. 12-5. Aortic stenosis (lateral projection). There is marked enlargement of the aortic arch cranial to the heart base *(arrows)*.

istic features include enlargement of the aortic arch (poststenotic dilatation) and left ventricle (Figs. 12-5 and 12-6).
    B. Left atrial enlargement will be present in advanced cases with concurrent mitral insufficiency.
  VI. Echocardiography
    A. Echocardiography is the most sensitive noninvasive method to diagnose and grade subaortic stenosis.
    B. This technique provides visualization of the defect and of secondary car-

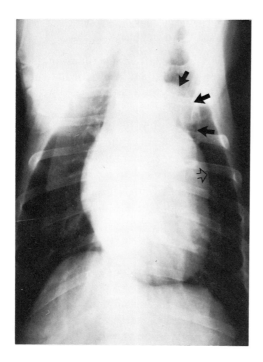

Fig. 12-6. Aortic stenosis (dorsoventral projection). The enlarged aortic arch extends craniolateral to the heart base *(arrows)*. The left auricle *(open arrow)* extends beyond the cardiac border, and there is slight left ventricular enlargement.

diac changes. In most cases, there is significant left ventricular hypertrophy. In severe or advanced cases the papillary muscles become hyperechoic (bright) secondary to calcium deposition.
C. Doppler echocardiography allows determination of the velocity of blood flow through the defect and provides reliable data regarding severity. The grading system is as for pulmonic stenosis.

VII. Cardiac catheterization
A. Cardiac catheterization may be used to confirm the diagnosis, although this procedure is usually unnecessary since the advent of echocardiography. Cardiac catheterization and angiography are occasionally used when multiple cardiac defects are suspected.
B. Angiography will illustrate the stenosis and poststenotic dilatation. Pressure measurements obtained during selective catheterization are used to determine the gradient across the stenosis. Unlike echocardiography, general anesthesia is required and has been shown to significantly lower pressure gradients.

Therapy and Prognosis

I. Surgery
A. There are several surgical techniques used to relieve left ventricular obstruction. There are only a limited number of institutions currently performing these techniques due to their complexity, special equipment requirements, and expense.
B. Surgery is not indicated for cases with mild stenosis (low gradients). Surgery should be considered for those cases with severe stenosis (>100 mmHg; ejection velocity >5 m/s) without evidence of irreversible myocardial damage.

II. Balloon dilatation
A. As in pulmonic stenosis, balloon valvuloplasty may be effective in alleviating outflow obstruction. This technique has much less morbidity than corrective surgery, since it requires insertion of an arterial catheter rather than a thoracotomy.
B. Studies have documented significant reductions in pressure gradients immediately following balloon dilatation. Although short-term (2 to 3 months) effects are favorable, long-term success is unknown.

III. Medical management
A. Beta-blockers (propranolol, atenolol) are used to reduce myocardial oxygen demands. They are probably of some benefit in reducing the frequency of arrhythmias.
B. Antibiotics should be administered when bacteremia is suspected or likely (e.g., dental procedures) to reduce the chance of endocarditis developing.
C. Treatment with various cardiac drugs, diuretics, low-salt diets, and rest is usually of minimal benefit in those severe cases that have developed congestive heart failure.

VENTRICULAR SEPTAL DEFECT

Introduction

I. Anatomy
   A. The interventricular septum separates the left ventricle and right ventricle. It is muscular at the apex, and tapers to a membranous portion at the heart base near the origin of the aorta. Septal defects may occur in any area of the septum, but are most commonly located in the membranous portion.
   B. Ventricular septal defects may occur as isolated defects, may coexist with concurrent defects (e.g., PDA and atrial septal defect), or may be a component of complex cardiac anomalies.
II. Pathophysiology
   There are two major factors that determine the consequences of a ventricular septal defect, the size of the defect and the relative pressures (or resistances) of the ventricles.
   A. Small defects may be of no hemodynamic significance, although they may predispose the animal to the development of endocarditis. In some cases, small defects close spontaneously. Moderately sized defects may allow significant shunting and do produce clinical signs. Very large defects may create a functional single ventricle with equilibration of left and right ventricular pressures.
   B. When left and right ventricular pressures are normal, blood will shunt left-to-right as the left ventricular systolic pressure is roughly 5 times greater than right ventricular systolic pressure. In the typical VSD (left-to-right shunting membranous defect), most of the blood is shunted into the right ventricular outflow tract or main pulmonary artery. This creates a large volume overload to the pulmonary circulation, the left atrium, and left ventricle. When pulmonary resistance remains relatively normal, the right ventricle is spared most of the effects of the shunting.
   C. If right ventricular resistance increases (e.g., pulmonic stenosis, pulmonary hypertension) right ventricular pressure will increase proportionally, thereby decreasing the shunt volume. If right ventricular pressure increases to a point where it exceeds left ventricular pressure, blood will shunt right-to-left and signs of cyanosis may develop.

Diagnosis

I. Etiology and breed predisposition
   A. Breed studies in the Keeshond have shown the defect to be polygenic.
   B. The English bulldog appears to have a higher incidence than other breeds, but the defect is seen in many purebred and mixed breed dogs.
   C. Breed incidence in the cat has not been determined.
II. History and clinical signs
   The clinical course of animals with ventricular septal defect is variable and to a large extent dependent upon the size of the defect and the ventricular

pressures. Small defects may cause little or no functional disturbances and may cause no clinical signs. Moderate-to-large defects usually produce signs of left-sided failure subsequent to the chronic left-sided volume overload. In cases that develop pulmonary hypertension, signs of of right-sided failure will predominate.

III. Physical examination
 A. Palpation
   In many cases, a precordial thrill is present at the right-heart base (third to fourth intercostal spaces, just above the costochondral junctions). Volume overloading of the left ventricle often accentuates the left-sided impulse. In cases with significant pulmonary hypertension, precordial thrills are unusual and the right apical impulse is accentuated.
 B. Auscultation
   1. Typically, the murmur is harsh, holosystolic, and heard best at the right sternal border, second through fourth intercostal spaces. Small defects may result in early systolic murmurs only, whereas larger defects produce holosystolic murmurs.
   2. A murmur of functional pulmonic stenosis may be heard over the pulmonic valve area. This is due to the extra volume of blood passing through the pulmonic valve and not to a structural valve problem.
   3. A split second heart sound occasionally is present due to slightly prolonged right ventricular ejection time.
   4. When the defect causes destabilization of an aortic valve cusp, a diastolic murmur of aortic insufficiency may be present in addition to the systolic murmur. This combination is referred to as to-and-fro murmur and is not a continuous murmur.
   5. In cases with progressive pulmonary hypertension, elevations in right ventricular resistance result in diminished shunting. With very large defects and/or severe pulmonary hypertension, a murmur may be absent because of the lack of a pressure differential across the septum.

IV. Electrocardiogram
 A. Electrocardiographic abnormalities usually parallel the degree of hemodynamic compromise.
 B. The ECG may be normal in a small defect.
 C. The ECG may show evidence of left, right, or biventricular enlargement, depending on hemodynamic consequences of the shunt.
 D. Right bundle branch block may also be observed.

V. Thoracic radiographs
 A. Small defects usually do not cause radiographic changes.
 B. Left ventricular enlargement, left atrial enlargement, and increased pulmonary artery prominence are seen with larger defects resulting in significant left-to-right shunting.
 C. Right ventricular enlargement accompanied by prominent tortuous pulmonary arteries may be present in cases of pulmonary hypertension and right-to-left shunting.

VI. Echocardiography
 A. The diagnosis of VSD can usually be confirmed by routine echocardiography. Typical findings include left ventricular and left atrial dilatation,

and a loss of the interventricular septum. It is important to distinguish the septal dropout normally present in the membranous septum from a ventricular septal defect. In most VSD cases, the interventricular septum is slightly blunted just apical to the defect, whereas the septum tapers gradually in normal animals.

   B. Contrast echocardiography will confirm the presence of a right-to-left shunting VSD. Agitated saline is rapidly injected into a peripheral vein, resulting in the appearance of microbubbles (contrast) within the heart. In the absence of a right-to-left shunt, all contrast remains right-sided. In *right-to-left shunting* VSD, microbubbles will be seen traversing the defect.

   C. Doppler echocardiography will confirm the shunting of blood through the defect.

VII. Other diagnostic procedures
   Cardiac catheterization and angiography may be used to confirm the diagnosis of VSD. As with other congenital defects, the use of cardiac catheterization has decreased with the availability of echocardiography. Determination of oxygen saturation of blood from each chamber may be used to confirm shunting. Left-to-right shunts produce a "step-up" in oxygen saturation in the right ventricle compared to the right atrium.

Therapy and Prognosis

The prognosis and need for therapy are dependent upon the severity of the defect. With small defects, spontaneous closure may occur within the first 2 years of life. Indications for surgical intervention include a large septal defect, the presence of clinical signs, or a calculated shunt ratio of 3:1 or greater.

   I. Surgery
   Open heart techniques have been used with reasonable success. Although curative, these techniques are only available at a very limited number of locations and often prohibitively expensive. Reduction of the shunt can be accomplished by pulmonary artery banding, a technique resulting in elevation of the right ventricular systolic pressure. As right ventricular pressure increases, the shunt volume decreases, and the pulmonary circulation is spared the deleterious effects of chronic volume overload.

  II. Medical management
   In patients where surgical correction or palliation is not an option, medical management of congestive heart failure may be required. Treatment should be tailored to the type and degree of failure (see Ch. 14). Animals with VSD should receive antibiotic prophylaxis prior to procedures likely to produce bacteremia (e.g., dental cleaning).

 III. Prognosis
   Prognosis is excellent for animals with small defects or for those with surgically corrected defects. Cases with moderate-to-large defects have a variable clinical course and prognosis, depending on shunt volume and pulmonary artery effects.

TETRALOGY OF FALLOT

Introduction

I. Tetralogy of Fallot is the most common cyanosis-producing defect and results from a combination of pulmonic stenosis, high ventricular septal defect, right ventricular hypertrophy, and varying degrees of dextroposition and overriding of the aorta.

II. The right ventricular hypertrophy is secondary to the obstruction in right ventricular outflow. The pulmonic stenosis compartment may be valvular, infundibular, or both.

Pathophysiology

I. The hemodynamic consequences of tetralogy of Fallot depend primarily on the severity of the pulmonic stenosis and the ventricular septal defect.

II. The direction and magnitude of the shunt through the septal defect is dependent upon the degree of right ventricular obstruction. If the pulmonic stenosis is mild and right ventricular pressures are only modestly elevated, blood will shunt primarily from left to right. Pathophysiologically, these cases are similar to VSD cases with pulmonary artery banding (i.e., the mild right ventricular obstruction protects the right ventricle from excessive shunting).

III. When pulmonic stenosis is severe, the elevated right ventricular pressures will result in right-to-left shunting. Consequences include reduced pulmonary blood flow (resulting in fatigue and shortness of breath) and generalized cyanosis (resulting in polycythemia and weakness).

IV. Due to the shunting of venous blood into the aorta and consequent hypoxia, the kidneys are stimulated to release erythropoietin. Chronic elevations in erythropoietin result in polycythemia. The increased blood viscosity associated with polycythemia can have significant hemodynamic effects, producing sludging of blood and poor capillary perfusion. Animals with severe polycythemia often have a history of seizures.

Diagnosis

I. Etiology and breed predisposition
   A. Breeds predisposed to tetralogy of Fallot include the Keeshond, English bulldog, miniature poodle, miniature schnauzer, and wire-haired fox terrier. This defect has been recognized in other breeds, and in cats.
   B. In the Keeshond, a polygenic trait has been found.

II. History and clinical signs
   Typical historical features include stunted growth, exercise intolerance, cyanosis, collapse, and seizure activity.

III. Physical examination
   A. Palpation

A precordial thrill may be felt in the third left intercostal space, near the costochondral junction.

  B. Auscultation

In most cases, a murmur of pulmonic stenosis is present. The intensity of the murmur is attenuated when severe polycythemia is present.

IV. Electrocardiogram
  A. A right ventricular enlargement pattern is usually present.
  B. Arrhythmias are not usually present.

V. Thoracic radiographs
  A. Variable right-heart enlargement is present.
  B. Pulmonary vessels are undersized, and the main pulmonary artery is often diminished.

VI. Echocardiography
  A. Echocardiography will confirm the diagnosis. Evident are malposition of the aortic root, right ventricular hypertrophy, and ventricular septal defect.
  B. Routine contrast echocardiography will demonstrate right-to-left shunting at the level of the VSD. Flow through the defect can also be determined by Doppler echocardiography.

VII. Cardiac catheterization
  A. Selective angiocardiography of the right ventricle demonstrates simultaneous filling of the aorta and pulmonary artery in cases with right-to-left shunts.
  B. Nonselective angiocardiography may support a diagnosis of tetralogy of Fallot, but this technique is much less sensitive than echocardiography.

Therapy and Prognosis

I. Surgery
  A. Surgical correction of tetralogy of Fallot is uncommonly performed because of the attendant mortality and expense. Palliative surgical options include the Blalock anastomosis and the Potts anastomosis. In the Blalock anastomosis, the left subclavian artery is anastomosed with the pulmonary artery in order to increase pulmonary blood flow. The Potts anastomosis consists of a side-to-side anastomosis of the aorta and pulmonary artery. These procedures are generally effective in reducing signs of pulmonary hypoperfusion and systemic hypoxia.
  B. In some cases, palliation can be provided by reducing pulmonic stenosis. Surgical valvuloplasty or balloon valvuloplasty are options.

II. Medical management
  A. Beta-adrenergic blockade has been used to reduce the dynamic component of right ventricular outflow obstruction, and to attenuate beta-adrenergic–mediated decreases in systemic vascular resistance. Increases in systemic vascular resistance will lower the magnitude of right-to-left shunting.
  B. Polycythemia should be controlled by periodic phlebotomy. When the PCV exceeds 68, intervention is indicated. Up to 20 ml/kg of blood can be re-

moved and replaced with a crystalloid solution, such as lactated Ringers or saline.

Mitral Valve Dysplasia

Introduction

Congenital malformation of the mitral valve complex (mitral valve dysplasia) is a common congenital cardiac defect in the cat. In addition, several canine breeds are predisposed: bull terrier, German shepherd, and Great Dane.

I. Anatomy
   A. Mitral valve dysplasia results in mitral insufficiency and systolic regurgitation of blood into the left atrium.
   B. Any component of the mitral valve complex (valve leaflet, chordea tendineae, papillary muscles) may be malformed. Often, more than one component is defective.
II. Pathophysiology
   A. Malformation of the mitral valve complex results in significant valvular insufficiency. Chronic mitral regurgitation leads to a volume overload to the left heart, which results in dilation of the left ventricle and atrium.
   B. When mitral regurgitation is severe, cardiac output decreases resulting in signs of cardiac failure.
   C. Dilatation of the left-sided chambers predisposes affected animals to arrhythmias.
   D. In some cases, malformation of the mitral valve complex causes a degree of valvular stenosis as well as insufficiency.

Diagnosis

I. History and clinical signs
   Clinical signs correlate with the severity of the defect. Affected animals usually display signs of left-sided heart failure including weakness, cough, and exercise intolerance.
II. Physical examination
   A. Palpation: affected animals may have a precordial thrill over the left cardiac apex.
   B. Auscultation: a holosytolic murmur of mitral regurgitation is prominent at the left cardiac apex. A diastolic heart sound (gallop rhythm) is present in some cases.
III. Electrocardiogram
   A. Atrial arrhythmias (APCs, atrial fibrillation) are common.
   B. Evidence of left atrial enlargement (widened P-waves) and left ventricular enlargement may be present.

IV. Thoracic radiographs

The most prominent abnormality is severe left atrial enlargement. Left ventricular enlargement is also present. Pulmonary veins are congested.

V. Echocardiography

A. Echocardiography demonstrates malformation of the mitral valve complex (fused chordae tendineae and thickened immobile valve leaflets) and left atrial and ventricular dilatation.

B. Doppler echocardiography demonstrates severe mitral regurgitation. If present, mitral stenosis can be identified.

Therapy and Prognosis

Prognosis for the affected animal with clinical signs is poor. Mildly affected animals may remain free of clinical signs for several years. Therapy for progressive left-sided heart failure is detailed in Chapter 14.

SUGGESTED READINGS

Birchard SJ, Bonagura JD, Fingland RB: Results of ligation of patent ductus arteriosus: 201 dogs (1969–1988). J Am Vet Med Assoc 196:2011, 1990

Bonagura JD: Congenital heart disese. p. 976. In Ettinger SJ (ed): Textbook of Veterinary Internal Medicine. 3rd Ed. WB Saunders, Philadelphia, 1989

Brownlie SE, Cobb MA, Chambers J, et al: Percutaneous balloon valvuloplasty in four dogs with pulmonic stenosis. J Sm Anim Prac 32:165, 1991

Cooper RC, Weber WJ, Goodwin JK: Symposium: The treatment of congenital heart defects. Part III: The surgical treatment of congenital heart defects. Vet Med 87(7):676, 1992

Goodwin JK, Lombard CW: Patent ductus arteriosus in adult dogs: Clinical features of 14 cases. J Am Anim Hosp Assoc 28:349, 1992

Jacobs G, Mahaffey M, Rawlings CA: Valvular pulmonic stenosis in four Boykin spaniels. J Am Anim Hosp Assoc 26:246, 1990

Moise NS: Doppler echocardiographic evaluation of congenital cardiac disease—an introduction. J Vet Int Med 3:195, 1989

Orton EC, Bruecker KA, McCracken TO: An open patch-graft technique for correction of pulmonic stenosis in the dog. Vet Surg 19:148, 1990

13

Cardiovascular Disorders in Systemic Diseases

Francis W. K. Smith, Jr.
John V. Cali, Jr.
Philip R. Fox

INTRODUCTION

Many systemic diseases produce associated disorders of cardiovascular structure and function (Table 13-1). The veterinarian may detect cardiovascular abnormalities as the predominant clinical sign, or systemic disease manifestations may overshadow cardiac abnormalities. Although cardiovascular disease may sometimes be of no clinical significance, at other times it may constitute the major medical concern. Detection of cardiovascular involvement may be based on clinical signs, radiographic changes, electrocardiographic or echocardiographic abnormalities, and laboratory findings. Emphasis will be given to diseases having the greatest cardiovascular effects or incidence in practice. The focus of discussion will be the cardiovascular effects and their treatment.

ENDOCRINE DISEASES

HYPERTHYROIDISM

Overview

I. Hyperthyroidism is the most common systemic disturbance to affect cardiac function in cats and is rare in dogs. Hyperthyroid heart disease can be a severe problem, leading to heart failure in some animals.
II. Hyperthyroidism is a disease of middle-aged to geriatric cats (range, 4 to 22 years; mean, 13 years) that is generally caused by a thyroid adenoma. Clinical evidence of thyrotoxic heart disease is unusual before the age of 7 years. Dogs generally develop nonfunctional thyroid adenocarcinomas.

Cardiac Pathophysiology

I. Direct effects of thyroid hormone
   A. Positive inotropic effects result from an increased Na^+-K^+ ATPase activity, increased mitochondrial protein synthesis, and increased synthesis

TABLE 13-1. CLASSIFICATION OF
IMPORTANT SYSTEMIC DISORDERS
THAT AFFECT THE HEART

Endocrine
    Thyroid gland
        Hyperthyroidism
        Hypothyroidism
    Adrenal gland
        Hyperadrenocorticism
        Hypoadrenocorticism
        Pheochromocytoma
    Pituitary
        Acromegaly (hypersomatatropism)
    Pancreas
        Diabetes mellitus (hyperglycemia)

Metabolic
    Hypercalcemia
    Hypocalcemia
    Hyperkalemia
    Hypokalemia
    Hypoglycemia
    Uremia
    Anemia

Neoplastic and infiltrative heart diseases

Physical and chemical agents
    Hyperpyrexia (heat stroke)
    Hypothermia
    Carbon monoxide
    Toad poisoning
    Oleander toxicity
    Chocolate (theobromine) toxicity
    Doxorubricin cardiotoxicity

Infectious inflammatory myocardial diseases
    Bacterial (Lyme disease)
    Viral (parvovirus)
    Mycotic
    Protozoal (trypanosomiasis)

Miscellaneous
    Systemic lupus erythematosis (SLE)
    Neurologic disease
    Gastric dilatation-volvulus (GDV)
    Pancreatitis

and enhanced contractile properties of myosin. Thyroid hormone favors the production of the alpha heavy chain myosin isoenzyme, which has the fastest ATPase activity. Thyroid hormone increases the number of slow calcium channels, improving the recycling of calcium by the sarcoplasmic reticulum. Systolic and diastolic performance are both altered.
  B. Positive chronotropic effects result from an increased rate of sinoatrial firing, decreased threshold of atrial activation, and shortened refractory period of the conduction tissue. The effect on atrial activation may increase the risk for atrial arrhythmias.
II. Indirect effects of thyroid hormone
  A. The effect of thyroid hormone on the adrenergic system is controversial. The number of myocardial B-adrenergic receptors and their affinity are

increased in hyperthyroid animals. However, this does not always explain or result in an increased responsiveness to catecholamines. Postreceptor effects of thyroid hormone are postulated. Circulating catecholamine levels are normal.

B. Hyperthyroidism results in an increased metabolic rate, and consequently an increased tissue oxygen demand. The need for increased tissue perfusion and oxygen delivery requires greater cardiac output. Peripheral vasodilation increases tissue perfusion and decreases afterload. As blood volume increases, increased venous return to the heart and increased preload result. The combination of increased preload, increased contractility, increased heart rate, and decreased afterload results in increased cardiac output. Chronic volume overload and high metabolic rate can result in heart failure even though the cardiac output is still greater than normal. This is referred to as high-output heart failure.

C. Hypertension is a frequent sequela of hyperthyroidism in cats, with one study showing an incidence of 87 percent. This occurs inspite of peripheral vasodilation, and probably reflects the increased stroke volume and heart rate in these animals. Increasing stroke volume and heart rate increases cardiac output. Blood pressure is a function of cardiac output and systemic vascular resistance.

D. The combination of volume and pressure overload alters myocardial protein synthesis and degradation, which results in myocardial hypertrophy and chamber dilation. These changes are most notable in the left heart. In rare cases, hyperthyroid cats with congestive heart failure develop a cardiomyopathy of overload that resembles dilated cardiomyopathy.

E. The net effects of hyperthyroidism on the cardiovascular system are increased cardiac contractility, increased heart rate, cardiomegaly, left ventricular hypertrophy, increased cardiac output, systemic hypertension, and occasionally high-output heart failure.

Diagnosis

I. History and physical examination
   A. Historical findings and clinical signs include weight loss, polyphagia, unkempt coat, polydipsia, diarrhea, nervousness, hyperactivity, vomiting, tremor, polyuria, lethargy, aggression, decreased appetite, weakness, episodic panting, and bulky, foul-smelling stool.
   B. Cardiovascular abnormalities that may be present on physical examination include tachycardia, premature heart beats, gallop rhythm, cardiac murmur, and muffled heart sounds.
   C. Noncardiac findings can include thinness, palpable thyroid gland, hyperactivity, dehydration, cachectic, easily stressed, small kidneys, depression, weakness, and ventral flexion of the neck.

II. Electrocardiography
   A. ECG findings in hyperthyroid cats are sinus tachycardia (34 percent), right bundle branch block (9 percent), tall R waves in lead II (7 percent), left anterior fascicular block (3 percent), ventricular premature complexes (3

percent), incomplete AV block (3 percent), and atrial premature complexes (2 percent).
   B. Sinus tachycardia and increased R wave voltage resolve with treatment of hyperthyroidism. APCs and VPCs may decrease in frequency or become abolished. Conduction disturbances may or not resolve. If arrhythmias or R wave amplitude changes persist after hyperthyroidism is controlled, idiopathic cardiomyopathy should be ruled out.
III. Radiography
   A. Moderate-to-severe cardiomegaly is seen in 40 percent of cases.
   B. Evidence of congestive heart failure (pulmonary edema or pleural effusion) is reported in 11 percent of cases.
IV. Echocardiography
   A. Common findings in hyperthyroidism include an increased left atrium: aorta ratio (LA:Ao), left ventricular wall hypertrophy, septal hypertrophy, left atrial dilatation, increased aortic amplitude, increased posterior wall amplitude, and increased fractional shortening.
   B. Hyperthyroid cats presenting in congestive heart failure may show evidence of left ventricular hypertrophy, left atrial dilation, regional hypokinesis, or, occasionally, eccentric left ventricular hypertrophy.
V. Clinical pathology
   A. Elevated serum values for alkaline phosphatase, lactate dehydrogenase, aspartate transaminase, and alanine transaminase can be recorded.
   B. Mild azotemia is present in approximately 25 percent of cases.
   C. T_4 and T_3 values are usually elevated. However, thyroid hormone levels fluctuate during the day and may dip into the normal range in mildly hyperthyroid animals.
VI. Specialized diagnostic tests
   A. Additional diagnostic tests may occasionally be needed to confirm hyperthyroidism in cats with normal resting T_4 values.
   B. T_3 suppression test
      1. Administer T_3 at 25 μg per cat PO TID for seven doses. Collect blood for a T_4 determination prior to the first dose of T_3 and 2 to 4 hours after the last dose.
      2. A normal cat's T_4 level will suppress to less than 20 nmol/L (~1.5 mg/dL); a hyperthyroid cat's T_4 level will remain above this value. T_3 values can be measured concurrently to assess owner compliance. T_3 values should rise regardless of the cat's thyroid status.
   C. TRH response test
      1. To perform the TRH response test, inject 0.1 mg/kg of TRH and obtain blood samples before and 4 hours after TRH injection.
      2. In normal cats, the post-TRH T_4 is at least 60 percent greater than baseline. A hyperthyroid cat's T_4 levels change less than 50 percent following TRH administration.
      3. The TRH response test takes less time to perform than the T_3 suppression test and does not depend on the owner's ability to medicate the cat. TRH can cause vomiting, salivation, tachypnea, and defecation following the injection. TRH is substantially more expensive than T_3.
   D. Thyroid imaging with radioactive technetium 99m will identify the affected

gland(s). This imaging study is recommended prior to surgery in any hyperthyroid cat with nonpalpable thyroid glands, because the thyroid glands can migrate into the chest, rendering them inoperable.

Therapy

I. Management of hyperthyroidism
   A. Medical management
      1. Administer methimazole (Tapazole) at 5 mg PO TID. Propylthiouracil (PTU) is rarely used because of a high incidence of side effects. These drugs inhibit the formation of thyroid hormones, but do not inhibit or block the release of already formed T_3 and T_4. Therefore, serum thyroid levels do not drop acutely.
      2. Inorganic iodine therapy is rarely used. Iodine blocks thyroid hormone synthesis and release, and thyroid levels rapidly drop. Rapid reduction of thyroid levels may benefit patients with severe congestive heart failure. Pre-operative use may decrease the vascularity of the thyroid gland. Administer one dose of methimazole prior to the iodine, so that the iodine is not incorporated into new thyroid hormone. Administer one drop of saturated solution of potassium iodide orally once a day for 7 to 10 days.
   B. Surgical treatment effectively cures the condition and eliminates the need for chronic medication. Medical management generally is instituted to stabilize the patient prior to surgery. The most frequent complication of surgery is transient postoperative hypocalcemia.
   C. Radioactive iodine also cures the condition and does not require anesthesia or surgery.
II. Management of arrhythmias
   A. The expedient way to manage tachyarrhythmias is to start methimazole therapy. Even before euthyroidism is restored, many arrhythmias improve or are abolished. In this fashion, ancillary therapy is usually unnecessary.
   B. Severe tachyarrhythmias (i.e., atrial tachycardia, multiform VPCs, ventricular tachycardia) in patients without heart failure are best managed with beta-blockers such as propranolol (2.5 to 7.5 mg TID) or atenolol (3.125 to 6.25 mg SID). Higher than normal doses of beta-blockers may be needed because of an increased rate of metabolism and elimination. Supraventricular arrhythmias in asthmatic cats should be managed with diltiazem (1.5 to 2.5 mg/kg TID).
   C. Supraventricular arrhythmias in patients with congestive heart failure can be managed with digoxin, beta-blockers, or diltiazem. In general, exercise caution when using beta-blockers in the presence of CHF, since these agents depress cardiac contractility and may exacerbate heart failure. Cats with hyperthyroidism almost always have increased contractility, so worsening or CHF with beta blockade is rare. Ideally, congestion should be treated and controlled with diuretics prior to prescribing a beta-blocker. Diltiazem also depresses contractility, but less so than beta-blockers. The

vasodilating effects of diltiazem usually offset its negative inotropic effects.
III. Management of hypertension is usually accomplished with control of the hyperthyroid state. The use of beta-blockers, vasodilators, and other agents is occasionally indicated.
IV. Management of congestive heart failure
   A. Diuretics are used to control pulmonary edema and pleural effusion.
   B. Nitroglycerin ointment can be used in patients with critical congestion, or in those refractory to diuretics alone. Enalapril (Enacard) also may be helpful in refractory cases.
   C. Treat arrhythmias as discussed above.
   D. Digoxin also may be useful in cases where chronic hyperthyroidism results in dilated cardiomyopathy.

Prognosis

I. The prognosis for remission of sinus tachycardia, voltage changes, arrhythmias, and congestive heart failure is generally favorable when the hypermetabolic state is controlled through the medical or surgical techniques discussed.
II. The prognosis is poor if dilated cardiomyopathy has developed secondary to chronic overload of the heart.

HYPOTHYROIDISM

Overview

 I. Hypothyroidism is a common endocrinopathy in dogs and is rarely encountered as a naturally occurring condition in cats.
 II. Hypothyroidism is most commonly diagnosed in middle-aged dogs. Many breeds are affected and there appears to be a breed predilection in the golden retriever, Doberman pinscher, dachschund, Irish setter, miniature schnauzer, Great Dane, poodle and boxer. There is no sex predilection. Hypothyroidism is rare in cats and generally limited to postoperative cases following surgical removal of unilateral or bilateral functional thyroid tumors.
III. The cardiac effects of hypothyroidism are generally the opposite of those found in hyperthyroidism. The cardiac effects of hypothyroidism rarely have severe consequences. However, hypothyroidism can aggravate heart failure and complicate the management of cardiac patients.

Cardiac Pathophysiology

I. Cardiac contractility is decreased as a result of decreased Na^+-K^+ATPase activity, decreased mitochondrial protein synthesis, and decreased synthesis and contractile properties of myosin.

II. Cardiac conduction is decreased as a result of a decreased rate of sinoatrial firing, increased threshold of atrial activation, and prolonged refractory period of the conducting tissue. Enhanced vagal tone in hypothyroidism also slows the heart rate and accentuates sinus arrhythmias. Evaluate the thyroid status in any dog in congestive heart failure with an inappropriately slow heart rate.

III. Thyroid hormone plays an important role in lipid and cholesterol metabolism. Hypothyroidism predisposes animals to increased levels of cholesterol and to a lesser extent, triglycerides. Although rare in dogs, hypercholesterolemia can result in atherosclerosis and myocardial infarction. Lipid abnormalities resolve with thyroid hormone supplementation.

IV. Hypothyroidism decreases the metabolic rate, thus lessening the required cardiac output. Correcting hypothyroidism increases the workload on the heart. This is important to remember when treating animals in congestive heart failure.

V. Hypothyroidism decreases digoxin clearance, predisposing patients to digoxin toxicity.

Diagnosis

I. History and physical examination
   A. Historical findings in hypothyroid animals include alopecia and other dermatologic problems, lethargy, weakness, depression, infertility, and diarrhea.
   B. Cardiovascular abnormalities noted on physical examination can include muffled heart sounds, weak apex heart beat, weak pulses, and bradycardia.
   C. Noncardiac physical findings can include symmetric alopecia, seborrhea, myxedema, pyoderma, hypothermia, depression, and lameness.

II. Electrocardiography
   A. ECG changes in hypothyroidism reflect decreased automaticity of pacemaker tissue and depressed conduction. Changes that reflect decreased automaticity may include sinus bradycardia, pronounced sinus arrhythmia, and atrial and ventricular arrhythmias. Changes that reflect depressed conduction may include AV block, widened QRS complexes, and inverted T waves. The most common findings reported in dogs are sinus bradycardia and inverted T waves.
   B. Low-voltage complexes are frequently seen in hypothyroid animals.
   C. Atrial fibrillation in giant breed dogs occasionally accompanies hypothyroidism, usually in association with dilated cardiomyopathy. Supplementation with thyroid hormone rarely causes conversion to sinus rhythm.

III. Radiographs are generally normal. In the rare instances where hypothyroidism leads to heart failure, there is evidence of cardiomegaly and pulmonary edema.

IV. Echocardiography may reveal mild decreases in indices of cardiac contractility and mild chamber enlargement. Always check thyroid status when depressed contractility is noted in an animal of a breed not predisposed to dilated cardiomyopathy.

V. Clinical pathology
  A. The hemogram may reveal a low-grade nonregenerative anemia.
  B. The most common abnormality on the serum chemistry profile is hypercholesterolemia and, occasionally, hypertriglyceridemia.
  C. A normal serum T_4 value generally is sufficient to rule out hypothyroidism. Unfortunately, a low serum T_4 does not confirm the diagnosis. Concurrent systemic ailments and numerous drugs can cause depressed serum T_4 values in animals with normal thyroid function (euthyroid sick syndrome). To make a diagnosis in these cases requires integration of the history, physical findings, and other blood test results, or confirmation by specialized diagnostic tests.
  D. Serum T_3 values are less reliable than T_4 values at diagnosing hypothyroidism.
VI. Specialized diagnostic tests
  A. Evaluation of free T_4 (fT_4), free T_3 (fT_3), reverse T_3 (rT_3) and autoantibodies to T_3 and T_4 has been used to try and increase diagnostic accuracy. In general, hypothyroid animals will have a low serum T_3, T_4, fT_3, fT_4, and rT_3, and may have increased levels of autoantibodies. The classic pattern in patients with euthyroid sick syndrome is low serum T_3 and T_4, normal fT_3 and fT_4, and increased rT_3. Not all animals follow these patterns.
  B. The TSH response test is currently the gold standard in veterinary medicine for diagnosing hypothyroidism. Animals with hypothyroidism have low baseline T_4 values and fail to increase their T_4 values above a predetermined level following administration of TSH. Animals with euthyroid sick syndrome will also have low baseline T_4 levels, but following TSH administration, their T_4 values will increase above an absolute cutoff value.

Therapy

I. Treatment of hypothyroidism is simple and inexpensive. L-thyroxin is administered at 20 µg/kg PO BID. After 1 month, evaluate a serum T_4 value 4 to 6 hours after a dose of L-thyroxin. If the post-pill T_4 value is normal and clinical signs have resolved, you can try decreasing the frequency to SID. Ideally, a post-pill T_4 value should then be obtained in another month at 4 to 6 and 24 hours after a dose of thyroxin. This is important to make sure that there is an adequate duration of effect with SID dosing.
II. Treatment in patients with congestive heart failure is more complicated. Supplementation will increase the metabolic rate and demand on the heart. If the failing heart is unable to meet these demands, heart failure will worsen. Therefore, implement thyroid hormone supplementation gradually in patients with cardiac disease, especially if they are already in failure. Start with one-fourth of the standard dose and increase it by a quarter-dose weekly.
III. The risk of digoxin toxicity is increased in hypothyroid states. Monitor hypothyroid animals closely for signs of digoxin toxicity, and consider assessing thyroid status in any animal with normal renal function that develops digoxin toxicity on reasonable doses of digoxin.

Prognosis

There are few complications in the treatment of hypothyroidism.

Hypoadrenocorticism (Addison's Disease)

Overview

I. Hypoadrenocorticism is a potentially life-threatening endocrinopathy that is uncommon in dogs and rare in cats. The disease is more common in female dogs and usually occurs in young to middle-aged animals. Approximately 90 percent of cases occur before 7 years of age, with an age range of 6 months to 15 years.

II. Primary hypoadrenocorticism (Addison's disease) results from destruction of the zona glomerulosa and zona fasciculata of the adrenal gland. These areas of the adrenal gland produce aldosterone and cortisol, respectively. Destruction is generally immune mediated, but also can occur secondary to infection, neoplasia, infarction, and drugs such as o,p'-DDD (Lysodren, Mitotane).

III. Secondary hypoadrenocorticism results from decreased production or release of ACTH from the pituitary gland. Secondary adrenal insufficiency may occur following acute withdrawal of long-term, high-dose glucocorticoid therapy resulting from suppression of the hypothalamic-pituitary-adrenal axis. These patients have normal mineralocorticoid activity, so electrolyte values are normal. Cortisol values are depressed.

IV. Adrenal destruction occurs gradually, so basal hormone levels remain normal. It is only when the animal is stressed that the adrenal reserve is inadequate, and signs develop. Eventually, the destruction proceeds to the point that basal hormone levels are depressed and clinical signs are present without stress.

Cardiac Pathophysiology

I. Cardiovascular effects of cortisol
   A. Cortisol is important in maintaining vascular integrity and responsiveness to catecholamines. Cortisol deficiency predisposes animals to hypotension.
   B. Cortisol has a positive inotropic effect on the heart.
   C. Cortisol is important in helping the body deal with stress. This is why so many Addisonian crises follow stress, and why glucocorticoid supplementation must be increased during periods of stress.
II. Cardiovascular effects of aldosterone
   A. Aldosterone acts on the distal renal tubule to enhance sodium retention and potassium elimination. Aldosterone deficiency results in hyponatremia and hyperkalemia.
   B. Hyponatremia decreases plasma osmotic pressure, causing fluid shifts

out of the vascular compartment. This contributes to hypovolemia and
hypotension.

  C. Hyperkalemia alters cardiac conduction, resulting in numerous arrhyth-
     mias. The cardiac effects of hyperkalemia are aggravated by low sodium,
     low calcium, and acidosis.
III. Net cardiovascular effects of hypoadrenocorticism are hypovolemia, sys-
     temic hypotension, altered cardiac conduction, depressed myocardial func-
     tion, and, rarely, heart failure. These changes can be fatal if not rapidly diag-
     nosed and aggressively treated.

Diagnosis

  I. History and physical examination
     A. A history of waxing and waning of clinical signs, with more severe signs
        during periods of stress, generally is present.
     B. Patients often present with history of decreased appetite, vomiting, diar-
        rhea, depression, weakness, and cardiovascular collapse. Hemorrhagic
        vomiting and diarrhea may be the prominent signs in some dogs. Other
        signs include weight loss, polyuria, polydipsia, and shivering.
     C. Transient improvement after intravenous fluid therapy or corticosteroid
        administration followed by subsequent relapse days or weeks later can
        occur.
     D. Findings on physical examination include depression, weakness, dehydra-
        tion, bradycardia, and weak femoral pulses. Hypothermia occurs infre-
        quently.
 II. Electrocardiography (Fig. 13-1)
     A. ECG changes vary with the magnitude of the hyperkalemia and are aggra-
        vated by hyponatremia, hypocalcemia, and acidosis. The following ECG
        findings are seen with experimentally induced hyperkalemia.
        1. Peaking of the T wave with a narrow base is the earliest ECG abnormal-
           ity and may be observed when serum K^+ exceeds 5.7 to 6.0 mEq/L.

A 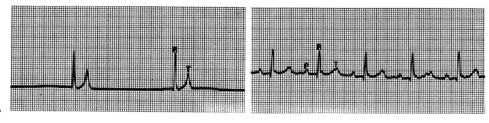 B

Fig. 13-1. (A) Hyperkalemia in a dog in cardiovascular collapse, consistent with an Addisonian crisis. P waves are absent (atrial standstill), and T waves are tall and peaked. Serum
potassium was 8.4 mEq/L. (B) After institution of therapy, P waves are present, and the
T wave is of smaller amplitude. Serum potassium is now 4.8 mEq/L. (From Tilley LP:
Essentials of Canine and Feline Electrocardiography. 3rd Ed. Lea & Febiger, Philadelphia,
1992, with permission.)

2. P wave morphology is altered, its amplitude reduced, intra-atrial conduction delayed, and PR interval prolonged when serum K^+ exceeds 7.0 mEq/L.
3. P waves become unrecognizable (atrial standstill) at plasma K^+ levels greater than 8.5 mEq/L.
4. The QRS widens uniformly at plasma K^+ levels greater than 9 mEq/L.
5. Sinoatrial exit block or junctional rhythms with and without escape complexes may be present.
6. Ventricular fibrillation and ventricular asystole may occur at plasma K^+ levels greater than 10 mEq/L.

B. In clinical cases, ECG changes do not correlate as closely with potassium concentrations as they do in published experimental studies.
C. The rhythm with atrial standstill secondary to hyperkalemia is generally slow and may be regular or irregular. It is a sinoventricular rhythm. The sinus node continues to fire and impulses are transmitted to the AV node and ventricles by internodal pathways. P waves are absent because atrial myocytes are not activated.
D. Hyperkalemia is the most common cause of atrial standstill. Atrial standstill also occurs with fibrous replacement of atrial muscle cells secondary to severe atrial distention (valve disease, cardiomyopathy) in dogs and cats, with cardiac arrest, and secondary to an atrial myopathy in dogs, most commonly seen in English springer spaniels.

III. Radiographs show microcardia and attenuated vasculature. These changes are the result of hypovolemia and rapidly resolve with steroid and volume replacement.

IV. Clinical pathology
A. A low-grade normocytic, normochromic nonregenerative anemia is usually present, but may be masked by the effects of hemoconcentration. Eosinophilia and lymphocytosis may also be present.
B. A serum chemistry profile frequently reveals azotemia, hyponatremia, and hyperkalemia. A sodium:potassium ratio of less than 27 supports hypoadrenocorticism, but is not pathognomonic for the disease. Hypercalcemia and hypoglycemia are not uncommon.
C. Mild-to-moderate metabolic acidosis is common during a crisis.
D. It is unusual for a dog with untreated Addison's disease to have a urine specific gravity greater than 1.030, and it is often less than 1.020.
E. In patients with secondary hypoadrenocorticism, sodium and potassium levels are normal. The other abnormalities described above may be present.

V. Specialized diagnostic tests
A. A tentative diagnosis is frequently obtained from the history and results of the CBC and serum chemistry profile. However, there are numerous causes of hyperkalemia, and acid-base and electrolyte changes associated with severe gastrointestinal disease and renal failure can cause an abnormal sodium:potassium ratio that would erroneously suggest Addison's disease.
B. An ACTH response test is helpful in confirming Addison's disease and essential for documenting secondary hypoadrenocorticism.

Therapy

 I. Addisonian crisis therapy
    A. Patients that present with cardiovascular collapse and atrial standstill re-
       quire aggressive therapy. Therapy is directed at rapidly correcting hypovo-
       lemia, correcting rhythm disturbances, correcting electrolyte imbalances,
       and replacing mineralocorticoids and glucocorticoids.
    B. Volume replacement and correction of hyponatremia and hypochloremia
       is initially achieved with rapid infusion of 0.9 percent saline at 40 to 90
       mL/kg/hr and then modified according to patient needs.
    C. Glucocorticoid deficiency is corrected with either hydrocortisone hemisuc-
       cinate or hydrocortisone phosphate (2 to 4 mg/kg IV QID), prednisolone
       sodium succinate (2 to 4 mg/kg IV QID), or dexamethasone sodium phos-
       phate (1 to 4 mg/kg IV BID). Hydrocortisone is preferred for its mineralo-
       corticoid properties. It should be noted that hydrocortisone and predniso-
       lone interfere with cortisol assays, so ideally should be started after the
       ACTH response test is performed. Dexamethasone has no mineralocorti-
       coid effects and does not interfere with the cortisol assay.
    D. Desoxycorticosterone acetate (DOCA) is no longer commercially avail-
       able, so mineralocorticoid deficiency is initially corrected with hydrocorti-
       sone injections, if available. If hypoadrenocorticism has been documented,
       desoxycorticosterone pivilate (DOCP) at 2.2 mg/kg IM can be adminis-
       tered. Fludrocortisone acetate (Florinef) at 0.02 mg/kg/day can be used as
       soon as vomiting stops (assuming therapy has not been instituted with
       DOCP).
    E. Hyperkalemia is corrected in several different ways
       1. Saline infusion results in rapid dilution of potassium and is often the
          only treatment needed.
       2. Severe hyperkalemia associated with significant cardiac conduction ab-
          normalities often requires more aggressive therapy. Treatment options
          include sodium bicarbonate (1 to 2 mEq/kg) given slowly IV over 5
          minutes *or* a combination of regular insulin (0.5 U/kg IV) and dextrose
          (1 g/kg IV). Dextrose can also be administered alone, as it will stimulate
          endogenous insulin secretion.
    F. If life-threatening cardiac arrhythmias are noted, administer calcium gluco-
       nate (10%) at 0.5 to 1 mL/kg slowly IV over 10 to 15 minutes. Monitor the
       ECG while administering calcium. Calcium will temporarily correct rhythm
       disturbances by countering the effect of potassium on the conduction tis-
       sue. Calcium has no effect on serum potassium levels. Calcium overdose
       can also cause severe cardiac disturbances, so careful monitoring is re-
       quired.
II. Maintenance therapy
    A. Mineralocorticoid replacement is initiated with either fludrocorticosterone
       acetate at 0.02 mg/kg/day given orally or DOCP at 2.2 mg/kg q 25 days given
       IM. These doses–and dose interval for DOCP—are adjusted as needed to
       maintain normal electrolyte balance. DOCP is not commercially available,
       but can be obtained from Ciba-Geigy. Therapy must be individualized to

the patient. A large trial with DOCP showed a dose and interval range of 1.5 to 2.2 mg/kg q 25 to 30 days.
   B. Glucocorticoid replacement is achieved with either prednisone at 0.2 mg/ kg PO SID or cortisone at 1.0 mg/kg PO SID. Some patients receiving fludrocorticosterone acetate or DOCP do not need glucocorticoid supplementation except during periods of stress.

Prognosis

   I. Excellent prognosis with therapy
  II. Many dogs appear to do better with a small daily maintenance dose of prednisone or cortisone. During illness or other stressful periods, however, larger doses of glucocorticoids are necessary to avoid relapse into acute adrenal crisis.

HYPERADRENOCORTICISM (CUSHING'S DISEASE)

Overview

   I. Hyperadrenocorticism is a common endocrinopathy in older dogs and is rarely reported in cats. The syndrome is associated with excessive levels of cortisol that result from excess pituitary adrenocorticotropic hormone (ACTH) or excess ACTH from ectopic nonendocrine tumors, functional adrenocortical adenoma, or carcinoma. Iatrogenic Cushing's syndrome occurs with excessive glucocorticoid administration.
  II. Pituitary-dependent hyperadrenocorticism accounts for 80 to 85 percent of cases of hyperadrenocorticism. It is a disease of middle-aged and older dogs (usually older than 6 years of age), although a few cases have been diagnosed under 1 year of age. There is no sex predilection. Poodles, dachshunds, and beagles may be at increased risk.
 III. Dogs with functional adrenocortical tumors tend to be older, ranging from 6 to 16 years of age with a mean age of 11 years of age. Females are affected more frequently. German shepherds, toy poodles, dachshunds and terriers are most commonly affected.
  IV. Hyperadrenocorticism rarely produces significant cardiac disease. However, signs and side effects of hyperadrenocorticism can mimic cardiac disease. Systemic effects of hyperadrenocorticism can also exacerbate underlying cardiac disease.

Pathophysiology

   I. Systemic hypertension
   A. Hypercortisolism increases vascular resistance by increasing smooth muscle sensitivity to catecholamines and increasing production of angioten-

sinogen. Mineralocorticoid properties of cortisol enhance the renal resorption of sodium and secondary fluid retention, resulting in an increased vascular volume. Hypertension is present in 57 to 82 percent of cushingoid dogs.

B. Systemic hypertension may cause myocardial hypertrophy.

C. Many affected dogs have coexisting atrioventricular valvular insufficiency and its associated cardiac changes. Hypertension might exacerbate underlying cardiac problems.

II. Pulmonary thromboembolism

A. Patients with hyperadrenocorticism are predisposed to pulmonary thromboembolism, with most cases diagnosed while the animal is being treated for Cushing's disease. Factors causing thromboembolism with Cushing's disease include obesity, increased hematocrit, hypertension, and increased levels of clotting factors.

B. Pulmonary thromboembolism should be suspected in any cushingoid patient with a history of acute onset of dyspnea or cyanosis.

III. Panting

A. Altered ventilation mechanics are often present due to weakness in the muscles of respiration, increased thoracic fat deposition (decreasing chest wall compliance), and increased diaphragmatic abdominal pressure resulting from adipose tissue and hepatomegaly. Mild respiratory distress or rapid respiratory rate at rest often results.

B. Many cushingoid dogs have variable degrees of lower airway disease or parenchymal disease.

IV. The triad of mitral/tricuspid insufficiency, respiratory disease, and Cushing's syndrome may create intractable dyspnea due to cardiopulmonary failure.

Diagnosis

I. History and physical examination

A. The major historical features are systemic manifestations of hypercortisolism; they include polydipsia, polyuria, polyphagia, panting, alopecia, anestrus, exercise intolerance, and lethargy.

B. Findings on physical examination may include abdominal enlargement, hepatomegaly, muscle weakness, testicular atrophy, symmetric alopecia, skin atrophy, hyperpigmentation, calcinosis cutis, bruising, and obesity.

II. Electrocardiograms show no characteristic changes. ECG evidence of left ventricular enlargement is often present in cushingoid dogs with mitral valvular insufficiency.

III. Radiography

A. Hypercortisolism causes changes on thoracic radiographs that include calcification of the tracheal and bronchial rings and osteoporosis of the thoracic vertebrae. Metastatic pulmonary lesions are seen infrequently with adrenal tumors.

B. Radiographic changes associated with pulmonary thromboembolism include hypoperfusion of the infarcted lung lobes, overcirculation within

the normal lung lobes, pleural effusion, and blunting and thickening of the pulmonary arteries. Thoracic radiographs may be normal.
IV. Echocardiography is rarely part of the work up of Cushing's disease.
V. Clinical pathology
  A. The excessive production of cortisol may result in neutrophilia, lymphopenia, eosinopenia, and erythrocytosis (females).
  B. Chemistry abnormalities include fasting hyperglycemia, increased serum alkaline phosphatase (sometimes extremely elevated), increased ALT, increased cholesterol, lipemia, and decreased BUN.
  C. Urinalysis shows specific gravity less than 1.015 and often less than 1.008. Proteinuria, glycosuria, and bacterial cystitis are sometimes noted.
VI. Specialized diagnostic tests
  A. A urine cortisol:creatinine ratio is a quick screening test for Cushing's disease. This test has a high sensitivity, but low specificity for Cushing's disease. The ACTH response test and low-dose dexamethasone suppression tests are the standard tests used to confirm the diagnosis.
  B. A high-dose dexamethasone suppression test or serum ACTH level are used to try and differentiate between adrenal tumors and pituitary-dependent Cushing's disease.
  C. Ultrasound or computed tomography (CT scan) can be used to try and differentiate pituitary-dependent Cushing's disease from adrenal tumors in patients that do not suppress with the high-dose dexamethasone suppression test.

Therapy

  I. Pituitary-dependent hyperadrenocorticism
  A. Chemotherapy using Lysodren is the standard treatment. Lysodren selectively, and usually reversibly, destroys the zona fasciculata (cortisol) and zona reticularis (sex hormones) of the adrenal gland. The zona glomerulosa (aldosterone) is occasionally affected.
  B. Ketoconazole (Nizoral) can be substituted in animals that do not tolerate Lysodren. Ketoconazole blocks an enzymatic step that is necessary for the production of cortisol.
  C. Patients need frequent monitoring with ACTH response tests so medications can be adjusted.
  D. Hypophysectomy and bilateral adrenalectomy with replacement hormone therapy are rarely used alternatives to medical management.
 II. Adrenocortical tumor
  A. Surgical removal of the affected adrenal gland(s) is recommended if possible.
  B. There is a high morbidity associated with surgery. Ideally, the patient is stabilized first by decreasing cortisol synthesis with ketoconazole.
  C. If the tumor is inoperable or metastasis is identified, manage the patient with either Lysodren or ketoconazole. Very high doses of Lysodren are

usually required in patients with adrenal tumors. Many dogs with adrenal tumors respond poorly to medical management.
   D. Replacement steroid therapy is necessary both intra- and postoperatively.
III. Management of heart failure and hypertension, if present, is undertaken through standard therapeutic protocols.

Prognosis

  I. Excellent prognosis is confirmed with resectable, benign adrenal tumors.
 II. Nonresectable or metastatic adrenal adenocarcinoma have a poor prognosis.
III. Chemotherapy with o,p′-DDD (Lysodren) or ketoconazole for pituitary dependent hyperadrenocorticism has potential side effects, but most treated dogs respond well to therapy. Average survival in one study was 2 years, with a range of 18 days to 7 years.

HYPERSOMATATROPISM (ACROMEGALY) IN CATS

Overview

  I. Acromegaly is a syndrome associated with increased levels of growth hormone (hypersomatatropism).
 II. In cats, acromegaly occurs secondary to a pituitary tumor. It is a rare endocrinopathy that is seen in middle-aged to old cats. It is most common in males and rarely seen in females.
III. In dogs, hypersomatatropism is associated with progestogen treatment or endogenous progestogens that are produced during diestrus. It does not cause clinically significant cardiac problems in dogs. The syndrome is seen in females and is reversible with discontinuation of progestogen therapy or resolves spontaneously with the end of diestrus.

Cardiovascular Pathophysiology

  I. The trophic effect of growth hormone results in generalized organomegaly, including the heart. Cardiac changes are those of myocardial hypertrophy. Heart failure is a common sequela of acromegaly in cats.
 II. Systemic hypertension is seen frequently in humans with acromegaly. Blood pressure measurements have not been reported in cats with this disease.

Diagnosis

  I. History and physical examination
     A. Most cats present with a history or polyuria, polydypsia, and weight gain.
     B. Cardiac abnormalities noted on physical examination may include a sys-

tolic murmur, gallop rhythm, and signs of CHF (dyspnea, cyanosis, muffled heart sounds, or crackles).
  C. Other abnormalities include hepatomegaly, nephromegaly, large head, arthritis, prognathism, pot belly, large tongue, and circling.
  II. Electrocardiographic abnormalities have not been observed in these patients.
 III. Radiographs of the thorax usually demonstrate cardiomegaly, and less commonly pulmonary edema or pleural effusion.
 IV. Echocardiograms generally reveal ventricular hypertrophy.
  V. Clinical pathology
  A. The hemogram is generally unremarkable, although some cats have erythrocytosis.
  B. All cases are hyperglycemic and glucosuric. Most cats are also hyperproteinemic, azotemic, and hyperphosphatemic. Hypercholesterolemia, increased alanine aminotransferase (ALT), increased serum alkaline phosphatase (SAP), and ketonuria are seen less frequently.
 VI. Specialized diagnostic tests
  A. A validated growth hormone assay is not currently available for cats.
  B. Computed tomography can be used to identify the pituitary tumor.
  C. Evaluate blood pressure in any suspected or confirmed cases.

Therapy

  I. Treatment options include hypophysectomy, radiation therapy, and medical management with bromocriptine or somatostatin. Hypophysectomy has not been reported in cats. Radiation therapy is difficult to obtain and has only resulted in transient improvement to date. Medical management is generally unsuccessful.
  II. Supportive medical care includes high doses of insulin for insulin-resistant diabetes mellitus and diuretics for congestive heart failure.

Prognosis

  I. Survival in cats with acromegaly ranges from 4 to 42 months.
  II. Most cats die or are euthanatized due to severe congestive heart failure, renal failure, or expanding pituitary tumor.
Note: Hypersomatatropism without acromegaly has been associated with hypertrophic cardiomyopathy in some cats. Thirty-one cats with hypertrophic cardiomyopathy were shown to have growth hormone levels that were four times the control levels. None of the cats that were examined post-mortem had pituitary tumors and none demonstrated hyperinsulinism or diabetes mellitus.

Pheochromocytoma

Overview

  I. These tumors of adrenal medullary origin are uncommonly detected in dogs. They are typically seen in old dogs (mean age 11 years, with range of 1 to 16 years) and extremely rare in cats.

II. Pheochromocytomas are catecholamine-producing tumors derived from chro-maffin cells.

III. In addition to important effects on the cardiovascular system, catecholamines have significant metabolic effects, stimulating glycogenolysis and gluconeo-genesis.

Cardiac Pathophysiology

I. The cardiovascular effects of pheochromocytomas result from the α_1, β_1 and β_2 effects of norepinephrine and epinephrine. Stimulation of alpha and beta adrenergic receptors generally causes opposite effects. The dominant effect varies with relative receptor density and activation thresholds. For example, in vascular smooth muscle, alpha adrenergic effects predominate. Thus, hypertension results when both alpha and beta adrenergic receptors are stimulated.

II. β_1 adrenergic effects include sinus tachycardia, increased cardiac conduction velocity, and increased contractility.

III. β_2 adrenergic effects on the cardiovascular system include venous and arteriole vasodilation.

IV. α_1 adrenergic effects on the cardiovascular system include venous and arteriole vasoconstriction. Approximately 50 percent of dogs with pheochromocytomas are hypertensive at the time of testing.

V. Myocardial injury may result from catecholamine excess (i.e., myonecrosis with subsequent fibrosis and interstitial inflammation is reported in some humans with pheochromocytomas).

Diagnosis

I. History and physical examination
   A. Historical observations include weakness, anorexia, vomiting, weight loss, panting, dyspnea, lethargy, diarrhea, whining, pacing, polyuria, polydypsia, shivering, and epistaxis.
   B. Cardiac abnormalities noted on physical examination include lethargy, tachypnea and dyspnea, arrhythmias, systolic murmur, and pulmonary crackles.
   C. Other physical findings are emaciation, peripheral edema, ascites, and abdominal mass.
   D. Many signs and physical findings are reported to be episodic because of the episodic release of catecholamines by the tumor.

II. Electrocardiography
   A. Nonspecific ST segment and T wave changes may be noted.
   B. Arrhythmias, especially ventricular premature complexes and paroxysmal ventricular tachycardia, can occur.

III. Radiography
   A. Generalized cardiomegaly and pulmonary edema can develop, probably due to sustained chronic hypertension.
   B. Adrenal tumors can be identified in one-third of the cases.

IV. Clinical pathology
   A. No consistent abnormalities are present on the hemogram or chemistry profile.
   B. Demonstration of elevated 24-hour urinary excretion of vanillylmandelic acid, total metanephrines, fractionated catecholamines, and plasma catecholamines is diagnostic in humans.
 V. Special diagnostic tests
   A. Abdominal ultrasound may be helpful as a localizing procedure.
   B. Angiography can be used in some situations to evaluate adrenal masses invading the caudal vena cava.
   C. Computed tomography, nuclear imaging, and provocative testing to induce hypertension (with histamine, tyramine, and glucagon) or hypotension (with phentolamine) may be useful, but rarely are practical or available in general practice.

Therapy

 I. Alpha and beta adrenergic blocking drugs may help control hypertension and arrhythmias, respectively. Always start with an alpha adrenergic blocker such as phenoxybenzamine (0.2 to 1.5 mg/kg PO BID). If a hypertensive crisis is identified, administer phentolamine at 0.02 to 0.1 mg/kg IV, followed by an intravenous infusion. If tachyarrhythmias remain a problem, then add a beta blocker such as propranolol. Using a beta blocker without alpha blockade can result in severe hypertension.
II. Surgical tumor removal is the only definitive treatment. This should be attempted after medical stabilization in patients without metastasis.

Prognosis

Dogs with inoperable lesions have a poor prognosis. Long-term alpha and beta adrenergic blockers may be used in these instances.

DIABETES MELLITUS

Diabetes mellitus causes devastating cardiovascular problems in humans. The cardiovascular systems of dogs and cats are remarkably immune to the effects of hyperglycemia. Studies reveal only a subclinical reduction of myocardial contractility.

METABOLIC DISTURBANCES

DISORDERS ASSOCIATED WITH HYPERKALEMIA

Overview

 I. Over 95 percent of body potassium is intracellular, with only 2 to 5 percent extracellular. Therefore, serum potassium values are not always reliable indicators of total body potassium stores.

II. Clinical causes of hyperkalemia include the following:
   A. Excessive administration of oral potassium supplements or potassium supplemented fluids.
   B. Decreased renal elimination associated with oliguric or anuric renal failure, hypoadrenocorticism (Addison's disease), and, rarely, drugs (potassium-sparing diuretics and ACE inhibitors).
   C. Ruptured urinary tract and urethral obstruction.
   D. Translocation from intracellular to extracellular space (metabolic acidosis, rapid release from tissue during severe injury).

Diagnosis, Therapy, and Prognosis

Identification and treatment of the underlying cause of hyperkalemia are essential. See section on hypoadrenocorticism (Addison's disease).

DISORDERS ASSOCIATED WITH HYPOKALEMIA

Overview

I. When severe potassium loss has occurred and the animal is symptomatic for hypokalemia, severe muscle weakness or paralysis may develop.
II. Clinical causes of hypokalemia include the following
   A. Decreased intake: Anorexia, especially when combined with potassium-deficient fluid administration.
   B. Excessive gastrointestinal loss
      1. Chronic vomiting
      2. Severe diarrhea
      3. Overuse of enemas, laxatives, or exchange resins.
   C. Excessive urinary loss
      1. Renal (renal tubular acidosis, postobstructive diuresis, chronic pyelonephritis
      2. Drugs (diuretics, amphotericin B)
      3. Secondary hyperaldosteronism (liver failure, congestive heart failure, nephrotic syndrome)
   D. Extracellular to intracellular transfer
      1. Metabolic alkalosis
      2. Insulin and glucose administration
      3. Hyperinsulinism (insulinoma)
      4. Ketoacidotic diabetes mellitus

Cardiac Pathophysiology

I. Severe hypokalemia causes hyperpolarization of nerve and muscle fiber membranes.

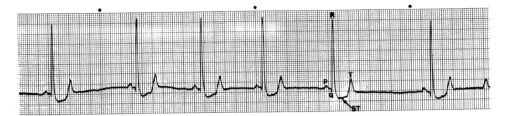

Fig. 13-2. ST segment depression in a dog with hypokalemia (serum potassium 3.3 mEq/L) secondary to respiratory alkalosis. (From Tilley LP: Essential of Canine and Feline Electrocardiography. 3rd Ed. Lea & Febiger, Philadelphia, 1992, with permission.)

II. Electrocardiographic changes are manifested in delayed and abnormal repolarization, increased automaticity, and increased duration of the action potential.

Diagnosis

   I. History and physical examination
      A. Muscle weakness may be mild or present as profound weakness and depression. Ventroflexion of the head is frequently seen in symptomatic cats.
      B. Polyuria and polydypsia may occur.
  II. Electrocardiography
      A. QT interval prolongation and U waves may occur.
      B. ST segment may become depressed (Fig. 13-2), with a gradual blending of T waves and what appears to be a tall U wave.
      C. Ventricular and supraventricular arrhythmias may occur.
 III. Clinical pathology may be reflective of the underlying disease process contributing to hypokalemia. Urine concentrating ability may be impaired.

Therapy

   I. Treat the primary disease process.
  II. Parenteral replacement with potassium chloride (KCl) is recommended when potassium loss is severe and the animal is symptomatic for hypokalemia (Table 13-2). Do not exceed 0.5 mEq/kg/hr.

TABLE 13-2. GUIDELINES FOR POTASSIUM SUPPLEMENTATION

Serum Potassium (mEq/L)	mEq KCl to Add to 250 ml Fluid	Maximum Fluid Rate (ml/kg/hr)
<2.0	20	6
2.1–2.5	15	8
2.6–3.0	10	12
3.1–3.5	7	18
3.6–5.0	5	25

(From Greene RW, Scott RC: Lower urinary tract disease. p. 1572. In Ettinger SJ (ed): Textbook of Veterinary Internal Medicine. WB Saunders, Philadelphia, 1975, with permission.)

III. Parenteral administration may initially decrease the serum K^+ level. This effect is minimized by avoiding dextrose-containing fluids, administering K^+ at correct rate and concentration, and starting oral potassium gluconate supplementation early.

IV. Return to alimentation and treatment of the primary disease responsible for hypokalemia will replace potassium deficits. Therefore, prolonged oral maintenance therapy is rarely indicated except when ongoing excessive loss of potassium due to diuretic administration or polyuric renal disease is present.

V. Hypokalemia markedly increases the likelihood of toxicity when digitalis is being administered. Serum potassium should be promptly checked and corrected when digitalis toxicity is suspected.

VI. Hypokalemia increases the risk of ventricle arrhythmias and decreases the responsiveness to class I antiarrhythmic agents (lidocaine, procainamide, quinidine). Serum potassium should be promptly checked and corrected when refractory ventricular arrhythmias are identified.

Prognosis

The prognosis is good if the underlying condition can be corrected or managed.

DISORDERS ASSOCIATED WITH HYPERCALCEMIA

Overview

I. Hypercalcemia occurs when serum calcium concentration consistently exceeds 12 mg/dl in mature dogs and 11 mg/dl in cats. Young, actively growing dogs may normally have calcium values of greater than 12.0 mg/dl.

II. Many different disorders can cause hypercalcemia. These include calcium bone resorption, increased gastrointestinal calcium absorption, increased serum protein-binding of calcium, increased calcium binding to anions, and decreased renal and intestinal calcium removal from serum.

III. The following conditions are associated with hypercalcemia
   A. Young growing puppy (normal)
   B. Paraneoplastic syndromes (lymphosarcoma, anal sac apocrine gland adenocarcinoma, occasionally other soft tissue tumors, primary and metastatic bony tumors).
   C. Hypoadrenocorticism
   D. Renal failure
   E. Skeletal lesions (septic osteomyelitis, disuse osteoporosis, hypertrophic osteodystrophy)
   F. Nutritional (hypervitaminosis D, hypervitaminosis A, calcium administration)
   G. Primary hyperparathyroidism
   H. Other (hemoconcentration, hyperproteinemia, severe hypothermia, laboratory error)

Cardiac Pathophysiology

I. Cardiovascular effects of experimentally induced acute hypercalcemia include raised systolic and diastolic blood pressure, especially with renal failure.

II. Clinically, elevated calcium levels have little if any direct adverse effect on cardiac function. In hypercalcemic crisis (>16 mg/dl serum calcium), cardiac arrhythmias or arrest may occur.

III. Animals with hypercalcemia may be more predisposed to complications of digitalis intoxication.

IV. Long-standing hypercalcemia may predispose to calcification to myocardium, blood vessels, and other soft tissues.

Diagnosis

I. History and physical examination
Regardless of its cause, hypercalcemia affects the kidney (renal dysfunction, polyuria, polydipsia, nocturia, nephrocalcinosis, renal failure, uremia), gastrointestinal system (anorexia, constipation, and vomiting from decreased gastrointestinal smooth-muscle excitability), and nervous system (generalized skeletal muscle weakness from decreased neuromuscular activity).

II. Radiography
A. Thoracic radiographs may indicate mediastinal mass(es), metastasis, abnormal bony densities, or osteolysis.
B. Abdominal radiographs may show organomegaly, abnormal bone density, sublumbar masses, or sublumbar lymphadenopathy.
C. Skeletal survey radiographs may exhibit isolated bony lesions that could account for hypercalcemia. Osteopenia, metastatic calcification, or focal bony lesions may be present.

III. Electrocardiography
A. The characteristic ECG finding is a short QT interval. In extreme cases, the ST segment may fuse with the upstroke of the T wave. ECG changes do not correlate closely with serum calcium concentration.
B. Hypercalcemia may predispose to arrhythmias of digitalis intoxication.
C. ECG changes resolve after correction of the serum calcium.

IV. Clinical pathology
A. Hypercalcemia often causes diminished urinary concentrating ability. The urine is usually hyposthenuric or isosthenuric.
B. Renal failure with azotemia may develop from progressive structural and functional alterations in the kidney.
C. Hypophosphatemia or hyperphosphatemia may be recorded, depending on the presence or absence of renal failure and the underlying etiology of hypercalcemia.
D. Serum alkaline phosphatase may be elevated if severe bone disease or concomitant hepatic disease is present.
E. A hemogram may be normal, display hemoconcentration or anemia, or occasionally show evidence for leukemia (when this disease is associated with the underlying etiology).

F. Bone marrow evaluation may be unremarkable or disclose evidence of lymphosarcoma, leukemia, or multiple myeloma.

Therapy

I. Initial treatment is directed at reducing the systemic effects of hypercalcemia.
   A. Pre-existing dehydration should be corrected and hydration maintained.
   B. Administration of 0.9 percent saline should be used to enhance the renal excretion of calcium.
   C. Furosemide (5 mg/kg initially and 5 mg/kg/hr thereafter) and/or sodium bicarbonate (1 to 4 mEq/kg) may also help in cases of moderate-to-severe hypercalcemia.
   D. Glucocorticosteroids may limit bone resorption, decrease intestinal calcium absorption, increase renal calcium excretion, and be cytolytic in certain neoplasms.
II. Definitive treatment is directed at the underlying etiology.

Prognosis

Prognosis depends on early detection, ability to establish a definitive diagnosis, and success of treatment. The prognosis of many causes of hypercalcemia is guarded to poor.

DISORDERS ASSOCIATED WITH HYPOCALCEMIA

Overview

I. Hypocalcemia, although infrequently encountered, can cause profound clinical signs. It occurs when serum calcium concentration is less than 8 mg/dl in the dog and less than 7 mg/dl in the cat (ionized calcium <5 in dogs and <4.5 in cats).
II. The following conditions may be associated with hypocalcemia
   A. Renal failure
   B. Eclampsia (puerperal tetany)
   C. Canine acute pancreatitis
   D. Hypoparathyroidism
      1. Idiopathic
      2. Postoperative (during bilateral thyroid surgery)
   E. Ethylene glycol toxicity
   F. Hyperphosphatemia
   G. Hypocalcemia due to hypoalbuminemia, where calcium values are not adjusted for serum protein concentration

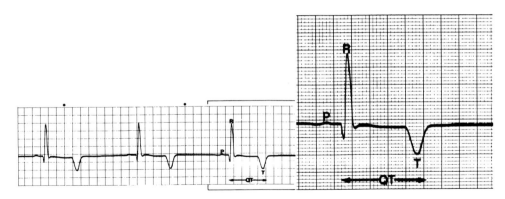

Fig. 13-3. Prolonged QT interval in a dog with severe hypocalcemia (2.2 mg/dl) secondary to ethylene glycol toxicity. (From Tilley LP: Essentials of Canine and Feline Electrocardiography. 3rd Ed. Lea & Febiger, Philadelphia, 1992, with permission.)

Cardiac Pathophysiology

I. Hypocalcemia causes an excitatory effect on nerve and muscle cells. Neuromuscular irritability, tetany, and seizures may result.

II. Animals with coexisting congestive heart failure may experience decreased cardiac function that improves with restoration of calcium levels (due to the augmenting effect of calcium on myocardial contractility).

III. Acutely induced hypocalcemia (i.e., treatment with chelating agents) can potentially cause sharp reductions in blood pressure and shock.

Diagnosis

I. History and physical examination
   A. Tetany, seizures, anorexia, vomiting, and abdominal discomfort are the predominant signs in affected animals.
   B. Handling or stress may precipitate tetany.

II. Electrocardiography (Fig. 13-3)
   The typical ECG manifestation of hypocalcemia consists of QT prolongation.

III. Clinical pathology
   Clinical pathology will reflect abnormalities associated with the underlying disease process. Hypocalcemia is usually diagnosed when low serum calcium levels are detected during clinical investigation of tetany, seizures, renal failure, pancreatitis, or other disorders through analysis of a serum biochemical profile.

Therapy

I. Severe hypocalcemia (<6 mg/dl) is a life-threatening emergency.
   A. Ten percent calcium gluconate is administered intravenously (0.5–1.5 ml/kg) slowly over a 15- to 30-minute interval. Calcium should be adminis-

tered slowly as ECG changes do not closely conform to serum calcium levels, especially when other electrolyte and acid/base disturbances are present.

   B. Electrocardiographic monitoring should accompany administration
      1. Calcium infusion should be temporarily interrupted if ST segment elevation or bradycardia occur, to be reinstated at a slower rate when these changes have abated.
      2. Gradual QT interval shortening from its prolonged state may accompany calcium infusion.
      3. Calcium is cardiotoxic if replaced too quickly; even a normal concentration of serum calcium may be toxic if replenished to that level too rapidly.

   C. Subsequent intravenous calcium administration may be repeated every 6 to 12 hours, or as needed.

  II. Clinical signs of hypocalcemia may abate slowly despite calcium infusion. Resolution of clinical signs may not provide a reliable guide as an end point of adequate calcium administration. Some hypocalcemic signs may persist (i.e., weakness, anorexia) when cardiotoxic effects of calcium infusion occur.

 III. Vitamin D therapy may be required in some disorders to maintain eventual control of hypocalcemia. In treatment of postoperative parathyroid insufficiency, care must be taken to detect recovery of parathyroid function in order to avoid vitamin D–associated hypercalcemia.

Prognosis

For most causes of hypocalcemia that are carefully managed, the prognosis is good to excellent.

HYPOGLYCEMIA

Overview

   I. Hypoglycemia may be caused by hyperinsulinism due to a functional islet-cell pancreatic carcinoma, or from insulin administered for the treatment of diabetes mellitus.

  II. Other clinical entities associated with hypoglycemia include nonpancreatic tumors, glycogen storage diseases, juvenile hypoglycemia, neonatal hypoglycemia, septic shock, Addison's disease, and hepatic disease.

Cardiac Pathophysiology

Irrespective of the etiology, hypoglycemia triggers catecholamine release, which causes tachycardia, increases in myocardial oxygen demand, and, potentially, arrhythmias.

Diagnosis

I. History and physical examination
Clinical manifestations of hypoglycemia range from lethargy to episodic weakness and seizures.
II. Electrocardiographic findings can include ST depression, T wave flattening, QT prolongation, and arrhythmias. ECG changes usually resolve with correction of hypoglycemia.
III. Laboratory findings
A. A low blood glucose level (<60 mg/dl) is usually present. A fasting blood glucose level may be needed to confirm hypoglycemia.
B. Elevated insulin levels or amended insulin:glucose ratio may be demonstrated with insulinomas.

Therapy

I. Hypoglycemic crisis, regardless of cause, is managed by slow, intravenous administration of 50 percent dextrose to effect.
II. Treat underlying disease or improve diabetic regulation.

Prognosis

I. Resolution of neurologic signs due to hypoglycemia is usually abrupt and virtually complete.
II. Prolonged, untreated hypoglycemia may result in cerebrocortical hypoxic damage. Lack of symptom amelioration after therapy may indicate cerebral hypoxia and edema.

UREMIA

Overview

I. Uremia is generally associated with renal failure.
II. Uremia is not uncommon in geriatric populations, and affects cardiac function, and renal failure reduces elimination of many cardiac drugs (digoxin, most ACE inhibitors, many beta blockers).

Cardiac Pathophysiology

A. Hypertensive cardiovascular disease, electrolyte imbalance, fluid overload, and anemia can contribute to the production of disturbances.
B. Renal failure can cause elevations or reductions of potassium and calcium; associated changes may register on the ECG.

C. Systemic hypertension is a common sequela of chronic renal failure in dogs and cats, and is reported to occur in 50 to 93 percent of dogs and 65 percent of cats.
D. Pericardial effusion has been reported as a sequela of uremia in cats and less commonly in dogs. The effusion may occur secondary to uremic serositis.
E. There is an increased incidence of pulmonary thromboembolism with protein-losing glomerulopathy.
F. Uremic toxins have a cardiodepressant effect.

Diagnosis

  I. History and physical examination
     A. Signs that may accompany uremia include polyuria, polydypsia, depression, anorexia, lethargy, vomiting, diarrhea and weight loss.
     B. Uremic pneumonitis and metabolic acidosis cause dyspnea or tachypnea that may be confused for signs of congestive heart failure.
 II. Electrocardiography
     A. Nonspecific ECG abnormalities may be attributed to hypertension, anemia, electrolyte abnormalities, and pericarditis.
     B. Conduction defects or arrhythmias may occur.
III. Clinical pathology may reveal abnormalities in the hemogram, urinalysis, and biochemistry profile consistent with uremia (increased BUN, creatinine, and phosphorus; nonregenerative anemia, and isosthenuria).

Therapy

  I. Treatment is directed at managing uremia and its underlying causes. Therapy generally includes parenteral fluids, protein and phosphorus restriction, phosphate binders, and sometimes calcitriol and erythropoietin.
 II. Management of congestive heart failure in patients with concurrent renal failure is extremely challenging and often frustrating. Guidelines include
     A. Confirm renal failure by checking the urine specific gravity prior to instituting fluid or diuretic therapy. Many sick animals with cardiac disease or dehydration will have poor renal perfusion and prerenal azotemia. These patients' azotemia generally resolves with appropriate cardiac or fluid therapy.
     B. Rehydrate cautiously with low-sodium fluids, such as half-strength saline and dextrose.
     C. Reduce doses or avoid cardiac drugs eliminated by the kidneys. If using ACE inhibitors or digoxin, monitor kidney function and electrolytes frequently. Monitor digoxin levels periodically. Digitoxin can be substituted for digoxin. Hydralazine and nitroglycerin can be substituted for ACE inhibitors.
     D. Monitor and control hypertension, electrolyte, and acid-base disturbances.

Prognosis

Resolution of the uremic state may improve ECG abnormalities, although arrhythmias may persist

ANEMIA

Overview

I. Anemia is a sign of a disease, not a disease entity.
II. Evaluation should emphasize history (drug or toxin exposure), clinical signs related to other disorders complicated by anemia (fever, lethargy, bleeding, weight loss), physical examination (petechiae, lymphadenopathy), and clinical pathology.
III. Symptoms of reduced cardiac reserve associated with anemia depend on the severity of anemia and on the presence and extent of underlying cardiac disease.

Cardiac Pathophysiology

I. The combination of tissue hypoxia and reduced blood viscosity leads to decreased systemic vascular resistance and is associated with increased cardiac output. When anemia is associated with increased viscosity (multiple myeloma or macroglobulinemia), cardiac output may fail to rise.
II. Physiologic consequences depend on the developmental rate of anemia.
   A. With acute blood loss (i.e., hemorrhage), hypovolemic shock may predominate.
      1. In normal dogs, left ventricular function can become depressed when the hematocrit level is reduced below 24 percent in acute anemia.
      2. When heart failure occurs, it usually suggests the presence of underlying heart disease that had been compensated until the burden of augmented cardiac output was added.
   B. With chronic anemia in which blood volume is maintained, cardiac output may rise due to tachycardia with little change in stroke volume.
   C. In severe chronic anemia, heart rate may be normal or only minimally elevated, and cardiac output is increased principally due to augmented stroke volume. This augmented stroke volume is associated with cardiac dilation and hypertrophy.
   D. Chronic anemia is usually well tolerated because of compensatory mechanisms that include increased cardiac output, redistribution of blood flow, and decreased oxygen affinity of red blood cells. As in thyrotoxicosis, most animals in which congestive heart failure with anemia develops have underlying heart disease aggravated by increased cardiac work caused by anemia.

E. Pulmonary thromboembolism may occur with autoimmune hemolytic anemia.

Diagnosis

I. History and physical examination
   A. Chronic anemia produces few symptoms, which may include fatigue and mild exertional dyspnea.
   B. The precordium may be hyperactive, with bounding or pistol shot arterial pulses, pale or icteric mucous membrane color, and prolonged capillary refill time.
   C. A medium-pitched, mid-systolic murmur at the left apex, generally grade I-III/VI, is common with severe anemia.
   D. Heart sounds may be accentuated.
II. Radiology
   Thoracic radiographs may display mild cardiac enlargement, but this will vary depending on the presence and extent of previously existing heart disease.
III. Electrocardiography
   A. Sinus tachycardia is often present. The heart rate varies with the rate of onset and degree of anemia. Ventricular premature complexes sometimes develop.
   B. Left ventricular enlargement (QRS wide or tall R waves) may occur secondary to systemic hypertension.
IV. Clinical pathology
   The laboratory database varies considerably depending on the cause of anemia.

Therapy

I. Treatment of anemia depends on the underlying cause.
II. In animals with anemia and congestive heart failure, correction of the anemia may be necessary before optimal response of the heart failure to pharmacotherapy can occur. Rapid infusion of whole blood to a severely anemic animal with severe underlying cardiac disease may precipitate heart failure.
III. A decision as to when to transfuse a patient is based on the clinical assessment, which includes the rate of anemia development, the patient's state of compensation, and progression of continued red blood cell loss.

Prognosis

Successful management of anemia and underlying causes confers a good prognosis.

NEOPLASTIC AND INFILTRATIVE HEART DISEASES

Overview

I. Primary tumors of the heart and pericardium are uncommon. Hemangiosarcoma may originate in the right auricle or right atrium, especially in German shepherd dogs.

II. Metastatic tumors invade the heart, pericardium, or both.
   A. Cardiac metastasis may occur with most types of primary tumors.
   B. Hemangiosarcoma frequently metastasizes to the heart.
   C. Lymphosarcoma is the most common tumor that metastasizes to the heart in cats.

III. Infiltrative myocardial disease involving non-neoplastic cells is rare in the dog and uncommon in the cat.

Cardiac Pathophysiology

I. Tumors from other tissues gain direct access to the heart by invasive growth from adjacent structures or spread by hematogenous or lymphatic vessels.

II. The relative infrequency of cardiac metastasis has been attributed to metabolic peculiarities of striated muscle, rapid coronary blood flow, efferent lymphatic drainage from the heart, and the vigorous kneading action of the myocardium.

III. Myocardial neoplasia may cause congestive heart failure due to diastolic dysfunction, obstruction to ventricular inflow or outflow, pericardial tamponade, or arrhythmias.

Diagnosis

I. History and physical examination
   A. Cardiac involvement may not display clinical manifestations. Signs depend on the site and extent of metastasis. Cardiac inflow or outflow obstruction and arrhythmias may cause signs of congestive heart failure and weakness.
   B. Pericardial involvement may cause pericardial effusion or tamponade. Physical findings include auscultating muffled heart sounds, jugular venous distention, ascites, and weakness (often acute).

II. Radiography
   A. Radiographic evidence of progressive cardiac enlargement may be observed.
   B. Pneumopericardiography or angiocardiography may assess the thickness and any irregularities of the pericardium, epicardium, and endocardium.

III. Electrocardiography
   A. Reduced QRS voltage on the ECG and electrical alternans occur in many, but not all, cases with pericardial effusion.
   B. Atrial or ventricular arrhythmias, conduction disturbances, and complete heart block can occur.
IV. Echocardiography
   A. Echocardiographic evidence of pericardial effusion may be demonstrated. Diastolic right atrial or right ventricular collapse signifies pericardial tamponade.
   B. Two-dimensional echocardiography may facilitate identification of intracavitary, intramural, and pericardial masses.
V. Pericardiocentesis may detect cytologic evidence of neoplasia.

THERAPY

I. Pericardiocentesis may offer temporary relief from cardiac tamponade.
II. Animals with myocardial infiltration of tumors sensitive to chemotherapy or radiotherapy may respond favorably.
III. Congestive heart failure and arrhythmias are often poorly responsive to pharmacotherapy.

PROGNOSIS

In most cases, antemortem diagnosis is not appreciated, etiology cannot be defined, or therapy is not effective.

PHYSICAL AND CHEMICAL AGENTS THAT AFFECT THE CARDIOVASCULAR SYSTEM

Many noninfectious stimuli can cause myocardial injury. Damage can be acute and transient or chronic and lead to permanent myocardial change. Effects are usually related to the severity, dose, and rate of exposure.

HYPERPYREXIA (HEAT STROKE)

Overview

I. Hyperpyrexia is usually associated with heat stroke when the rectal temperature rises to 41° to 44°C (106° to 111°F). Experimentally, signs of heat stroke develop consistently at temperatures above 43°C (109°F) in dogs.
II. Heat stroke develops in animals exposed to high environmental temperatures.

It commonly occurs in animals left in unventilated automobiles during the summer months.

III. High humidity reduces evaporation of water from the oral and nasal cavities, and reduces the ability of small animals to regulate their temperatures.

IV. Animals that are obese, brachycephalic, very young or old, or having cardiopulmonary disease are predisposed to heat stroke.

V. Malignant hyperthermia is a rare but potentially fatal abnormal response to anesthetic agents. It is characterized by an acute, rapid rise in body temperature and severe biochemical changes accompanied by muscle rigidity.

Cardiac Pathophysiology

I. Heat-induced vasodilation results in hypotension and decreased organ perfusion.

II. Respiratory alkalosis may result from panting.

III. Dehydration with hemoconcentration may occur, as well as mild hyperkalemia and hypophosphatemia.

IV. Tachyarrhythmias and cardiogenic shock can occur due to myocardial hemorrhage, ischemia, and necrosis.

V. Disseminated intravascular coagulopathy (DIC) may develop due to destruction of clotting factors.

VI. Right-heart dilation may occur.

VII. Mechanisms suggested for myocardial injury include direct thermal effects, circulatory collapse with secondary myocardial hypoxia, decreased coronary blood flow, and secondary metabolic injury.

VIII. Animals that recover from heat stroke may be prone to subsequent occurrences due to heat-induced damage to the thermoregulatory zone of the hypothalamus.

Diagnosis

I. History and physical examination
   A. The diagnosis is usually made on the reported history of an animal being exposed to high environmental temperatures. However, some cases have more subtle history.
   B. Depending on the duration and severity of the heat stroke, clinical signs may include panting, sinus tachycardia, bright red oral mucous membranes, and hyperthermia. Extremities become hot to the touch.
   C. Red mucous membranes may turn pale because of diminished circulation or vasoconstriction.
   D. Watery diarrhea may occur, which can progress to bloody diarrhea.
   E. Stupor and coma with respiratory arrest can follow.
   F. With malignant hyperthermia, an acute, profound temperature elevation may be the first noticeable sign to the surgeon.

    1. If the heart rate is monitored, tachycardia may be the earliest indication.

    2. Skeletal muscle hypertonus may occur.

II. Electrocardiogram may show tachycardia, extrasystoles (especially if DIC develops), and ST segment and T wave abnormalities.

III. Clinical pathologic alterations relate to the stage and severity of the hyperpyrexia.

Therapy

I. Therapy should begin with lowering body temperature. Submergence in cool water or wetting the extremities with rubbing alcohol are useful techniques. Rectal temperature should be recorded every 5 to 10 minutes. Discontinue cooling when the body temperature drops below 39.5°C (103°F), to avoid hypothermia.

II. Supportive care should include isotonic fluid therapy (0.45 percent saline or half-strength lactated Ringer's solution, with 2.5 percent dextrose), correction of acid-base and electrolyte abnormalities, and treatment for DIC.

III. Nonsteroidal anti-inflammatory drugs or antipyretics (i.e., aspirin, flunixin meglumine) are contraindicated. The use of glucocorticoids remains controversial, but they are often used when cerebral edema is suspected.

IV. When malignant hyperthermia is anesthetic related, all inhalation agents and relaxants should be discontinued. Hyperventilation with 100 percent oxygen should be started.

V. Administer mannitol (2.0 g/kg of a 20 percent solution over 10 to 15 minutes) if cerebral edema is suspected or if stupor or coma develops.

VI. The patient should be monitored for several days for the development of complications such as renal failure and DIC.

Prognosis

I. Prognosis for heat stroke is guarded to good if detected and treated early.

II. Malignant hyperthermia is rare but seems to offer a worse prognosis.

III. Coagulopathy and renal failure confer a worse prognosis.

HYPOTHERMIA

Overview

I. Lowering of body temperature can occur accidentally, due to deep cooling from external cold, drugs, or interference with thermoregulatory centers during anesthesia.

II. Physiologic lesions of hypothermia depend on the extent and duration of exposure.

Cardiac Pathophysiology

I. Cardiac dilation with epicardial and subendocardial hemorrhage can result from severe hypothermia. Microinfarcts can occur in myocardial tissue.
II. Lesions may result from circulatory collapse, hemoconcentration, sludging of blood in capillaries, or decreased cellular metabolism.

Diagnosis

I. History and physical examination
   A. Signs vary with the degree of hypothermia (reduction in core temperature), mild (32° to 35°C or 89.6° to 95°F), moderate (28° to 32°C or 82.4° to 89.6°F) and severe (<28°C or 82.4°F).
   B. Signs include lethargy, ataxia, stupor, shivering and bradycardia. Cardiopulmonary arrest may occur with severe hypothermia.
II. Electrocardiography
   A. Mild hypothermia results in prolongation of the PR interval, QRS, and QT interval; atrial premature complexes; and inverted T waves.
   B. Moderate hypothermia produces atropine-resistant bradycardia and ventricular arrhythmias.
   C. Severe hypothermia may cause cardiac arrest secondary to ventricular fibrillation or asystole.

Therapy

I. Treatment initially involves warming the patient.
   A. Active external warming with warm water blankets is recommended for mild-to-moderate hypothermia. External warming causes vasodilation of skin vessels, which may initially transfer cooled blood to the body core, further decreasing internal temperature. This is rarely a significant clinical complication with mild-to-moderate hypothermia.
   B. Internal (core) warming is recommended if the rectal temperature is less than 30°C (86°F) or the cardiovascular status is unstable. This is accomplished by peritoneal analysis with dialysate fluids warmed to 45°C (113°F).
II. Appropriate supportive care (e.g., intravenous fluids, ventilation) must be administered. Severe hypothermia can cause cardiopulmonary collapse. Keep these patients well oxygenated and administer warmed IV fluids.
III. Cardiac output and ECG abnormalities improve after warming.
IV. Evaluation of the patient for underlying systemic disorders that could have predisposed it to hypothermia should be made once normothermia has been achieved.

CARBON MONOXIDE

Overview

The most common source of carbon monoxide (CO) is the exhaust of gasoline-burning engines.

Cardiac Pathophysiology

CO competes with oxygen for binding sights on hemoglobin, diminishing oxygen transport capacity. This results in myocardial hypoxia. Myocardial hemorrhage and necrosis may occur.

Diagnosis

    I. History and physical examination
       A. The history often supports exposure to fumes from a gasoline-burning engine.
       B. Clinical signs are often associated with cardiac hypoxia (sudden death) or hypoxia to the brain (convulsions, disorientation, coma).
       C. The physical exam is often unremarkable. A blood sample will be cherry red.
   II. Electrocardiography
      ECG abnormalities can include ST segment changes, conduction abnormalities, or arrhythmias.
 III. Specialized diagnostic test
      Carboxyhemoglobin blood levels can be measured.

Treatment

    I. One hundred percent oxygen should be administered.
   II. Any arrhythmias should be treated accordingly.
 III. Supportive care should include control of electrolytes and acid-base imbalances.

Prognosis

Clinical recovery usually occurs if the situation is detected and treated early.

TOAD POISONING

Overview

    I. The Colorado river toad *(Bufo alvaritus)* and the marine toad *(Bufo marinas)* secrete toxins from the parotid glands that can cause profound cardiotoxicity.

II. The animal does not have to ingest the toad to become poisoned. Toxic parotid secretions can be absorbed by the dog's or cat's oral mucous membranes just by the patient holding the toad in its mouth.

Cardiac Pathophysiology

The bufotoxin has digitalis-like effects on the heart.

Diagnosis

  I. History and physical examination
      A. The pet is often observed playing with the toad.
      B. Clinical signs occur within minutes and may include hypersalivation, vomiting, diarrhea, weakness, pulmonary edema, and seizures. Coma and death can occur within 30 minutes.
 II. Electrocardiography
      A. The digitalis-like effect of the toxin may result in any type of arrhythmia, therefore, an ECG should be monitored.
      B. Arrhythmias can occur and gradually worsen to ventricular fibrillation.

Therapy

  I. The patient's mouth should be rinsed immediately. Atropine may help decrease salivation.
 II. Provide supportive care, including anticonvulsive and antiarrhythmic medication as needed.
      A. Pentobarbital anesthesia will control seizures.
      B. Propranolol is quite effective for tachyarrhythmias. In patients without asthma or preexisting heart disease, doses of 0.5 to 2 mg/kg can be given slowly IV, to effect.

OLEANDER TOXICITY

Overview

Oleander *(Nerium oleander)* is an ornamental shrub found mostly in the southeast United States.

Cardiac Pathophysiology

The toxin of oleander is a digitalis-like glycoside.

Diagnosis

  I. History and physical examination
      Signs of vomiting and diarrhea occur within 2 to 3 hours

II. Electrocardiography may reveal any type of arrhythmia due to the digitalis-like compounds.

Therapy

I. Supportive care that includes fluid therapy, electrolyte replacement, and control of vomiting and diarrhea is recommended.
II. Arrhythmias should be treated accordingly.

CHOCOLATE TOXICITY

Overview

I. Toxic effects of chocolate are due to theobromide.
II. The LD_{50} of theobromide is 250 to 500 mg/kg (0.66 to 1.33 oz of baking chocolate/kg).

Cardiac Pathophysiology

I. Theobromide increases cyclic AMP, causes release of catecholamines, blocks adenosine receptors, and increases calcium uptake by the sarcoplasmic reticulum.
II. The net effect is to increase heat rate and the force of contractions.

Diagnosis

I. History and physical examination
   A. Clinical signs associated with chocolate toxicity include vomiting and diarrhea, hyperactivity, ataxia, hyperthermia, muscle tremors, coma, and death.
   B. Tachycardia is frequently noted, with bradycardia rarely reported.
II. Electrocardiogram findings may include sinus tachycardia and ventricular arrhythmias.

Treatment

I. Symptomatic therapy should include prevention of absorption, increasing elimination, maintenance of life support, and control of cardiac arrhythmias and seizures.
II. Arrhythmia management
   A. Lidocaine is used for rapid control of ventricular arrhythmias. Beta block-

ers are then added for additional control and maintenance therapy, if needed.
  B. Treat supraventricular tachycardia with beta blockers (i.e., propranolol, metoprolol, atenolol).

DOXORUBICIN CARDIOTOXICITY

Overview

  I. Doxorubicin is an anthracycline antibiotic used for its antineoplastic properties. Its mechanism of action as a chemotherapeutic agent is inhibition of nucleic acid synthesis.
 II. Cardiotoxicity manifested as arrhythmias or dilated cardiomyopathy usually develops after cumulative doses of 240 mg/m^2 in dogs, but toxicity can occur at dosages as low as 130 mg/m^2 (Dog range: 135 to 265 mg/m^2; Cat range: 130 to 320 mg/m^2).
III. Acute cardiotoxicity is manifested by arrhythmias during or shortly after administration. Dilated cardiomyopathy (DCM) may develop with chronic treatment. Although histologic lesions and echocardiographic changes may develop, clinical signs of congestive heart failure are uncommon in cats treated with doxorubicin.

Cardiac Pathophysiology

  I. The mechanism by which doxorubicin causes cardiotoxicity is unknown, but free radical generation and lipid membrane peroxidation may be involved in the pathogenesis. The heart rate at the time of drug administration may also determine the degree of cardiac toxicity, with slower heart rates associated with less toxicity.
 II. Histologic lesions consist of myocyte vacuolization, myocytolysis, and, occasionally, interstitial fibrosis.

Diagnosis

  I. History and physical examination
     Clinical signs and physical findings are associated with DCM and include exercise intolerance, dyspnea and coughing, hepatomegaly, and ascites. Congestive heart failure usually develops acutely.
 II. Radiography
     With DCM, chest radiographs show cardiomegaly with pulmonary edema and/or pleural effusion.
III. Electrocardiography
     A. In dogs, electrocardiographic abnormalities include ST segment and T wave changes, decreased QRS voltages, intraventricular conduction ab-

normalities, and atrial and ventricular arrhythmias. ECG changes are rare in cats treated with doxorubicin.

   B. ECG changes can occur acutely during drug administration. In this situation, stopping the drip and then reinstituting it at a slower rate may resolve the problem.

IV. Echocardiography
   The most consistent abnormalities with doxorubicin cardiotoxicity are increased left ventricular end-systolic internal dimensions and decreased fractional shortening.

Therapy

  I. If congestive heart failure develops, the patient should be treated accordingly. Unfortunately, the therapeutic response is poor.

 II. An ECG is recommended prior to each doxorubicin treatment, especially in dogs. If arrhythmias develop, doxorubicin treatment should be discontinued. An echocardiogram is recommended after the third cycle in dogs or fifth cycle in cats, and every 1 to 3 cycles thereafter. Doxorubicin treatment should be discontinued if contractility is impaired.

INFECTIOUS INFLAMMATORY DISEASES

Introduction

Overview

  I. The heart can be involved in an inflammatory process due to many infectious agents.
 II. Myocardial cells, interstitium, or vessels may be affected.

Cardiac Pathophysiology

  I. Myocardial injury can occur from direct myocardial invasion of an infectious agent, from a myocardial toxin produced by the agent, or as a resultant immune-mediated reaction.

 II. Important causes of myocardial injury in small animals include the following
   A. Bacterial myocarditis
      1. Pyogenic bacteria originate in septicemic states or from other septic foci.
      2. Clinical signs range from subclinical and nonspecific (weight loss, lethargy) to apparent and specific (arrhythmias, congestive heart failure).
   B. Viral myocarditis has been associated with canine parvovirus and distemper virus in dogs, and with suspected but not yet identified viral pathogens in cats. Clinical abnormalities include cardiomegaly, arrhythmias, and non-

specific ECG abnormalities. The severity of the cardiac changes ranges from congestive heart failure with canine parvovirus to subclinical myocarditis with canine distemper virus.

C. Fungus and algae can infect the heart secondary to a disseminated disease process, often in conjunction with reduced host defense.

D. Protozoal myocarditis can occur in dogs with canine trypanosomiasis *(Trypanosoma cruzi)* or in dogs and cats with toxoplasmosis *(Toxoplasma gondii)*.

    1. Trypanosomiasis is discussed below.

    2. Toxoplasmosis can produce signs dominated by the extent and severity of multiorgan system involvement.

Therapy

Treatment is often supportive and usually focused on the most prominent systemic manifestation of the disease process.

BORRELIOSIS (LYME DISEASE)

Overview

  I. Borreliosis is caused by the spirochete *Borrelia burgdorferi*. Transmission is via ticks of the *Ixodes* species.

 II. The incidence of cardiac involvement is unknown in animals. In man, 10 percent of patients with borreliosis have cardiac involvement.

III. Borreliosis in animals is usually acute and cured by antibiotics. However, the prognosis may be poor if second-stage disease involving the heart, kidneys, or central nervous system develops.

Cardiac Pathophysiology

  I. Spirochetes have been isolated from myocardial biopsies in humans.

 II. Dilated cardiomyopathy has been reported in a few humans with Lyme disease. Cardiac damage may involve an immune-mediated mechanism.

Diagnosis

  I. History and physical examination

    A. Ticks may be found on the dog, or the owners may report recent exposure to ticks in an endemic area.

    B. Although nonspecific, clinical signs include anorexia, depression, and lameness.

    C. Physical examination reveals fever, joint pain, and lymphadenopathy.

II. Electrocardiography
  A. The most common ECG finding in humans and dogs is AV block.
  B. Ectopic beats and ST segment abnormalities have also been reported in humans.
III. Specialized diagnostic tests
  Commercial test kits are available, but titers should be interpreted in view of the history, physical exam, and clinical signs. False-positive and false-negative titers are not uncommon.

Treatment

  I. Antibiotics are the treatment of choice for borreliosis. Tetracycline, doxycycline, ampicillin, or amoxicillin appear to be the most effective first-line agents.
 II. Humans with cardiac involvement are frequently treated with intravenous ceftriaxone or cefotaxime.
III. A 5 to 7 day course of anti-inflammatory doses of corticosteroids may be helpful for heart block that does not rapidly resolve with appropriate antibiotic therapy.

TRYPANOSOMIASIS (CHAGAS DISEASE)

Overview

  I. Trypanosomiasis is a rare disease caused by the protozoan *Trypanosoma cruzi*. It usually occurs in young dogs in the southeastern United States.
 II. Transmission is via the bite of a reduviid bug.

Cardiac Pathophysiology

  I. During the acute stage (2 to 4 weeks after infection), cardiac damage occurs when trypomastigotes rupture from myocardial cells. This causes myocardial failure, conduction disturbance, and arrhythmias.
 II. If animals survive the acute stage, they may remain asymptomatic for months. During this time, myocardial degeneration occurs and dilated cardiomyopathy develops. Myocardial damage during this stage may be related to immune mechanisms or the release of toxic parasitic products.

Diagnosis

  I. History and physical examination
  A. Clinical signs during the acute stage are related to left- and right-heart failure (mainly right). Collapse and sudden death may be noted in a previ-

ously healthy dog. Gastrointestinal signs of anorexia and diarrhea are also common. The lymph nodes will be enlarged during the acute stage.
  B. Clinical manifestations during the chronic stage are associated with dilated cardiomyopathy, with signs of right-sided heart failure often predominating. Various cardiac arrhythmias also occur. The cardiomyopathy is not curable and responds poorly to treatment.
  C. Physical findings associated with heart failure—such as pale mucous membranes, weak femoral pulses, and ascites—can be seen during both the acute and chronic stages.
II. Electrocardiography
    Conduction disturbances, ectopic beats, and sustained arrhythmias can be seen during the acute and chronic stages.
III. Radiography may show cardiomegaly, pulmonary edema, pleural effusion, hepatomegaly, and ascites.
IV. Echocardiography is normal during the acute phase. As the disease becomes chronic, ventricular contractility and wall thickness decrease, and cardiac chambers dilate.
V. Specialized diagnostic tests
  A. Trypomastigotes may be seen on a blood smear during the acute stage. The patient becomes aparasitemic 2 to 4 weeks after infection.
  B. Indirect fluorescent antibody, direct hemagglutination, and complement fixation tests confirm antibodies to *T cruzi*.
  C. Blood cultures can be performed, but they are time consuming.

Therapy

I. Treatment of this disease is very unrewarding. By the time the diagnosis is made, the disease is often no longer responsive to antiprotozoal medication.
II. Various therapeutic recommendations include oral benzimidazole (5 mg/kg once daily for 2 months), allopurinol (600 to 900 mg/day for 60 days) or nifurtimox (2 to 7 mg/kg every 6 hours for 3 to 5 months).
III. Alert owners and veterinary staff to potential zoonotic risk.

PARVOVIRUS

Overview

Parvovirus has caused cardiac disease when it infected puppies less than 2 weeks of age. Current cases of parvoviral myocarditis are very rare.

Cardiac Pathophysiology

Viral multiplication occurs in rapidly dividing myocardial cells, resulting is cell death and scarring.

Diagnosis

I. History and physical examination
  A. The cardiac form of parvovirus often results in sudden death.

B. Some puppies surviving the acute phase have developed heart failure weeks to months later, and died from cardiac arrhythmias or dilated cardiomyopathy 6 to 12 months later.
II. Electrocardiography revealed atrial or ventricular arrhythmias.
III. Echocardiography may revealed abnormalities in some infected dogs, consistent with dilated cardiomyopathy, including decreased fractional shortening, left atrial and ventricular enlargement, and increased E-point septal separation.

Therapy

I. Heart failure is managed with diuretics, digoxin, and ACE inhibitors.
II. Arrhythmias should be treated accordingly.

MISCELLANEOUS DISEASES

SYSTEMIC LUPUS ERYTHEMATOSUS

Overview

I. Cardiac disease due to systemic lupus erythematosus (SLE) is a common finding in humans, rare in dogs, and not reported in cats.
II. Pericarditis is the most common cardiac abnormality associated with SLE in humans. Other abnormalities in humans include myocarditis, congestive heart failure, and valvular heart disease. Ventricular arrhythmias were reported in two dogs and heart failure in one dog diagnosed with SLE.

Cardiac Pathophysiology

I. Pericarditis occurs secondary to vasculitis.
II. Myocarditis and endocarditis can also occur.

Diagnosis

I. History and physical examination
   A. Clinical signs associated with heart disease are usually overshadowed by the systemic signs of SLE.
   B. Clinical findings associated with arrhythmias or heart failure may be present.
II. Electrocardiography may reveal ventricular arrhythmias.
III. Echocardiographic abnormalities have not been reported in dogs or cats with SLE.
IV. Specialized diagnostic tests

A diagnosis of SLE can be made with a positive ANA titer in conjunction with clinical signs.

Therapy

I. Immunosuppressive doses of prednisone (2 mg/kg twice daily) is advised. If there is no improvement after 7 days, more aggressive immunosuppressive therapy should be considered.
II. Pericardiocentesis is recommended if pericardial effusion is present.

NEUROGENIC CARDIOMYOPATHY

Overview

I. Central nervous system (CNS) disease has been associated with myocardial lesions in clinical cases in all domestic species except the cat. Experimentally, stimulation of specific areas of cats' brains can cause myocardial necrosis.
II. Most cases involve trauma to the brain or spinal cord. CNS neoplasia, infection, encephalomalacia, and ruptured intervertebral discs can also result in myocardial damage.

Cardiac Pathophysiology

I. Histologic lesions include degeneration or disintegration of myocardial cells, with necrosis and mineralization. Scar formation may develop. The endocardium is most frequently involved, with occasional involvement of the subepicardium.
II. Myocardial necrosis may be evident as early as 3 days after the CNS damage, and generally is present within 5 to 10 days in affected animals. Cardiac arrhythmias are the most frequent clinical sequela.
III. The myocardial lesions probably occur due to increased sympathetic tone and release of catecholamines.

Diagnosis

I. History and physical examination
   Clinical signs are usually referable to the CNS disease and sometimes arrhythmias.
II. Electrocardiography
   Atrial and ventricular arrhythmias, ST segment depression, prolonged QT interval, and T wave abnormalities have been reported.
III. The diagnosis is often made on necropsy.

Therapy

Appropriate therapy for the CNS disease is advised. Treat arrhythmias as necessary.

GASTRIC DILATATION-VOLVULUS COMPLEX

Overview

  I. Gastric dilatation-volvulus complex (GDV) is a life-threatening emergency in the dog. It is most common in large, deep-chested dogs. No specific etiology has been determined, but GDV is often associated with exercise following a large meal.
 II. Cardiac arrhythmias occur in up to 40 percent of patients with GDV. Most arrhythmias are ventricular in origin. Atrial arrhythmias have also been reported. Arrhythmias usually occur within 36 hours of admission.

Cardiac Pathophysiology

The exact mechanism for the arrhythmias is unknown. Theories include acid-base imbalances, autonomic imbalances, myocardial hypoxia, electrolyte imbalances or a myocardial depressant factor.

Diagnosis

   I. History and physical examination
     A. Clinical signs are restlessness, pacing, lethargy, weakness, attempts to vomit, and abdominal distention.
     B. The physical examination often shows pale mucous membranes, rapid heart rate, weak femoral pulses, pain upon abdominal palpation and a distended, tympanic stomach, and signs associated with shock.
  II. Electrocardiography
     A. The ECG may reveal ventricular and occasionally atrial arrhythmias.
     B. ST segment and T wave changes may be evident.
 III. Radiography
     A. The stomach is gas filled, distended, and often rotated.
     B. The cardiac silhouette may be small due to decreased venous return.

Treatment

  I. Treatment should be directed toward gastric decompression and shock therapy.
 II. Any arrhythmias should be treated accordingly.

PANCREATITIS

Overview

Pancreatitis is a disease most frequently diagnosed in middle-aged, obese dogs and cats. Although many factors have been associated with pancreatitis, the etiology is often unknown.

Cardiac Pathophysiology

I. A myocardial depressant factor is released from the pancreas, which can result in decreased myocardial contractility and arrhythmias.
II. Activated pancreatic enzymes may also damage the myocardium directly or play a role in thrombus formation, resulting in myocardial ischemia.
III. Acid/base and electrolyte imbalances may also contribute to arrhythmias.

Diagnosis

I. History and physical examination
   A. Clinical signs are nonspecific and include vomiting, diarrhea, anorexia and depression.
   B. Physical examination may show abdominal pain, fever, dehydration, and shock.
   C. Sudden death associated with cardiac complications can occur.
II. Electrocardiography
   Atrial and ventricular arrhythmias and ST segment changes have been reported.
III. Radiography
   Abdominal radiographs reveal an increased density, calcification, or gas in the area of the pancreas.
IV. Clinical pathology
   Leukocytosis, hyperglycemia, increased liver enzymes, and increased amylase and lipase in serum and peritoneal fluid are common findings in animals with pancreatitis.

Therapy

I. It is important to decrease pancreatic secretions by withholding food and water.
II. Supportive care should include fluid and electrolyte replacement along with antibiotics.
III. Cardiac arrhythmias should be treated accordingly.

SUGGESTED READINGS

Appel MJ: Lyme disease in dogs and cats. Compend Cont Ed 12:617, 1990

Atkins C: The role of non-cardiac disease in the development and precipitation of heart failure. Vet Clin North Am (Small Anim Pract) 21:5, 1991

Barr SC: American trypanosomiasis in dogs. Compend Cont Ed 13:745, 1991

Carson TL: Toxic gases. p. 203. In Kirk RW (ed): Current Veterinary Therapy IX. WB Saunders, Philadelphia, 1986

Chew DJ, Nagode LA, Carothers M: Disorders of calcium: Hypercalcemia and hypocalcemia. p. 116. In DiBartola SP (ed): Fluid Therapy in Small Animal Practice. WB Saunders, Philadelphia, 1992

DiBartola SP, deMorais HSA: Disorders of potassium: Hypokalemia and hyperkalemia. p. 89. In DiBartola SP (ed): Fluid Therapy in Small Animal Practice. WB Saunders, Philadelphia, 1992

Feldman EC, Nelson RW: Canine and Feline Endocrinology and Reproduction. WB Saunders, Philadelphia, 1987

Fisch C: Electrolytes and the heart. p. 1599. In Hurst JW (Ed): The heart. 5th Ed. McGraw-Hill, New York, 1982

Fox PR: Canine myocardial disease. p. 467. In Fox PR (Ed): Canine and Feline Cardiology. Churchill Livingstone, New York, 1988

Fox PR, Nichols CER: Cardiac involvement in systemic disease. p. 565. In Fox PR (ed): Canine and Feline Cardiology. Churchill Livingstone, New York, 1988

Hooser SB, Beasley VR: Methylxanthine poisoning (chocolate and caffeine toxicosis). p. 191. In Kirk RW (ed): Current Veterinary Therapy IX. WB Saunders, Philadelphia, 1986

King JM, Roth L, Haschek WM: Myocardial necrosis secondary to neural lesions in domestic animals. J Am Vet Med Assoc 180:144, 1982

Loar AS, Susaneck SJ: Doxorubicin-induced cardiotoxicity in five dogs. Seminars in Vet Med and Sur 1:68, 1986

Mount ME: Toxicology. p. 456. In Ettinger SJ (ed): Textbook of Veterinary Internal Medicine. 3rd Ed. WB Saunders, Philadelphia, 1989

Muir WM: Gastric dilatation-volvulus in the dog, with emphasis on cardiac arrhythmias. J Am Vet Med Assoc 180:739, 1982

O'Keefe DA, Sisson DD, Gelberg HB et al: Systemic toxicity associated with doxorubicin administration in cats. p. 309. J Vet Int Med 7:5, 1993

Palumbo ME, Perri SF: Toad poisoning. p. 160. In Kirk RW (ed): Current Veterinary Therapy VIII. WB Saunders, Philadelphia, 1983

Peterson ME, Taylor RS, Greco DS et al: Acromegaly in 14 cats. p. 192. J Vet Int Med 4:4, 1990

Rosenthal DS, Braunwald E: Hematologic-oncologic disorders and heart disease. p. 1742. In Braunwald E (ed): Heart Disease. 4th Ed. WB Saunders, Philadelphia, 1992

Ruslander D: Heat stroke. p. 143. In Kirk RW (ed): Current Veterinary Therapy XI. WB Saunders, Philadelphia, 1992

Tilley LP, Bond BR, Patnaik AK, Liu S-K: Cardiovascular tumors in the cat. JAAHA 17:1009, 1981

Williams GH, Braunwald E: Endocrine and nutritional disorders and heart disease. p. 1827. In Braunwald E (ed): Heart Disease. 4th Ed. WB Saunders, Philadelphia, 1992

Yates RW, Weller RE: Have you seen the cardiopulmonary form of parvovirus infection? Vet Med April: 380, 1988

14

Pathophysiology and Treatment of Heart Failure

Mark D. Kittleson

INTRODUCTION

DEFINITION

Heart failure is a clinical syndrome caused by a cardiac disease that results in systolic or diastolic cardiac dysfunction (or a combination of both) severe enough to produce clinical signs of congestion/edema, inadequate perfusion, or both.

PATHOPHYSIOLOGY

I. Systolic function (the ability of the heart to contract and pump blood into an arterial system) is determined by myocardial contractility, preload, afterload (systolic myocardial wall stress), heart rate, heart size, and the presence or absence of leaks (shunts or regurgitant leaks) in the system (Fig. 14-1).
   A. The most common causes of systolic dysfunction are decreased myocardial contractility (myocardial failure), regurgitant leaks, and left-to-right shunts (leaks). Less commonly, systolic dysfunction can occur because of a decrease in venous return (mitral stenosis), an increase in afterload (aortic stenosis), or a decrease in heart rate (e.g., third-degree atrioventricular block).
   B. The pathophysiology of systolic dysfunction leading to congestive heart failure can be demonstrated by examining a theoretic situation in which a myocardial disease gradually results in worsening myocardial failure (decreased myocardial contractility).
      1. Start with a 3-year-old Doberman pinscher with early dilated cardiomyopathy (primary idiopathic myocardial failure). For the purposes of illustration, let us assume that the initial decrease in contractility produced by the myocardial disease is severe enough to cause problems and sudden enough that compensatory mechanisms have not had time to alter the initial course of events. In reality, the dog has had the disease since birth and contractility has gradually decreased to this point. The initial net result of the decrease in contractility is a decrease

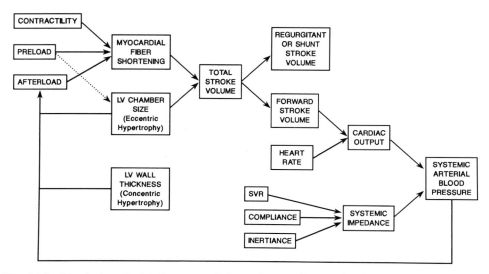

Fig. 14-1. The factors that influence and determine cardiovascular function and their relationships. LV, left ventricle; SVR, systemic vascular resistance.

in the amount of blood pumped with each beat (stroke volume). Since heart rate has not had time to increase, cardiac output also decreases (heart rate × stroke volume = cardiac output). Since the arterioles have not had time to constrict and increase resistance, the systemic arterial blood pressure decreases (pressure = cardiac output × resistance). The baroreceptors sense this and immediately engage the sympathetic nervous system.

2. The increase in sympathetic drive to the heart and blood vessels increases heart rate, contractility, and peripheral vascular resistance. This combination raises blood pressure back to normal and brings cardiac output back toward normal. The β_1 receptors, however, downregulate after 24 to 72 hours, and the ability of the sympathetic nervous system to counter the decrease in contractility disappears relatively rapidly.

3. At this time blood pressure is normal, mostly because of systemic arteriolar constriction, and cardiac output is reduced (hypoperfusion). The cardiovascular system must now find some way to increase cardiac output to normalize blood flow to the body. To compensate, the system increases the end-diastolic volume of the left ventricle by growing larger (eccentric or volume-overload hypertrophy).

4. The volume-overload hypertrophy (commonly called dilation) is stimulated by increased venous return to the heart, which increases the stretch on the myocardium in diastole. The increased venous return is brought about by the increased blood volume that is caused by renal salt and water retention. The kidneys sense a decrease in blood flow through them (decreased sodium presented to the macula densa) and ultimately release renin from the juxtaglomerular apparatus. Renin re-

sults in angiotensin II formation, which stimulates aldosterone release from the adrenal glands. Aldosterone acts on the distal tubules to increase sodium retention. Other mechanisms also result in salt and water retention, but the renin-angiotensin-aldosterone system appears to be the most important pathophysiologically and clinically.

5. The volume-overload hypertrophy compensates for the decrease in myocardial contractility, allowing the ventricle to pump a normal quantity of blood even though it does not contract as well (shortening fraction = 25 percent).

6. As myocardial contractility continues to decrease over time, volume-overload hypertrophy continues to increase to compensate. By the time the dog is 5 years old, the shortening fraction (the amount of wall motion or contraction) on this dog has decreased to 18 percent (normal, 30 to 40 percent), but the heart is still able to pump a normal quantity of blood.

7. When this imaginary dog is 7 years old, the shortening fraction has decreased to 10 percent. At this stage, it takes marked volume-overload hypertrophy to compensate completely; the ability of the ventricle to grow is reaching its limit. The kidneys, however, continue to retain salt and water in an attempt to produce further growth. At this time, the salt and water retention becomes detrimental as it forces more blood into the ventricle than the ventricle can accept, increasing the diastolic pressure. The increase in left ventricular diastolic pressure backs up into the left atrium (since the mitral valve is open, the left atrium and left ventricle essentially form one chamber), pulmonary veins, and ultimately the pulmonary capillaries. This creates pulmonary edema. The pulmonary edema may be mild to moderate at this stage, in which case the owner may still not notice anything wrong with the dog. If the pulmonary edema becomes severe—and it can do so within a short period of time—the dog presents with severe respiratory distress, which may appear as an acute problem to the owner.

8. If the edema remains mild to moderate, the disease may continue to progress until the dog finally presents with a shortening fraction of 5 percent, a markedly volume-overloaded ventricle, and signs of pulmonary edema and low cardiac output. This is end-stage disease, where the ventricle can no longer compensate for the severe depression in myocardial contractility.

C. Mitral regurgitation progresses similarly, except that the decrease in stroke volume is brought about by a backward leak of blood into the left atrium while myocardial contractility remains normal. The left ventricle develops volume-overload hypertrophy in this disease in order to allow the ventricle to eject a larger quantity of blood than normal, which compensates for the loss of stroke volume into the left atrium.

II. Diastolic dysfunction
Primary diastolic dysfunction can result from diseases that cause massive myocardial hypertrophy (e.g., hypertrophic cardiomyopathy), that result in endocardial or myocardial fibrosis (e.g., restrictive cardiomyopathy), or that

result from pericardial diseases (e.g., constrictive pericarditis, chronic pericardial tamponade). All result in abnormal filling of the ventricles during diastole. These disease processes generally produce chambers that are stiffer than normal, so that diastolic pressures are increased, resulting in congestion and edema. If filling is impeded to the point of producing a decreased end-diastolic volume of the ventricle, stroke volume may be decreased. In hypertrophic and restrictive cardiomyopathies, mitral regurgitation is a common complicating factor that contributes to the development of heart failure.

III. The cardiovascular system has three basic functions: to maintain a normal arterial blood pressure, to maintain normal blood flow (cardiac output), and to maintain these two at normal venous and capillary pressures. When the heart fails for whatever reason, these functions fail. The system is set up such that when the heart fails these functions fail sequentially, working within a system of priorities:

   A. *The first priority* is to maintain systemic arterial blood pressure to ensure flow and oxygen delivery to the critical vascular beds (brain, heart, kidneys). The high pressure is needed because these organs have high innate vascular resistance. Without adequate flow to these organs, death will occur within a short period of time.

   B. *The second priority* is to maintain cardiac output at an amount high enough to supply the entire body with an adequate amount of oxygen. If cardiac output becomes inadequate, death can occur in hours to days.

   C. *The third priority* is to maintain normal venous blood pressures. Death can occur in hours to weeks with high venous pressures.

   D. In heart failure, these cardiovascular functions are lost sequentially, with the lesser priority functions being lost first.

      1. When an acute disease results in systolic dysfunction, cardiac output initially decreases. This causes a decrease in systemic arterial blood pressure. The immediate response is peripheral vasoconstriction in an effort to increase systemic blood pressure back toward normal. However, this is done at the expense of cardiac output, since increasing blood pressure increases afterload and will serve to further decrease cardiac output.

      2. To compensate for an inadequate cardiac output, the body increases intracardiac diastolic volumes by increasing blood volume and by constricting systemic veins. The increase in blood volume is brought about by renal salt and water retention and increased thirst. The increased intracardiac volumes increase cardiac output but, if severe enough, also cause increased diastolic ventricular and so venous and capillary pressures, resulting in congestion and edema. The increased blood volume compensates for the systolic dysfunction and helps maintain cardiac output, which helps maintain systemic blood pressure. This may be at the expense of edema formation, however.

      3. When acute, overwhelming systolic dysfunction is present, the body does not have time to compensate. Cardiac output drops precipitously, resulting in a decrease in systemic arterial blood pressure. This is called cardiogenic shock. Cardiogenic shock is rare in chronic heart failure.

CLASSIFICATIONS OF HEART FAILURE

Congestive versus Low-Output Heart Failure

I. Congestive (backward) heart failure is defined as tissue congestion and edema due to increased capillary hydrostatic pressures that result from increased diastolic intraventricular pressures or increased atrial pressures. It can be due to primary diastolic dysfunction or to an increased blood volume occurring secondary to a disease that causes a primary low of systolic function.

II. Low-output (forward) heart failure is defined as clinical or laboratory evidence of inadequate tissue oxygen delivery due to a poor cardiac output. It is usually seen in the later stages of diseases that cause primary systolic dysfunction. It can be provoked in earlier stages with exercise.

Right- versus Left-Heart Failure

I. Right-sided congestive heart failure may result in hepatic congestion, ascites, and hydrothorax. Right-sided low-output heart failure decreases right ventricular cardiac output. It can result in a decreased amount of blood flow to the left ventricle, resulting in inadequate systemic blood flow.

II. Left-sided congestive heart failure is due to increased left ventricular diastolic and/or left atrial blood pressures that cause increased pulmonary venous and capillary pressures. In dogs this causes pulmonary congestion and edema. In cats this also produces pulmonary edema. It may also produce pleural effusion. In humans, it is thought that the visceral pleural veins drain into the pulmonary veins, with the result that left-heart failure can increase pleural venous pressure and so produce pleural effusion. The same appears to occur in the cat. Left-sided low-output failure is poor left ventricular cardiac output, resulting in inadequate tissue blood flow.

TYPES OF HEART FAILURE

Myocardial Failure

I. Myocardial failure is defined as a decrease in myocardial contractility. It results from diseases that cause a decrease in myocardial contractility. It can be due to a primary myocardial disease (idiopathic dilated cardiomyopathy, myocarditis) or secondary to prolonged increases in myocardial workload (e.g., aortic regurgitation, mitral regurgitation in large dogs). The most frequently diagnosed disease that results in myocardial failure is dilated cardiomyopathy. When myocardial failure is present, systolic function is poor, resulting in a low cardiac output and secondary fluid retention.

II. The myocardial disease can also result in a decrease in ventricular compliance, and thus altered diastolic ventricular function. Mitral regurgitation is also frequently present secondary to the left ventricular volume overload.

Heart Failure Due to Leaks

I. Mitral and tricuspid regurgitation result in a loss of forward stroke volume back into the left and right atria, respectively. The increased systolic atrial blood flow results in increased atrial pressure, which, when severe, can cause congestion and edema and increased atrial size. To compensate for the forward stroke volume loss, fluid retention occurs, producing volume overload hypertrophy (larger end-diastolic volume) of the affected ventricle. Since myocardial contractility remains relatively normal, the end-systolic volume of the ventricle remains normal while the volume overload hypertrophy produces an increase in end-diastolic volume. Consequently, total stroke volume (end-diastolic volume minus end-systolic volume) of the left ventricle is increased (whereas it is decreased in dilated cardiomyopathy). The increase in total stroke volume compensates for the amount of blood that leaks back into the left atrium. In late stages of the disease, salt and water retention increases diastolic intraventricular and atrial pressures, which can cause congestion and edema. When volume-overload hypertrophy can no longer compensate for the loss in forward stroke volume, cardiac output becomes inadequate and signs of low-output heart failure become evident. Myocardial failure may develop very late in the course of the disease in small dogs with mitral regurgitation. Atrial fibrillation may also develop late in the course of the disease. Large dogs routinely develop myocardial failure earlier in the course of their disease, which results in earlier development of heart failure.

II. Congenital left-to-right shunts share many characteristics with regurgitant lesions, such as a loss of forward stroke volume (i.e., the stroke volume that travels to the tissues) through the leak (in this case a shunt), which is compensated for by fluid retention and increased blood volume in the affected chamber(s) and blood vessels. Myocardial failure may develop, exacerbating the heart failure.

Heart Failure Due to Pressure Overload

I. Congenital stenotic lesions of the pulmonic or aortic valves cause increased systolic intraventricular pressures. If extremely severe (critical stenosis) at birth, these lesions probably produce peracute heart failure and death.

II. With lesser degrees of stenosis (noncritical), it is very unusual to see heart failure unless a concomitant leak—for example, mitral regurgitation due to mitral valve dysplasia—is also present. Instead the affected ventricle compensates with pressure-overload (concentric) hypertrophy. This compensation is usually so effective that ventricular function (stroke volume, shortening fraction) is normal.

III. Myocardial failure occasionally is seen secondary to pressure-overload hypertrophy. Much more commonly, these dogs die suddenly, presumably from severe ventricular tachyarrhythmias.

Heart Failure Due to Decreased Ventricular Compliance

I. Hypertrophic cardiomyopathy (HC) results in decreased ventricular compliance (increased stiffness) because of concentric hypertrophy.

II. Restrictive cardiomyopathy is caused by fibrosis of ventricular endocardium or myocardium, which increases ventricular stiffness. The increased ventricular stiffness can result in higher than normal diastolic intraventricular pressures, whether the diastolic volume is normal or even decreased.

III. The high diastolic intraventricular pressure may result in pulmonary congestion and edema (left-sided congestive heart failure).

IV. Probably more commonly these diseases also result in some degree of mitral regurgitation. The combination of this leak and the stiff ventricle results in the production of edema and effusion.

Heart Failure Due to Pericardial Disease

I. Constrictive pericarditis is caused by diseases that result in pericardial and epicardial scarring. The scarring results in cardiac constriction. This constriction results in increased diastolic intraventricular pressures. Since the right ventricle is thinner than the left ventricle, the diastolic pressure is usually higher in the right than in the left. In addition a diastolic pressure of 15 mmHg on the right side will produce severe ascites; on the left side it will only produce very mild pulmonary edema (apparently the systemic capillaries leak more readily than do the pulmonary capillaries). Consequently, dogs with constrictive pericarditis present with ascites.

II. Cardiac tamponade (compression of the heart due to fluid in the pericardial sac, causing signs of right-heart failure) can be acute or chronic.

A. Acute tamponade is usually due to hemorrhage into the pericardial space (e.g., left atrial rupture secondary to prolonged mitral regurgitation). The acute impediment to ventricular filling causes a decreased stroke volume, which will result in a decreased cardiac output, hypotension, shock, and death if untreated. Diastolic intraventricular and venous pressures are increased, especially on the right side, resulting in jugular venous distention and an elevated central venous pressure.

B. Chronic tamponade is seen with chronic pericardial effusion. The effusion increases intrapericardial pressure, as in acute tamponade, but in chronic tamponade the body has time to compensate. Cardiac output is frequently normal, but systemic venous pressure is increased secondary to the increased intrapericardial pressure; thus, signs of right-sided congestive heart failure (usually ascites) predominate.

DIAGNOSIS

History

A thorough history should be obtained from a client whose animal is being examined for heart disease. Clinical signs not evident on physical examination, previous medications and responses, and history of cardiovascular diseases may then be recorded. In this manner, an assessment of the progression of disease and the presence of any pre-existing complicating disease can be made.

 I. Cough

 Cough is often the presenting complaint in a dog with left-sided congestive heart failure. It is less common in the cat and may be confused with vomiting by the owner (in this situation the trachea should be manipulated to produce a cough, so that the owner can identify what is actually occurring). The clinician must remember that cough is not specific for heart failure, so that other diseases capable of producing a cough must be ruled out—or pulmonary edema as the cause must be ruled in—before therapy is initiated. Older small dogs with mitral regurgitation commonly have tracheal collapse, chronic pulmonary disease, compression of the left mainstem bronchus by an enlarged left atrium, or pulmonary edema. Such problems singularly or collectively can cause a cough.

 II. Tachypnea

 Tachypnea is defined as increased respiratory rate. This is a common sign that occurs with left-heart failure. It is commonly missed or ignored by the owner, since so many things can cause tachypnea normally. Since many dogs pant when they are being examined by a veterinarian, tachypnea is often times missed by veterinary clinicians. Respiratory rate can be used very effectively to monitor a left-heart failure patient's progression at home. Respiratory rate should be taken by the owner when the dog is lying quietly or sleeping in a cool environment. Respiratory rate should be less than 30 breaths per minute. If the respiratory rate increases in a dog with known left-heart failure, the owner should see a veterinarian or increase the diuretic dose, as this is usually a sign of increasing pulmonary edema.

 III. Dyspnea

 Dyspnea is defined as difficult breathing. By the time dyspnea is usually seen by an owner, severe pulmonary edema or severe hydrothorax is frequently present. Consequently, it is usually a late sign of heart failure in the dog and cat. Dyspnea can be more easily detected during exercise, if the patient exercises. By contrast, dyspnea is an earlier clinical sign of heart failure in humans, as it is experienced by the patient as difficulty in breathing.

 IV. Orthopnea

 Orthopnea is defined as difficult breathing when recumbent. An owner may notice that the animal is reluctant to lie down (because lying down makes it more difficult to breathe) or that the animal breathes heavily when lying down. Orthopnea may be present before dyspnea.

 V. Paroxysmal nocturnal dyspnea/coughing

 This occurs after an animal has been sleeping for a period of time. The owner complains that the dog wakes up coughing or dyspneic and that it then has to walk around before becoming comfortable again and going back to sleep. This sign is caused by a shift in blood volume from systemic veins to the heart and pulmonary circulation, resulting in higher diastolic ventricular pressure and pulmonary edema when the animal is recumbent. It is not a sign sensitive for heart failure, because many dogs with heart failure more commonly cough during the day and after exercise or excitement. It is also not specific for heart failure since dogs with other diseases may also cough at night.

VI. Ascites, hydrothorax, and peripheral edema

Ascites is a common finding in dogs with right-heart failure. When severe, it can be detected readily by visualization and/or ballottement. Small amounts of ascites may be detected with abdominal radiography or ultrasonography. Hydrothorax and peripheral edema are other clinical signs of right-heart failure. Systemic venous congestion may be evident. Central venous pressure is increased to greater than 10 cm H_2O.

VII. Exercise intolerance

Exercise intolerance can be one of the first signs of heart failure. However, since many pets do not exercise, this clinical sign is often not observed. Exercise intolerance occurs because cardiac output is inadequate for the increased tissue oxygen demand created by exercise. This results in tissue hypoxia, lactic acidemia, and muscle fatigue. Dyspnea is also present and is probably related to elevated pulmonary capillary pressure.

PHYSICAL EXAMINATION: CARDIOVASCULAR FINDINGS

Arrhythmias

I. Atrial fibrillation is a common finding in dogs with dilated cardiomyopathy but may also be present in dogs with chronic mitral regurgitation or long-standing patent ductus arteriosus. It may also occur in cats with cardiomyopathy. The heart rate is almost invariably increased in patients with heart failure and atrial fibrillation. This occurs because of high circulating catecholamine concentrations. The fast heart rate by itself may cause further myocardial failure (experimental dogs who have their hearts paced at 210 to 240 bpm develop myocardial failure severe enough to cause heart failure within 2 to 3 weeks). Consequently heart rate reduction is of paramount importance in patients with atrial fibrillation.

II. Atrial arrhythmias, other than atrial fibrillation, are also common in many different cardiovascular diseases that can lead to or are associated with heart failure.

III. Ventricular arrhythmias are common in boxers and Doberman pinschers with cardiomyopathy, but can be detected in many different cardiac diseases. Ventricular arrhythmias in conjunction with myocardial failure commonly predispose the animal to sudden death.

Gallop Sounds

Gallop sounds are common in patients with severe left ventricular volume overload and/or decreased myocardial compliance. Especially prevalent in cats with cardiomyopathy, they are caused by low-frequency vibrations and appear to originate from the left ventricle. They occur during early diastole with rapid ventricular filling (S_3) and late diastole during atrial systole (S_4). In cats with fast heart rates,

S_3 and S_4 commonly occur simultaneously (summation gallop). The type of gallop sound does not predict the type of heart disease present.

Signs and Diagnosis of Congestive Heart Failure

I. Pulmonary edema may occasionally be detected by auscultation, but auscultation is neither a sensitive (edema is commonly present when no auscultatory abnormalities are present) nor a specific (abnormal lung sounds are commonly present in animals without pulmonary edema) diagnostic test for this condition. Fine end-expiratory crackles are described in people with pulmonary edema. In people, these are heard after the patient takes a deep breath and then is told to breathe all the way out. This cannot be accomplished in veterinary medicine, which probably explains our inability to hear edema well in many animals. If pulmonary edema is suspected because of cough, dyspnea, or tachypnea, chest radiographs should be evaluated.

II. Systemic veins may or may not be distended with right-heart failure. The jugular veins should be examined for distension in a patient with right-heart disease and suspected right-heart failure. Examination of hepatic veins for distension is a more accurate means of demonstrating venous congestion. Manual compression of the cranial abdomen may demonstrate exaggerated jugular venous distention (hepatojugular reflux). In addition, ascites, hydrothorax, or peripheral edema may be present.

III. Pleural effusion is a common abnormality associated with right- and/or left-heart failure. Chest radiographs should be evaluated to determine if pleural effusion is present or not, except in patients with severe dyspnea. In patients with severe dyspnea, positioning for radiography may be stressful enough to cause death. Consequently thoracentesis should be performed first in these patients to confirm or exclude pleural effusion and to relieve the dyspnea.

Signs of Low-Output Heart Failure

I. Mild or moderate heart failure
Signs of low-output heart failure are usually only present when the animal exercises. Clinical signs are those of fatigue and dyspnea.

II. Severe heart failure
Cardiac output may be low when the patient is at rest, which may cause the extremities to be cold and sometimes will cause pale mucous membranes and a prolonged capillary refill time. Lactic acidemia at rest or with mild exercise and a low venous oxygen tension (<30 mmHg in a sample taken from free-flowing jugular venous blood) may be demonstrated.

ELECTROCARDIOGRAM

The electrocardiogram may indicate atrial and/or ventricular arrhythmias, atrial and/or ventricular enlargement, or conduction disturbances in association with cardiac disease. The ECG does not provide any definitive criteria for diagnosing heart failure.

Thoracic Radiographs

I. Signs of heart failure on thoracic radiographs are limited to those of pulmonary edema and pleural effusion.
   A. The earliest sign of left-heart failure is pulmonary venous congestion (engorged or enlarged pulmonary veins). This occurs when the pulmonary capillary pressure is 15 to 20 mmHg.
   B. As pulmonary venous and capillary pressures increase, interstitial (20 to 30 mmHg) and then alveolar edema (30 to 40 mmHg) appear. The edema may be centrally located around the base of the heart (perihilar), but may also be generalized. Pleural effusion may also be present, especially in cats with left- or left- and right-heart failure and in dogs with concomitant left- and right-heart failure.
   C. The cardiovascular silhouette is usually enlarged in heart failure.
      1. The enlargement can be due to atrial distension, ventricular volume overload hypertrophy, ventricular pressure overload hypertrophy, or pericardial effusion.
      2. Cardiac enlargement is not a sign of heart failure per se and may be absent in diseases such as constrictive pericarditis and restrictive cardiomyopathy.
II. Pleural effusion, hepatomegaly, and ascites may be present with right-sided congestive heart failure.

Echocardiography

Echocardiography is extremely helpful in differentiating cardiac diseases that cause heart failure and in identifying types of diseases that lead to heart failure, such as myocardial failure, heart failure due to a leak in the cardiovascular system, and heart failure due to decreased ventricular compliance. Although an echocardiogram cannot be used to definitively diagnose heart failure, it is very unusual to see left-sided congestive heart failure without moderate-to-severe left atrial enlargement or right-sided congestive heart failure without moderate-to-severe right atrial enlargement (in the absence of pericardial effusion). In right-sided congestive heart failure, hepatic venous congestion visualized with ultrasonography is a more sensitive diagnostic test of elevated systemic venous pressure than is observing distended peripheral veins.

Cardiac Catheterization

I. This diagnostic tool can be used to determine the underlying heart disease, to confirm the presence of heart failure (by measuring diastolic intraventricular pressures and cardiac output), and to assess the severity of heart failure. It has been used less commonly as less invasive tests have become more accurate and more available.
II. Since most animals with heart failure are anesthetic risks, it is desirable to either avoid cardiac catheterization, do the procedure with sedation and local

anesthesia or do it with light anesthesia and keep the procedure as short as possible.

III. In dogs that require invasive testing to assess the severity of cardiac disease, catheterization of the right side of the heart with a balloon-tipped thermodilution catheter (Swan-Ganz catheter) is preferred. This type of catheter can be placed with the dog awake or lightly sedated, and the catheter can be maintained in place to monitor the disease or response to therapy if necessary. The catheter is used to measure cardiac output and filling pressures of the right and left ventricles (the pressures that cause edema and effusion).

PROTOCOL FOR THE DIAGNOSIS OF HEART FAILURE

I. Confirmatory tests
   A. Left-sided congestive failure is absolutely confirmed by measuring pulmonary capillary pressure, but is usually more loosely confirmed by identifying pulmonary edema on a chest radiograph in association with left-heart disease and/or left-heart enlargement on a chest radiograph or an echocardiogram.
   B. Right-sided congestive heart failure is confirmed by identifying ascites, hydrothorax, or peripheral edema and either excluding other causes or confirming increased systemic venous pressure (either measured or observed as venous distension). More loosely it can be confirmed by identifying an enlarged right heart.
   C. Low-output heart failure may be difficult to confirm. If heart failure is mild to moderate, cardiac output may only be inadequate when the animal exercises. Exercise testing is rarely done in veterinary medicine. If low-output heart failure is present at rest, it can be documented by determining that a low cardiac output is responsible for causing tissue oxygen delivery to drop below the amount required by tissue oxygen consumption. This can be done by first assessing the adequacy of tissue oxygen delivery through measuring the difference in oxygen content between arterial and mixed venous blood, or by measuring mixed venous oxygen tension. A low-cardiac output as the cause for decreased tissue oxygen delivery then can either be confirmed by measuring cardiac output, or other causes can be excluded by determining hemoglobin concentration and arterial oxygen saturation. Such determinations are clinically difficult. The author generally substitutes a jugular venous sample or a mixed venous sample for determination of the venous oxygen tension, and then rules out arterial hypoxemia and anemia as causes of poor tissue oxygen delivery.

II. Differential diagnoses
   A. Noncardiac pulmonary disease frequently mimics heart failure. Both can cause coughing and dyspnea. It is not unusual for heart disease and pulmonary disease to be present in the same patient. One or both may be responsible for clinical signs. Thoracic radiographs are usually the best diagnostic test to differentiate the causes of cough and dyspnea, but false-negative and false-positive results do occur for all diseases assessed in this manner.

Although measurements of left ventricular end-diastolic or pulmonary capillary wedge pressure are the ideal means of confirming pulmonary edema due to left-sided heart failure, they cannot be done routinely on a practical basis.

B. Ascites, peripheral edema, and hydrothorax can be caused by diseases other than congestive heart failure. Usually the measurement of central venous pressure will confirm whether or not right-heart failure is the cause. Evaluation of the size of the hepatic veins is a good substitute.

THERAPY

MEDICAL THERAPY

Medical management is directed at treating and improving the clinical signs associated with heart failure and so improving the quality of life. Signs of congestion and edema can be treated with diuretics, a low-salt diet, positive inotropic agents, venodilators, arteriolar dilators, and ACE inhibitors. Signs of inadequate cardiac output can be treated with positive inotropic agents and arteriolar dilators. The appropriate treatment regimen for a given dog or cat depends on the clinical signs present, the severity of the clinical signs, and the underlying disease. The disease causing the heart failure rarely can be treated and reversed. Examples are taurine administration in cats with dilated cardiomyopathy, taurine and carnitine administration in American cocker spaniels with dilated cardiomyopathy, and carnitine administration in some boxer dogs with dilated cardiomyopathy.

THERAPY FOR DECREASING CONGESTION AND EDEMA

Low-Sodium Diets

I. Low-sodium diets can effectively decrease blood volume and reduce congestion and edema, especially in mild and moderate heart failure.
A. Unfortunately, many low-salt diets are not very palatable. As a result, owner and patient compliance with this form of therapy can be poor. Salt substitutes containing potassium chloride (KCl) can be added to improve flavor.
B. Commercial low-salt diets have a very low sodium content (30 to 50 mg/ 100 g dry weight) and probably are most appropriate as the sole caloric source for dogs with severe heart failure. In dogs with mild-to-moderate heart failure, dog food with a sodium content on the lower end of the range (350 to 400 mg/100 g dry weight) can be mixed 50:50 with a commercial low-sodium diet for the pet. Alternatively, the animal's normal diet can be fed and the edema treated medically.
C. Booklets can be obtained from the American Heart Association, its local chapters, or the USDA, detailing the sodium content of various foods or

listing those foods recommended for the patient on a low-salt diet. Many pet owners enjoy cooking a low-salt diet for their pet.

Diuretics

I. Diuretics used in heart failure increase urinary sodium excretion by decreasing sodium retention within renal tubules. By doing so they decrease blood volume and so decrease diastolic pressures within the heart. The choice and dose of diuretic depend on the severity of clinical signs. Oral doses for the only diuretics used by the author are listed in Table 14-1.

   A. If only congestion or mild edema is present, low-dose furosemide is generally used.

   B. Moderate-to-severe edema is usually also treated with furosemide. The dose and frequency depend on the severity of the edema and need to be titrated to produce the desired effect. If a patient is refractory to furosemide, the drug can be combined with a thiazide diuretic to promote additional diuresis. One study has documented that serum potassium concentration does decrease about 10 percent with chronic furosemide administration in dogs with heart failure. This degree of hypokalemia is generally clinically insignificant. This study also suggested that some dogs do develop clinically significant hypokalemia while on chronic furosemide therapy. In the author's experience, it is unusual for a dog or cat to develop clinically significant hypokalemia or dehydration as a result of chronic diuretic administration as long as the pet is eating and drinking, even when the upper end of the dosage range is used. Consequently, potassium supplementation is generally not required, although this type of supplementation is benign and may be used at the discretion of the clinician and owner. Regardless, owners should be warned that if their pet stops eating and drinking, problems with hydration and electrolyte balance may develop rapidly and the veterinarian should be informed promptly.

   C. Life-threatening pulmonary edema may be treated aggressively with intravenous furosemide. Doses up to 8 mg/kg may be administered to dogs as frequently as every hour until diuresis is evident and respiratory rate is decreasing. Intravenous doses in cats should not exceed 2 mg/kg. Although hyponatremia, hypokalemia, and dehydration are common with this intensive therapy, these result only rarely in death, whereas severe pulmonary edema that is not treated aggressively is a frequent cause of death.

TABLE 14-1. DIURETICS COMMONLY USED IN DOGS WITH HEART FAILURE

Generic Name	Trade Name	Route of Administration	Dosage
Hydrochlorothiazide	Hydrodiuril	PO	2–4 mg/kg BID
Chlorothiazide	Diuril	PO	20–40 mg/kg BID to TID
Furosemide	Lasix	PO	1–4 mg/kg SID to TID
		IV; IM	2–8 mg/kg up to every hour (see text)

THERAPY FOR INCREASING MYOCARDIAL
CONTRACTILITY

Positive inotropic therapy (therapy to increase contractility) should ideally be used only to treat heart failure when myocardial failure is present. As myocardial function is usually difficult to assess in a clinical situation, clinical decisions are generally made on the basis of population characteristics.

I. Dogs and cats with dilated cardiomyopathy always have poor myocardial contractility and probably should always be treated with positive inotropic drugs.
II. Small dogs with mitral regurgitation usually have normal or relatively normal myocardial function for at least 6 months to 1 year after they start showing signs of heart failure severe enough to require diuretic therapy, and may not require digitalis during this period.
III. Large dogs with primary mitral regurgitation, on the other hand, routinely develop myocardial failure with significant mitral regurgitation.
IV. In some diseases, such as hypertrophic cardiomyopathy where myocardial contractility is normal and left ventricular function is enhanced, the use of positive inotropes is contraindicated.

Digitalis Glycosides

I. The digitalis glycosides are the only positive inotropic agents available for long-term oral use. Newer positive inotropic agents may become available for clinical use and may replace digitalis in some situations and augment the use of digitalis in others.
   A. The use of digitalis glycosides is indicated in dogs and cats with signs of low output or congestive heart failure due to myocardial failure. The myocardial failure may be primary (e.g., dilated cardiomyopathy) or secondary to increased cardiac workloads (e.g., patent ductus arteriosus). Digitalis is also indicated as an antiarrhythmic agent when supraventricular arrhythmias are present, and to slow the ventricular response to atrial flutter and fibrillation.
   B. Digoxin is the most commonly used cardiac glycoside. Digoxin has a half-life of 24 to 36 hours in the dog and approximately 33 to 58 hours in the cat. Digoxin binds poorly to protein, and is excreted via glomerular filtration. About 60 percent of the digoxin in tablets is absorbed from the gastrointestinal tract and 75 percent of the elixir is absorbed (doses of digoxin should be reduced by 20 percent when the elixir is used).
   C. Digoxin usually should be administered as chronic oral maintenance doses. Parenteral administration and loading doses may result in toxicity. Doubling the maintenance dose for the first two doses may be done in emergency situations, such as when trying to control a supraventricular arrhythmia.
   D. The dosage of digoxin is 0.22 mg/m² of body surface area BID for large (>20 kg) dogs and 0.011 mg/kg BID for small dogs. Body surface area can either be calculated (BSA = 0.67×0.112) or the conversion from body weight to body surface area can be found in standard veterinary medicine texts.

E. Every time digoxin is administered to a patient, a pharmacologic experiment is carried out. Pharmacokinetics are so variable from patient to patient and so many factors affect digoxin pharmacokinetics that one cannot predict exactly what the digoxin dosage will be for a given case. Consequently one should start with a standard dosage and then measure the serum digoxin concentration 3 to 5 days later to determine if the dosage being administered is appropriate. The sample for measuring serum digoxin concentration should be taken 6 to 8 hours after the last dose. If the serum concentration is within the therapeutic range (1.0–2.0 ng/ml) and no signs of toxicity are present, the dosage should be maintained. If the serum concentration is greater than 2.5 ng/ml, digoxin should be discontinued for 1 to 2 days and the dosage reduced. If the serum concentration is less than 1.0 ng/ml, the dosage should be increased.

F. Digoxin dosage in cats is 0.005 to 0.01 mg/kg given once a day or divided BID for tablets. Cats dislike the taste of the elixir.
   1. One-fourth of 0.125 mg digoxin tablet every other day for cats weighing 2 to 3 kg
   2. One-fourth tablet daily for cats weighing 4 to 6 kg
   3. One-fourth tablet BID for cats weighing 7 or more kg).

G. Numerous factors alter digitalis dosages.
   1. Dogs or cats with hypernatremia, hypokalemia, or hypercalcemia require less digitalis.
   2. Both hyper- and hypothyroid animals need less digitalis.
   3. Animals with myocardial failure can be more sensitive to digitalis, so their doses must be titrated carefully.
   4. Dogs or cats with renal failure excrete less digoxin, resulting in a high serum concentration and toxicity. Patients with renal failure can be treated with digoxin, but must be treated cautiously, starting with low doses and titrating carefully upward while monitoring the serum concentration.
   5. Digoxin does not diffuse into fat, so estimates of lean body weight in obese patients should be used to calculate dosage.
   6. The largest body store of digoxin is in skeletal muscle. Consequently, cachexic dogs have a relative decrease in volume of distribution and so dosage must be decreased.
   7. Digoxin does not distribute well into ascitic fluid. As a general rule, digoxin dosage should be decreased by 10 percent in dogs with mild ascites, 20 percent in dogs with moderate ascites, and 30 percent in dogs with severe ascites.
   8. Quinidine, verapamil, and drugs that inhibit hepatic microsomal enzymes (chloramphenicol, tetracycline) should not be administered concurrently with digoxin. If quinidine and digoxin must be administered concomitantly, the digoxin dosage should be halved to start with.

H. Patients that receive an adequate amount of digitalis and that respond with an increase in myocardial contractility show improvement in clinical signs. Perfusion and exercise tolerance improve, and congestion and edema decrease. The heart rate usually decreases in animals treated for supraventricular tachyarrhythmias. ECG changes are insensitive and nonspecific indica-

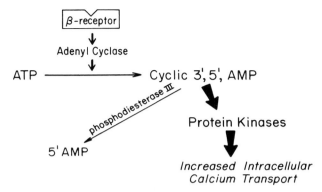

Fig. 14-2. The cascade of events that results in increased myocardial contractility after myocardial beta-adrenergic receptor stimulation. A similar cascade can be induced by phosphodiesterase III inhibition.

tors of adequate serum digitalis concentrations. About 80 percent of dogs with dilated cardiomyopathy do not respond to digoxin administration. Dogs with DC that do not respond have an average survival time of 6 weeks, as compared with 6 months for those that do respond. It is unusual for dogs with myocardial failure secondary to mitral regurgitation to have a clinically significant increase in contractility following digoxin administration.

I. Digitalis toxicity
   1. Mild digoxin intoxication produces anorexia and vomiting and can be treated by drug withdrawal.
   2. Severe toxicity may produce many different cardiac arrhythmias. Ventricular tachyarrhythmias are the most common and the most serious, as they can result in death. Lidocaine is the antiarrhythmic of choice in this situation. Digoxin should be discontinued for at least 48 hours, and the dose reduced based on the serum concentration achieved and the time it took to achieve it.

Bipyridine Compounds

I. Amrinone and milrinone* are agents that have potent positive inotropic and mild arteriolar dilating properties. They act by inhibiting the type of phosphodiesterase found in canine myocardium (phosphodiesterase F-III). Phosphodiesterases are responsible for breaking down intracellular cyclic AMP. Phosphodiesterase inhibition results in increased intracellular cyclic AMP, similar to the effects of beta receptor stimulation (Fig. 14-2). When beta receptors are chronically stimulated, they down-regulate and become less responsive to stimulation. By bypassing the beta receptor, the bipyridine compounds are able to maintain an increase in contractility chronically. Because they can increase contractility to degrees similar to the effects of catecholamines in dogs and cats, the bipyri-

---

* Milrinone is an experimental drug not yet approved for use in dogs or cats.

dine compounds are much more effective than digoxin. They appear to be less potent in their positive inotropic effects in humans. The bipyridines are much safer than digitalis. Amrinone is currently available for intravenous administration. Milrinone is experimental, but may be marketed in the future for chronic oral use in the dog.

A. Amrinone can be used in critical care situations to increase contractility for anywhere from hours to a few days. It is initially administered as a loading dose of 1 to 3 mg/kg. A constant rate infusion of 10 to 100 μg/kg/min is then administered to maintain the desired effect.

B. Milrinone, if marketed, will be used as an oral agent. When administered orally, the effects of milrinone can be observed within 30 minutes. Drug effect lasts at least 12 hours, but the positive inotropic effect is less than half the initial effect at 12 hours. Dogs with milder signs of heart failure may require dosing only every 12 hours. Dogs with severe heart failure may require dosing every 6 to 8 hours. The oral dose ranges from 0.5 to 1.0 mg/kg.

C. The positive inotropic properties of milrinone, along with its arteriolar dilating properties, make it a very attractive drug for treating myocardial failure. In clinical studies, milrinone appears to be effective in 70 to 80 percent of patients with severe heart failure. The drug may also be beneficial in treating dogs with chronic mitral valve degeneration because of the arteriolar dilation produced. The drug should probably only be used in mitral regurgitation patients refractory to other drugs, since the increase in force generated by the left ventricle may rupture chordae tendineae in about 4 percent of patients.

D. Milrinone has exacerbated ventricular arrhythmias in a small number of dogs with myocardial failure. Electrocardiographic monitoring is advised when the drug is first administered. If a ventricular arrhythmia is present before milrinone administration, it should be treated appropriately. If a ventricular arrhythmia develops after milrinone administration, the drug should be discontinued or the arrhythmia treated.

Dobutamine and Dopamine

I. The sympathomimetics are only used in acute situations to treat heart failure. Their short half-life (1 to 2 minutes) and extensive hepatic metabolism make them inappropriate for oral use. This class of drugs stimulates various adrenergic receptors, so that drug effects can vary markedly from one drug to another.

A. Dobutamine increases myocardial contractility by stimulating β_1 receptors. Both β_2 and α_1 receptors are stimulated in peripheral vasculature, so there is no major change in blood pressure.

1. Dobutamine can be used to treat dogs with acute myocardial failure resulting from anesthetic overdose, severe metabolic abnormalities, or myocardial depression following cardiac arrest. It can also be used to stabilize patients with chronic heart failure while waiting for other drugs to render support. As an example, a dog with severe heart failure due to dilated cardiomyopathy may benefit from short-term dobutamine ad-

ministration while maintenance doses of ACE inhibitors are administered.

   2. Dobutamine, like other sympathomimetics, should be administered as a constant-rate infusion. Usual infusion rates range from 5 to 20 μg/kg/min. Heart rate usually increases at infusion rates of greater than 20 μg/kg/min.

B. Dopamine acts similarly to dobutamine, with three major differences.

   1. Dopamine dilates renal and mesenteric vasculature, favoring flow to these vascular beds, and dobutamine favors flow to myocardial and skeletal muscle.

   2. The infusion rate for dopamine is 1 to 10 μg/kg/min, and infusion rates greater than 10 μg/kg/min produce vasoconstriction.

   3. There is some evidence that dopamine may increase diastolic intraventricular pressures in chronic heart failure patients, so dobutamine may be favored in this group.

VASODILATOR THERAPY

I. Vasodilators can be used to treat acute or chronic heart failure. Vasodilators dilate systemic arterioles, systemic veins, or both. Selected vasodilators may also have effects on the pulmonary vasculature.

A. Types of vasodilators

   1. Arteriolar dilators (e.g., hydralazine) decrease aortic input impedance (systemic vascular resistance), usually lower systemic arterial blood pressure in heart failure patients, and so decrease systolic myocardial wall stress (afterload). This may result in an increased myocardial fiber shortening (shortening fraction) and an increased stroke volume. In mitral regurgitation, the decreased resistance to forward direction flow induced by arteriolar dilators results in less regurgitant (backward) flow and greater aortic (forward) blood flow. This results in lowered left atrial pressures (decreased pulmonary edema), along with an increased forward stroke volume (improved perfusion).

   2. Venodilators (e.g., nitroglycerin) decrease diastolic intracardiac volumes by redistributing blood away from the heart and pulmonary circulation into the peripheral veins (Fig. 14-3). These agents may be used to treat signs of congestion and edema.

   3. Combination vasodilators (e.g., nitroprusside, prazosin) decrease congestion and edema and increase cardiac output.

   4. Angiotensin converting enzyme (ACE) inhibitors (e.g., captopril, enalapril) act as arteriolar dilators and venodilators, but in addition they decrease circulating plasma aldosterone concentration and so decrease renal sodium and water retention.

B. ACE inhibitors act by blocking the conversion of angiotensin I to angiotensin II (Fig. 14-4). Angiotensin II is a potent arteriolar constrictor and venoconstrictor. Consequently, ACE inhibitors act as arteriolar dilators and venodilators. Angiotensin II also stimulates aldosterone secretion in the zona glomerulosa of the adrenal gland, thus, ACE inhibitors decrease

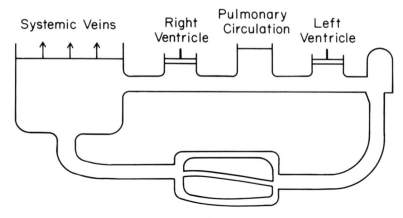

Fig. 14-3. The circulatory system, with the effect of venodilation depicted.

plasma aldosterone concentration, resulting in decreased salt and water retention. ACE inhibitors are the most commonly used vasodilators in veterinary medicine. They are relatively easy to use, the incidence of side effects is generally low, and they are reasonably effective. Neither captopril nor enalapril needs to be titrated to an effective endpoint and determining dosage is easy. Major side effects consist of hypotension and functional azotemia but are relatively uncommon. Gastrointestinal upset is relatively common with captopril. This side effect appears to be less common with enalapril. The ACE inhibitors have been documented to prolong survival in human heart-failure patients. This also appears to be the case in dogs.

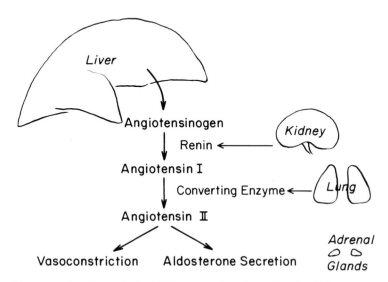

Fig. 14-4. The cascade of events that follows renin release by the kidneys in response to a decrease in renal blood flow.

The clinical impression of many veterinary cardiologists is that ACE inhibitors stabilize patients with heart failure, and that heart-failure stability appears to be better and more prolonged when ACE inhibitors are being administered. Neither drug is very effective in emergency situations.

1. Captopril, when administered acutely, decreases peripheral vascular resistance by about 25 percent in patients with myocardial failure. This increases cardiac output, but does not decrease edema formation. This effect is apparent within 1 hour and is gone within 4 hours. Doses of 0.5 to 1.0 mg/kg are effective both acutely and chronically. Chronic administration of captopril is effective in decreasing edema formation. When given chronically, captopril is effective when administered every 8 hours. About 50 percent of the drug is excreted unchanged in the urine, so renal failure can significantly increase the half-life of the drug. Consequently,the dose of captopril should be reduced in patients with renal failure.

2. Enalapril is an inactive drug that is converted to the active form of the drug, enalaprilat, in the liver. Almost all of the enalaprilat is excreted via the kidneys. Consequently enalapril should be used very cautiously in patients with renal failure. Captopril may be preferred in this situation. Otherwise, enalapril has two potential advantages over captopril. First, its duration of effect is longer, 12 to 14 hours. This decreases dosing frequency to once every 12 to 24 hours. Second, dogs appear to have fewer gastrointestinal disturbances than with captopril.

3. Both captopril and enalapril can induce functional azotemia. Renal blood flow is compromised in heart failure. To maintain normal glomerular filtration rate, angiotensin constricts the renal efferent arterioles (the arteriole exiting the glomerulus) to maintain intraglomerular pressure and increase filtration fraction. ACE inhibitor administration results in some efferent arteriolar dilation. In some cases, ACE inhibitor administration results in relatively profound efferent arteriolar dilation, which decreases glomerular filtration and results in azotemia. Because of this, it is recommended that renal function be examined before the onset of ACE inhibitor administration and again 4 to 7 days after initiating therapy. If azotemia develops and is relatively mild to moderate, decreasing the diuretic dose may result in reductions in serum urea nitrogen and creatinine concentrations. If the azotemia is severe or unresponsive to this maneuver, discontinuing the ACE inhibitor should be considered.

4. Once a patient is established on an ACE inhibitor, any withdrawal of the drug should be done very cautiously. The author has noted fulminant pulmonary edema within 24 hours of withdrawing captopril from dogs that were in heart failure.

C. Hydralazine can be used as primary therapy in patients with mitral regurgitation, as alternative therapy in patients with mitral regurgitation that are refractory to ACE inhibition, or as adjunctive therapy in mitral regurgitation patients refractory to ACE inhibition. Hydralazine is particularly effective at reducing mitral regurgitation in dogs with primary mitral valve

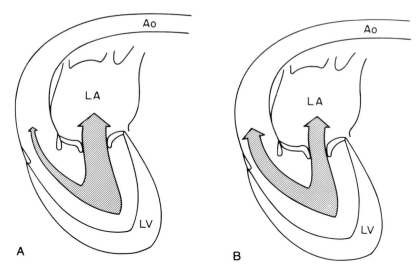

Fig. 14-5. Schematic diagrams of the left ventricle and left atrium in a dog with severe mitral regurgitation (**A**) before and (**B**) after arteriolar dilator therapy. Arteriolar dilation results in a decrease in systemic vascular resistance to flow into the aorta while resistance to flow through the mitral valve orifice remains constant. The net results are an increase in blood flow into the aorta and systemic circulation and a decrease in regurgitant flow into the left atrium.

disease (Fig. 14-5). When switching a patient from an ACE inhibitor to hydralazine, care must be taken to ensure that hydralazine's effects are evident within hours after the ACE inhibitor's effects have dissipated (captopril's effects are gone after 4 hours; enalapril's effects are gone after about 12 hours in dogs). Hydralazine and an ACE inhibitor may be used concomitantly, but extreme care must be taken to avoid hypotension in this situation. To avoid hypotension and to identify an appropriate dose, blood pressure must be monitored while hydralazine is titrated to a patient already receiving an ACE inhibitor.

1. Hydralazine's arteriolar dilating effects lasts 11 to 13 hours. Its dosage ranges from 0.5 to 3 mg/kg and must be titrated to an effective endpoint. Administering 1 mg/kg hydralazine to all dogs will result in ineffective doses being administered to approximately 60 percent of these dogs.
2. Before drug administration, baseline thoracic radiographs should be taken. Mucous membrane color should be evaluated carefully. Jugular venous oxygen tension should be evaluated if possible. If systemic arterial blood pressure (either systolic blood pressure from a Doppler machine or mean blood pressure) can be obtained, it may be recorded.
3. An initial dose of 1 mg/kg hydralazine should be administered to dogs PO. To determine whether this dose is effective, blood pressure measurement can be repeated in 1 hour and venous blood gas measurement in 3 hours, or clinical signs can be reevaluated anywhere from 5 hours to 1 day later.

4. If mean systemic arterial blood pressure has decreased between 15 and 20 mmHg or is less than 70 mmHg, the titration is complete and the 1 mg/kg dose should be continued at 12-hour intervals. The same is true if the venous P_{O_2} was less than 35 mmHg and has increased to more than 35 mmHg. If the mucous membrane color has improved dramatically, or if pulmonary edema has decreased (generally within 24 hours), the dosage administered was effective.

5. If no improvement has occurred, drug titration should continue and another 1 mg/kg dose (total dose, 2 mg/kg) administered if less than 8 hours have passed since the last dose. If more than 12 hours have passed, a 2 mg/kg total dose should be administered. The dog should be reevaluated as appropriate.

6. If there is still no response, a total dose of 3 mg/kg can be administered.

7. The total dose should be administered every 12 hours.

8. Side effects of hydralazine include hypotension and tachycardia. Clinically significant hypotension (i.e., mean systemic arterial blood pressure <60 mmHg,) is usually manifested as profound weakness. This should generally not be treated. Instead the dog should be observed for the 12 hours that the drug effect lasts. At the end of the 12-hour time period, the dog usually recovers very quickly without sequelae. The author has observed one dog that received 10 times the recommended dose that recovered uneventfully. A death secondary to hydralazine administration has never been recorded in humans, where the dosage record for an individual is 10 gm.

9. If heart rate is more than 180 bpm, use of a digitalis glycoside and/or propranolol may be considered to decrease the heart rate. Some dogs and cats have gastrointestinal disturbances associated with hydralazine use. This complication may be severe enough to preclude further therapy.

10. Dosage titration for cats should start at a total dose of 2.5 mg and can go as high as 10 mg.

D. The nitrates are vasodilators that are less commonly used in veterinary medicine. Examples include nitroglycerin, isosorbide dinitrate and mononitrate, and nitroprusside.

1. Nitroglycerin is administered transcutaneously to patients with heart failure. At low serum concentration, nitroglycerin produces venodilation; and at higher serum concentration, it produces venodilation and arteriolar dilation. When administered transcutaneously, low serum concentration is achieved, and thus only venodilation is evident. No studies of the clinical efficacy of nitroglycerin have been performed in veterinary medicine. One limited study by the author has suggested that nitroglycerin cream is not absorbed across canine thoracic skin. Nitroglycerin may be absorbed from other areas on the body where the skin is thinner. A major problem with chronic nitroglycerin administration in humans is tolerance to the drug.

2. Isosorbide is a venodilator that has not been studied clinically in the dog or cat. A recent experimental study has documented that isosorbide mononitrate, when administered at a dose of approximately 2

TABLE 14-2. VASODILATORS USED IN DOGS WITH HEART FAILURE

Generic Name	Trade Name	Mechanism of Action	Route of Administration	Dosage
Isosorbide dinitrate	Isordil	Venodilation	PO	1.0–1.5 mg/kg TID to QID
Nitroglycerin ointment	Nitro-BID	Venodilation	Cutaneous	0.25–2.0 inches TID to QID
Hydralazine	Apresoline	Arteriolar dilation	PO	0.5–3.0 mg/kg BID
Prazosin	Minipress	Arteriolar and venodilation	PO	1.0 mg TID (<15 kg body weight) 2.0 mg TID (>15 kg body weight)
Nitroprusside	Nipride	Arteriolar and venodilation	IV	1.0–5.0 µg/kg/min
Enalapril	Enacard	Arteriolar and venodilation ↓ Aldosterone	PO	0.5 mg/kg SID to BID
Captopril	Capoten	Arteriolar and venodilation ↓ Aldosterone	PO	0.5–1.0 mg/kg TID

mg/kg BID, is effective at reducing left ventricular volume-overload hypertrophy in dogs with experimental myocardial failure. Tolerance to isosorbide is a major problem in humans, although in the aforementioned study, isosorbide mononitrate appeared to be effective for at least 16 weeks.

    3. Nitroprusside is a potent arteriolar dilator and venodilator that must be administered intravenously. It is used only in emergency or intensive care situations when life-threatening heart failure is present. Systemic arterial blood pressure must be monitored when titrating nitroprusside to an effective endpoint.

  E. Suggested doses for other vasodilators are listed in Table 14-2. With any drug possessing arteriolar dilating properties, a low dose should be administered initially and the dose titrated to an effective endpoint.

II. Restriction of physical activity decreases tissue oxygen consumption, placing less demand on the heart for supplying oxygen delivery. The dog with mild heart failure may need only to curtail hunting activity or be confined to the yard. Dogs with severe heart failure may require cage rest. Dogs with life-threatening heart failure should be placed on cage rest and usually cannot tolerate even the slightest amount of physical activity. Even struggling during restraint or fighting oxygen administration given by mask may cause death. Dogs in these situations may benefit from sedation.

THERAPEUTIC STRATEGIES FOR TREATING HEART FAILURE

  I. Management of dogs with chronic degenerative mitral valve disease (see Ch. 6).

A. If a murmur only is present, but no signs of heart failure exist (class I), no treatment generally should be administered. Low-sodium diets are not beneficial at this time. ACE inhibitor administration may be indicated in dogs with marked cardiac enlargement but without objective evidence of heart failure, but studies to document this have not been completed.

B. Mild heart failure (class II)
   1. If signs are present only with heavy exercise, this activity should be curtailed.
   2. If exercise cannot be curtailed or if even light exercise causes coughing, dyspnea, or fatigue, low-dose furosemide or ACE inhibitor administration may be warranted.

C. Moderate heart failure (class III)
   1. If normal activity produces clinical signs, low-to-moderate doses of furosemide can be administered. Use of digitalis may be indicated if myocardial failure is present.
   2. Administration of an ACE inhibitor is usually indicated.

D. Severe heart failure (class IV)
   1. Administer moderate-to-maximum doses of furosemide when signs of heart failure are present at rest.
   2. Administer an ACE inhibitor.
   3. Administer digoxin if myocardial failure is present.
   4. Consider the use of a low-salt diet.

E. Emergency heart failure
   1. High-dose furosemide (up to 8 mg/kg up to every hour) or nitroprusside administration may be used if blood pressure can be monitored. In addition, hydralazine may be very effective in conjunction with lower-dose furosemide administration. Oral hydralazine produces effects within 30 minutes. The author generally starts emergency patients at 2 mg/kg rather than 1 mg/kg. This dose should be effective in more than 80 percent of patients and produce clinically significant hypotension in less than 30 percent. Even when clinically significant, the systemic hypotension is usually not life-threatening.
   2. Cage rest to avoid stress is of paramount importance. Such maneuvers as taking chest radiographs, placing jugular catheters, and administering oxygen by mask often prove fatal, especially when the animal struggles.
   3. If fluid therapy is needed, half-strength saline with 2.5 percent dextrose or 5 percent dextrose solutions should be used unless severe hyponatremia is present. Slow administration is advised, with careful monitoring, to prevent fluid overload.

F. Refractory heart failure
   1. When furosemide and an ACE inhibitor are no longer effective, consider adding a thiazide diuretic or replacing the ACE inhibitor with hydralazine or adding hydralazine along with the ACE inhibitor. In general, the addition of hydralazine should only be done by an individual who can monitor blood pressure and who has experience using hydralazine (see precautions above).
   2. When replacing captopril with hydralazine, start hydralazine titration 4 to 6 hours after the last dose of captopril and finish titration within

3 to 6 hours. When replacing enalapril with hydralazine, administer the evening dose and start the hydralazine titration the next morning. Titration, again, should be completed within 3 to 6 hours. If these protocols are not adhered to, the patient is essentially removed acutely from the ACE inhibitor, which can lead to acute and severe worsening of pulmonary edema and death.

II. Management of dogs or cats with dilated cardiomyopathy (see Chs. 7 and 8)
  A. Mild heart failure
    1. It is unusual to see this stage in the dog and rare to see it in the cat.
    2. Exercise restriction, diuretic administration, and ACE inhibitor administration may be beneficial.
  B. Moderate and severe heart failure
    1. Administer an ACE inhibitor.
    2. Furosemide dosage should be adjusted so that edema is controlled (respiratory rate <30 breaths/minute in patients with pulmonary edema), but dehydration and poor perfusion are not produced (these rarely occur as long as the patient is eating and drinking).
    3. Administer digoxin.
    4. Consider the use of a low-salt diet.
  C. Life-threatening heart failure
    1. Administer up to 8 mg/kg furosemide intravenously (4 mg/kg in cats) up to every hour until diuresis is established and the respiratory rate is decreasing. Then decrease the dose to 4 mg/kg (2 mg/kg in cats) every 2 to 8 hours depending on the patient's clinical condition. If the patient develops profound electrolyte disturbances or severe dehydration, treat cautiously with intravenous fluid therapy. Alternatively, administer nitroprusside with or without dobutamine intravenously while monitoring blood pressure. Nitroprusside dose should be high enough to decrease mean or systolic arterial blood pressure by 15 to 30 mmHg. Administer adjunctive therapy.
    2. Administer oxygen (oxygen cage if possible).
    3. ACE inhibitors are not good emergency drugs, as they only produce mild arteriolar dilation acutely. Consequently, even though their administration should be started early, one cannot depend on them to produce beneficial results.
    4. Digoxin also cannot be depended on to produce acute beneficial effects.

III. Management of cats with hypertrophic cardiomyopathy
  A. Mild-to-moderate heart failure
    1. Administer diltiazem (7.5 to 15 mg/cat TID) or propranolol (2.5 to 5.0 mg BID to TID).
    2. Low doses of furosemide may be needed to control pulmonary edema.
  B. Severe heart failure
    1. Administer furosemide (1 to 2 mg/kg PO BID to TID).
    2. Administer diltiazem or propranolol.
  C. Life-threatening heart failure
    1. Cats with hypertrophic or intermediate cardiomyopathy should be stressed as little as possible; should have a thoracentesis to rule out pleural effusion; should be placed in an oxygen-enriched environment;

and should have furosemide (1 to 4 mg/kg IV or IM) administered. Nitroglycerin cream may be used as an adjunct to help clear pulmonary edema.

    2. Administer diltiazem or propranolol.

IV. Management of dogs with heartworm disease and heart failure (see Ch. 11)

    A. Cage rest, diuretics, and arsenical therapy are the mainstays of therapy for this condition. Digoxin administration is controversial.

    B. Dogs should receive cage-rest for at least 1 week before arsenical therapy.

    C. Heart-failure therapy can often be discontinued 4 to 8 weeks after arsenical administration if the dog survives.

V. Management of dogs with chronic pericardial effusion and tamponade

    A. Echocardiography should be performed prior to pericardiocentesis to establish a diagnosis.

    B. If the prognosis is favorable, pericardiocentesis should be performed to decrease intrapericardial and right ventricular end-diastolic pressure.

    C. Furosemide may be administered after pericardiocentesis to hasten the removal of ascites.

SUGGESTED READINGS

Bright JM, Golden AL: Evidence for or against the efficacy of calcium channel blockers for the management of hypertrophic cardiomyopathy in cats. Vet Clin North Am (Small Anim Pract) 21:1023, 1991

Clemmer TP: Oxygen transport. Int Anesth Clin 19:21, 1981

DeLellis LA, Kittleson MD: Current uses and hazards of vasodilator therapy in heart failure. p. 700. In Kirk RW, Bonagura JD (eds): Current Veterinary Therapy XI. WB Saunders, Philadelphia, 1992

Kittleson MD: Dobutamine. J Am Vet Med Assoc 177:642, 1980

Kittleson MD: Concepts and therapeutic strategies in the management of heart failure. p. 279. In Kirk RW (ed): Current Veterinary Therapy VII. WB Saunders, Philadelphia, 1983

Kittleson MD: The efficacy and safety of milrinone for treating heart failure in dogs. Vet Clin North Am (Small Anim Pract) 21:905, 1991

Kittleson MD, Hamlin RL: Hydralazine pharmacodynamics in the dog. Am J Vet Res 44: 1501, 1983

Kittleson MD, Eyster GE, Knowlen GG et al: Myocardial function in small dogs with chronic mitral regurgitation and severe congestive heart failure. J Am Vet Med Assoc 184:455, 1984

Kittleson MD, Eyster GE, Knowlen GG et al: Efficacy of digoxin administration in dogs with idiopathic congestive cardiomyopathy. J Am Vet Med Assoc 186:162, 1985

Kittleson MD, Johnson LJ, Olivier NB: Acute hemodynamic effects of hydralazine in dogs with chronic mitral regurgitation. J Am Vet Med Assoc 187:258, 1985

Kittleson MD, Johnson LJ, Pion PD, Mekhamer YE: The acute haemodynamic effects of captopril in dogs with heart failure. J Vet Pharm Ther 16:1, 1993

Kittleson MD, Knowlen GG: Positive inotropic drugs in heart failure. p. 323. In Kirk RW (ed): Current Veterinary Therapy IX. WB Saunders, Philadelphia, 1986

Knowlen GG, Kittleson MD: Captopril therapy in dogs with heart failure. p. 334. In Kirk
    RW (ed): Current Veterinary Therapy IX. WB Saunders, Philadelphia, 1986
Knowlen GG, Kittleson MD, Nachreiner RF, Eyster GE: Comparison of plasma aldoste-
    rone concentration among clinical status groups of dogs with chronic heart failure. J Am
    Vet Med Assoc 183:991, 1983
Singhvi SM, Peterson AE, Ross JJ Jr, et al: Pharmacokinetics of captopril in dogs and
    monkeys. J Pharm Sci 70:1108, 1981

15

Treatment of Cardiac Arrhythmias and Conduction Disturbances

Michael S. Miller
Larry Patrick Tilley

INTRODUCTION

DEFINITION

Arrhythmias are defined as abnormalities of cardiac impulse formation, conduction, rate, and regularity. Other terms such as dysrhythmia and ectopic rhythm are also used to describe electrophysiologic cardiac disturbances. Many cardiac arrhythmias are benign and clinically insignificant and require no specific therapy. Other arrhythmias may cause severe clinical signs or degenerate into malignant arrhythmias leading to cardiac arrest and sudden death. In the latter case, immediate therapeutic intervention may be life saving.

GENERAL MECHANISMS

The current view on the mechanisms for cardiac arrhythmias includes isolated or concurrent abnormalities in impulse initiation (automaticity), propagation (including reentry), triggered activity (early and delayed after depolarizations) and anisotropy (different conduction velocity longitudinally versus horizontally). At the turn of the century, arrhythmias were documented using arterial and venous pulse spygmograms. However, electrograms were soon found to be superior in accurately identifying arrhythmias. The interested reader should consult the Suggested Readings list at the end of this chapter for further information about the mechanisms of cardiac arrhythmias. Arrhythmias can be classified according to the mechanism underlying the arrhythmias (Table 15-1).

GENERAL ETIOLOGY

Cardiac arrhythmias may occur in either the presence or absence of specific cardiac disease (Table 15-2). Numerous systemic disorders may be correlated with abnormal cardiac rhythms. Specific arrhythmias are more likely to occur in pa-

TABLE 15-1. CLASSIFICATION OF CARDIAC ARRHYTHMIAS

Normal sinus impulse formation
  Normal sinus rhythm
  Sinus arrhythmia
Disturbances of sinus impulse formation
  Sinus bradycardia
  Sinus tachycardia
Disturbances of supraventricular impulse formation
  Atrial premature complexes
  Sinus arrest and/or block
  Atrial tachycardia
  Atrial flutter
  Atrial fibrillation
  Atrioventricular (AV) junctional rhythm
Disturbances of ventricular impulse formation
  Ventricular premature complexes
  Ventricular tachycardia
  Ventricular asystole
  Ventricular fibrillation
Disturbances of impulse conduction
  Atrial standstill
  First-degree AV block
  Second-degree AV block
  Complete AV block (third degree)
Disturbances of both impulse formation and impulse conduction
  Sick sinus syndrome
  Ventricular pre-excitation and the Wolff-Parkinson-White (WPW) syndrome

tients with heart disease (e.g., atrial fibrillation associated with dilated cardiomyopathy in large-breed dogs) and may be useful as clues to the underlying disease. The amount of structural damage to the heart is not always correlated with the type and severity of any arrhythmia.

INITIAL INTERPRETATION OF CARDIAC ARRHYTHMIAS

INITIAL EVALUATION

  I. Review all pertinent clinical data: age, breed, medical history, physical examination, previous ECG strips, and all laboratory tests.
 II. Make a general inspection of the ECG.
     A. Is normal sinus rhythm or a cardiac arrhythmia present?
     B. If an arrhythmia is present, does it occur rarely, frequently, intermittently, or continuously? Is it uniform or multiform?
     C. Is the arrhythmia clinically insignificant or significant? Does it correlate with specific clinical signs?
     D. Are provocative maneuvers (e.g., exercise, ocular or carotid sinus pressure) or pharmacologic intervention (e.g., intravenous lidocaine) required to further evaluate an arrhythmia?

TABLE 15-2. ETIOLOGIES OF CARDIAC ARRHYTHMIAS

I. Cardiac
   A. Dog
      1. Heredity (genetics not documented in all cases)
         a) Doberman (His bundle degeneration)
         b) English springer spaniel (persistent atrial standstill)
         c) Miniature schnauzer, dachshund, cocker spaniel (sick sinus syndrome)
         d) Pug and Dalmatian (sinus node disease)
         e) Pug (stenosis and degeneration of the His bundle)
         f) Wolff-Parkinson-White syndrome
         g) Golden retriever (Duchenne muscular dystrophy)
         h) German shepherd (ventricular tachyarrhythmia)
      2. Atrial and/or ventricular arrhythmias
         a) Atrial enlargement, secondary to congenital defects or acquired disease
         b) Cardiomyopathy
         c) Congenital heart disease
         d) Congestive heart failure
         e) Mitral valve disease (congenital and acquired)
         f) Myocarditis, endocarditis, ischemia
         g) Neoplasia
         h) Trauma
         i) Drugs
      3. Conduction system disease
         a) Acquired sinus and AV node disease (sick sinus syndrome)
         b) Cardiomyopathy
         c) Neoplasia
         d) Surgical damage to conduction tissue
         e) Trauma
         f) Vascular (e.g., microscopic intramural myocardial infarction)
         g) Ventricular septal defect and other congenital defects
         h) Infection (e.g., Lyme disease)
         i) Drugs
         j) Degeneration
   B. Cat
      1. Heredity (rare)
            Wolff-Parkinson-White Syndrome
      2. Atrial and ventricular arrhythmias
         a) Cardiac enlargement secondary to congenital heart defects
         b) Cardiomyopathy
         c) Neoplasia
         d) Trauma
         e) Systemic disease
      3. Conduction system disease
         a) Cardiomyopathy
         b) Neoplasia
         c) Degenerative
         d) Idiopathic fibrosis in older cats
II. Noncardiac in dog and cat
   A. Acidosis or alkalosis
   B. Autonomic nervous system imbalance (parasympathetic or sympathetic); central nervous system (e.g., pain, excitement, fear); respiratory, gastrointestinal or organic brain disease
   C. Drug toxicity (e.g., digitalis, preoperative sedatives, or anesthetic agents, catecholamines, antiarrhythmic agents, bronchodilators)
   D. Electrolyte disorders (e.g., hyperkalemia, hypercalcemia, hypokalemia, hypocalcemia, hypomagnesemia)
   E. Endocrinopathies (e.g., hypothyroidism, hyperthyroidism, Addison's disease, pheochromocytoma)
   F. Hypothermia
   G. Hypovolemia
   H. Hypoxia
   I. Mechanical stimulation (e.g., cardiac catheterization, intravenous catheter)
   J. Neoplasia
   K. Shock
   L. Toxemia or sepsis
   M. Trauma

SYSTEMATIC APPROACH TO THE ECG STRIP

  I. Sinus rhythm or arrhythmia?
 II. Heart rate rapid, slow, or normal?
III. Do the P (atrial) waves occur at regular or irregular intervals? What is the height, width, direction?
IV. Do the QRS (ventricular) complexes occur with regularity and uniformity? What is their morphology?
 V. What is the relationship between the P waves and the QRS complexes? The PR interval is a measurement of atrioventricular (AV) conduction time. Is the PR interval of normal duration, regular or irregular, or is there no consistent relationship between the P wave and QRS complex?
VI. In summarizing the above findings, is the predominant rhythm sinus, atrial, AV junctional, or ventricular? Is the arrhythmia a disorder of impulse formation, conduction, or both?

FINAL INTERPRETATION OF A CARDIAC ARRHYTHMIA

  I. What is the possible mechanism for the arrhythmia?
     A. Is there an abnormal impulse formation?
     B. Is it atrial, AV junctional, or ventricular in origin?
     C. Is there a conduction abnormality?
 II. Is the P wave present? Where does it start? Is it related to the QRS complex? If the P wave is not related to the QRS complex, what is the abnormality causing the AV dissociation?
III. What reason or abnormality explains the absence of the P wave?
     A. Is the P wave superimposed on a portion of the QRS complex, ST segment, or T wave?
     B. Is the arrhythmia atrial standstill, atrial fibrillation, atrial flutter, AV junctional escape rhythm, or atrial tachycardia?
IV. If AV dissociation is present, where does the QRS complex evolve from? Is there an AV junctional and/or purkinje or idioventricular foci involved?
 V. Is the wide and bizarre QRS complex due to a ventricular arrhythmia or caused by a premature atrial impulse that is aberrantly conducted (refer to atrial premature complexes, P: QRS characteristics)?
     What are the differential possibilities of the arrhythmia?
VI. What is the clinical significance of the arrhythmia?
     A. Is specific therapy required?
     B. What is the best immediate therapy?

THERAPEUTIC APPROACH

  I. Have a precise diagnosis for the arrhythmia, if possible.
 II. Eliminate noncardiac causes (e.g., acid-base and electrolyte abnormalities, hypothermia, hypovolemia, hypoxemia, and other systemic problems) be-

fore using an antiarrhythmic drug, unless hemodynamic or electrical instability is present.

  A. Stop other drug therapy that may be the cause of the arrhythmia (e.g., digitalis, quinidine, procainamide, xylazine, and acetylpromazine).
  B. Correct electrolyte disturbances or metabolic abnormalities with appropriate fluid and supportive therapy (e.g., hypokalemia or acid-base disturbances may predispose to an arrhythmia that is refractory to therapy).

III. The purpose of drug therapy for cardiac arrhythmias is to prevent clinical signs such as weakness, syncope, seizures, personality changes, and congestive heart failure. Drug therapy also may decrease electrical instability and the likelihood of progression to a malignant arrhythmia (e.g., ventricular fibrillation).

IV. Select the antiarrhythmic drug best suited to the underlying cause of the arrhythmia (e.g., phenytoin for digitalis-induced tachyarrhythmias, lidocaine to terminate supraventricular arrhythmias, or atrial fibrillation over an anomalous pathway in the Wolff-Parkinson-White syndrome (WPW) rather than digoxin or propranolol).

 V. Be familiar with recommended dose ranges of the various antiarrhythmic drugs (see section on antiarrhythmic therapy).

VI. Be aware of synergistic effects of antiarrhythmic drugs (e.g., digoxin and propranolol may additively delay AV conduction) and antagonistic effects (e.g., quinidine may increase serum digoxin levels, increasing the possibility of digoxin toxicity). Refractory arrhythmias may require a combination of antiarrhythmic agents, although the possibility of drug-related toxicity may increase (e.g., digoxin and propranolol, procainamide and propranolol, quinidine and propranolol, Mexiletine or tocainide and propranolol, procainamide and diazepam, and quinidine and diazepam).

VII. Be aware that some arrhythmias may require antiarrhythmic drugs in addition to other therapeutic modalities (e.g., sick sinus syndrome patients with bradyarrhythmia-tachyarrhythmias may require a permanent cardiac pacemaker for the bradyarrhythmia and an antiarrhythmic drug for the tachyarrhythmia). For ventricular tachycardia due to quinidine or procainamide toxicity, conventional antiarrhythmic drugs may worsen this arrhythmia. Stopping the drug and administering sodium bicarbonate, isoproterenol, or dopamine may prove effective in controlling this toxic arrhythmia.

GENERAL MANAGEMENT OF ARRHYTHMIAS

Premature Complexes

  I. Treat the underlying problem (e.g., surgical correction of a pyometra with toxic myocarditis).
 II. If premature complexes are frequent (>20 to 30 per minute) repetitive, and/or correlated with clinical signs or underlying cardiac disease (e.g., chronic valvular disease, cardiomyopathy), antiarrhythmic agents should be considered.

III. Digitalis may be effective when atrial premature complexes (APCs) or ventricular premature complexes (VPCs) are associated with congestive heart failure (CHF). If digitalis is used for congestive heart failure complicated by frequent VPCs, the ECG should be monitored every few days to determine whether the arrhythmia is worsening or resolving.

MANAGEMENT OF SUPRAVENTRICULAR TACHYARRHYTHMIAS

I. A vagal maneuver (e.g., ocular or carotid sinus pressure) is often effective in terminating paroxysmal atrial or AV junctional tachycardia. The dive reflex (i.e., immersing the head in cool water) may also be an effective maneuver. A vagal maneuver increases parasympathetic stimulation to the sinus and AV nodes and reduces the sinus node discharge rate, slows AV node conduction, or terminates junctional reentry.

II. Digitalis is the drug of choice for atrial fibrillation, producing a rapid ventricular response in the dog and cat, although diltiazem can be started simultaneously to rapidly reduce the ventricular rate.

III. If digitalis toxicity is a consideration, the drug should be stopped immediately. Phenytoin may be effective in terminating the arrhythmia in the dog.

IV. Intravenous or oral propranolol diltiazem, or adenosine may be effective in terminating a supraventricular tachyarrhythmia not complicated by congestive heart failure (beware of hypotension, bradycardia, and AV block).

V. Verapamil, diltiazem, and beta blockers are effective for the treatment of supraventricular tachyarrhythmias with a reentrant mechanism in the dog. Intravenous adenosine has been found to be effective for this purpose in humans and possibly dogs.

VI. Direct current (DC) shock (cardioversion) is reserved for a severe tachyarrhythmia that is refractory to antiarrhythmic therapy in a patient that remains symptomatic. Use of a cardioverter synchronized to the QRS complex of the ECG is mandatory. This method should not be used by an inexperienced clinician. Electrical shock administered during the electrical vulnerable period (QT interval on the ECG) will likely result in ventricular fibrillation. Digoxin toxicity is a contraindication for DC shock.

VII. The use of temporary pacemakers and premature electrical stimulation or overdrive suppression of the arrhythmia is another therapeutic modality, although not one commonly used in veterinary medicine. Specialized equipment is again required.

VENTRICULAR ARRHYTHMIAS

I. Intravenous lidocaine without epinephrine is the drug of choice for the treatment of ventricular tachycardia in the canine patient. Procainamide and quinidine are the next most commonly used drugs.

II. Electrolyte and metabolic abnormalities must be treated with appropriate fluid therapy.

III. Mexiletine, tocainide, and propranolol are less commonly used for the treatment of ventricular tachycardia.
IV. Lidocaine and phenytoin are the drugs of choice for ventricular tachycardia induced by digitalis toxicity. Mexiletine or tocainide may also be useful for this purpose.
 V. Underlying problems (e.g., congestive heart failure, endocarditis) must also be treated.
VI. DC shock should be reserved for refractory ventricular arrhythmias in patients that are symptomatic, and should be administered by clinicians experienced with cardioversion.

SPECIFIC CARDIAC ARRHYTHMIAS

SUPRAVENTRICULAR RHYTHMS

Normal Sinus Rhythm

  I. Location
Impulses are generated from the sinus node.
 II. Heart rate and rhythm
   A. 60 to 160 beats/min (bpm) dog (up to 180 bpm in toy breeds and 220 bpm in the pup); 120 to 240 bpm in the cat
   B. The rhythm is regular, with a less than 10 percent variation in the RR interval.
III. P: QRS characteristics
There is a normal P wave for each QRS complex, with a constant PR interval (Fig. 15-1).
IV. Differentials
None
 V. Significance
This is a normal cardiac rhythm in the dog and cat.
VI. Treatment
None

Sinus Arrhythmia

  I. Location
Impulses are generated from the sinus node.
 II. Heart rate and rhythm
60 to 180 bpm dog; 120 to 240 bpm in the cat. The rhythm is irregular with a greater than 10 percent variation in the RR interval.
III. P: QRS characteristics
There is a normal P wave for each QRS complex, with a constant PR interval. A wandering pacemaker (P waves vary in shape) is often present.

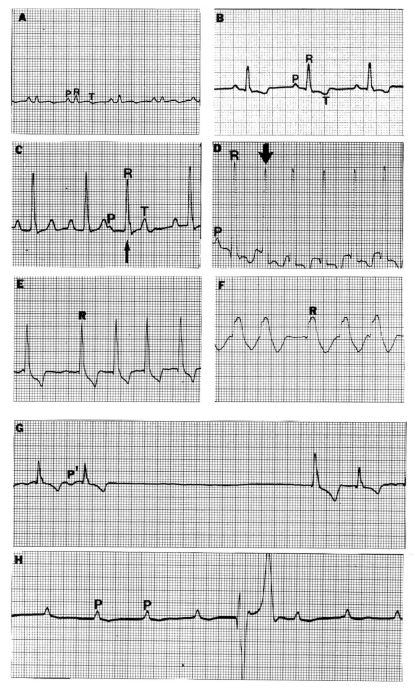

Fig. 15-1. Selected sinus and supraventricular rhythms. Lead II rhythm strips, paper speed = 50 mm/sec; 1 cm = 1 mV. **(A)** Normal sinus rhythm, cat. **(B)** Normal sinus rhythm, dog. **(C)** Atrial premature complex *(arrow)*, dog. **(D)** Paroxysmal atrial tachycardia *(begins at arrow)*, dog. **(E)** Atrial fibrillation, dog. **(F)** Atrial fibrillation with left bundle branch block, dog. **(G)** AV junctional rhythm (negative P′ waves) with a period of sinus block and/or arrest with a low AV junctional or ventricular escape beat, dog. **(H)** Complete AV block, dog.

VI. Differentials

Atrial premature complexes (APCs)

V. Significance

    A. Sinus arrhythmia is a normal cardiac rhythm in the dog, but is very unusual in the cat (e.g., some cats with respiratory disease).

    B. Sinus arrhythmia is correlated with a variation in vagal tone, usually in synchronization with respiration. This rhythm may be coupled with a wandering pacemaker (alteration in P-wave morphology due to a change in the site of impulse origination or conduction through the atria).

    C. A wandering pacemaker is also a normal variation in the dog.

VI. Treatment

None, unless associated with a symptomatic sinus bradycardia.

Sinus Bradycardia

  I. Location

Impulses are generated in the sinus node, but at a slower than normal frequency.

 II. Heart rate and rhythm

    A. Less than 70 bpm in the dog (less than 60 bpm in very large breeds) and less than 120 bpm in the cat.

    B. The rhythm is regular, with a slight variation in the RR interval.

III. P : QRS characteristics

    A. There is a normal P wave for each QRS complex. The PR interval is constant.

    B. AV junctional or ventricular escape complexes may occur, as well as atrial or ventricular premature complexes.

IV. Differentials

Marked sinus arrhythmia

 V. Significance

Sinus bradycardia is associated with

    A. Various clinical abnormalities including hypothermia, endocrinopathies (e.g., hypothyroidism, Addison's disease)

    B. Drugs (e.g., acetylpromazine, xylazine, digoxin, propranolol, edrophonium chloride, pilocarpine, general anesthesia)

    C. Diseases associated with an increase in vagal stimulation (e.g., neurologic, pharyngeal, gastrointestinal, respiratory)

    D. Sick sinus syndrome (sinus node disease).

VI. Treatment

    A. Sinus bradycardia is usually self-limiting and often does not require therapy; it is important to correct any underlying disorders.

    B. If clinical signs such as weakness or syncope develop, parenteral atropine or glycopyrrolate (intramuscular or subcutaneous route is preferred) is used initially.

    C. Theophylline blocks endogenous adenosine, found to be a cause of sinus node depression in humans.

    D. Sympathomimetic agents, such as epinephrine, isoproterenol, dopamine,

or dobutamine, may be used in emergency (cardiac arrest) situations, although other severe arrhythmias may be triggered by these drugs.
   E. Artificial pacing is sometimes necessary with symptomatic bradycardia that remains unresponsive to drug therapy.

Sinus Tachycardia

   I. Location
   Impulses are generated in the sinus node but at a faster than normal frequency.
  II. Heart rate and rhythm
      A. The rate is greater than 180 bpm in the dog and 240 bpm in the cat.
      B. The rhythm is regular.
 III. P: QRS characteristics
      A. There is a normal P wave for each QRS complex with a constant PR interval.
      B. The P waves may be partially or completely fused with preceding T waves.
  IV. Differentials
      A. Paroxysmal atrial tachycardia, atrial flutter with 2: 1 AV block, and AV junctional tachycardia are included.
      B. A vagal maneuver (e.g., ocular or carotid sinus pressure for 5 to 10 seconds) may clarify identification by temporary slowing, but not abrupt termination.
   V. Significance
   Sinus tachycardia may occur with stress, anxiety, pain, shock, anemia, fever, congestive heart failure, hyperthyroidism, drugs (e.g., atropine, sympathomimetic agents), functional pheochromocytoma, light anesthesia, and numerous other causes.
  VI. Treatment
   Depending on the patient's clinical status, the specific cause of the rapid heart rate should be established and treated. Although there are exceptions, antiarrhythmic agents generally are not required. For congestive heart failure, digitalis and diuretic therapy may improve cardiac output, improve baroreceptor function, and lessen sympathetic tone to the sinus node. For hyperthyroidism without congestive heart failure, propranolol may be useful in decreasing the cardiac rate. The calcium channel blocker diltiazem may reduce the heart rate in cats with hypertrophic or restrictive cardiomyopathy.

SUPRAVENTRICULAR RHYTHMS

Atrial Premature Complexes

   I. Location
   Impulses originate from an atrial focus other than the sinus node (ectopic focus).

II. Heart rate and rhythm

The heart rate varies depending on the intrinsic sinus node rate and frequency of the APCs; the rhythm is irregular.

III. P: QRS characteristics

There is usually an abnormal P′ wave (premature P wave) followed by a normal QRS complex; the P′R interval of the APC may vary from the sinus rhythm PR interval. The P′ wave may have various morphologies and may be fused with the T wave of the preceding beat. The P′ wave may occur so early in the cardiac cycle that it will find the AV conduction system refractory and the impulse will not be conducted to the ventricles (e.g., APC with physiologic AV block). The pause following the APC is often less than fully compensatory (R wave before and after R wave of APC is equal to two normal RR intervals) due to premature depolarization and resetting of the sinus node (Fig. 15-1C). The QRS complex is usually normal, but an early APC may find the ventricular conduction system in a relative refractory period and result in a bizarre (abnormal shape or direction) QRS complex. This abnormality is termed an APC with aberrant ventricular conduction. This aberrant QRS complex is often confused with a VPC (quicksand of electrocardiography). Aberrant ventricular conduction commonly occurs in humans with a long R wave to R wave interval preceding an APC with a prolonged PR interval; it is termed *Ashman's phenomenon*. A short coupling interval (duration between previous normal P wave and ectopic P′ wave) to the APC also favors aberrant conduction.

IV. Differentials

A. Marked sinus arrhythmia and VPCs when aberrant ventricular conduction follows an APC.

B. A P′ wave preceding the abnormal QRS complex and a similarity of the initial deflection of the QRS complex with a preceding normal beat would support aberrant conduction.

C. In humans, about 90 percent of aberrantly conducted beats have the pattern of a right bundle branch block.

V. Significance

A. APCs often indicate underlying cardiac disease (e.g., chronic valvular fibrosis, cardiomyopathy, congenital defect, or cor pulmonale).

B. Other causes include electrolyte disturbances, hypoxia, drug toxicity (e.g., digitalis), toxemias, increased sympathetic tone, and myocarditis.

C. APCs may progress to other supraventricular arrhythmias such as paroxysmal atrial tachycardia and atrial fibrillation.

VI. Treatment

A. Infrequent APCs may be a normal variation and do not require treatment.

B. If this arrhythmia is correlated with congestive heart failure, digoxin and diuretic therapy is used initially. If the APCs are correlated with poor hemodynamic status without congestive heart failure, then digoxin, diltiazem, propranolol, quinidine, or procainamide may be considered in the above order of preference.

C. If congestive heart failure is not present, digoxin may increase the frequency of the atrial premature contractions due to its effect of shortening the atrial myocardial cell refractory period, as well as by other complex mechanisms.

Sinus Arrest and/or Block

I. Location

A primary disorder in the sinus node resulting in lack of generation of the cardiac impulse or its poor propagation through surrounding tissue may cause sinus arrest and/or sinus block. It is not possible to distinguish between sinus block or arrest in the dog due to the normal variation in the RR interval (sinus arrhythmia).

II. Heart rate and rhythm

   A. The rate is variable and is often correlated with a bradycardia or slow sinus arrhythmia.

   B. The rhythm is regularly irregular or irregular with pauses.

III. P: QRS characteristics

There is a normal P wave for each QRS complex, with a pause equal to or greater than two times the normal RR interval (Fig. 15-1G). The P wave may vary in shape if a concurrent wandering pace-maker is present. The PR interval is constant.

IV. Differentials

Marked sinus arrhythmia and sinus bradycardia are included.

V. Significance

   A. Sinus arrest may be consistent with an increase in vagal tone (e.g., ocular pressure, brachycephalic breeds, irritation of the vagus nerve).

   B. Pathology of the atria including fibrosis, cardiomyopathy, neoplasia, and drug toxicity (e.g., digitalis, propranolol, quinidine, xylazine, and acetylpromazine) may result in sinus arrest.

   C. Release of perinodal endogenous adenosine may also cause sinus block and/or sinus arrest.

   D. Sinus arrest is one of the complex arrhythmias in the sick sinus syndrome (SSS) that affects small breed dogs, including the miniature schnauzer, dachsund, pug, and cocker spaniel. Often there is concurrent AV nodal disease producing AV block and/or paroxysmal atrial tachycardia (i.e., bradycardia-tachycardia syndrome).

VI. Treatment

   A. Asymptomatic dogs or cats require no specific therapy.

   B. When correlated with signs of weakness or syncope, an atropine response test should be performed (0.04 mg/kg IM) followed by a follow-up ECG in 15 to 30 minutes.

   C. If there is a decrease in the sinus pauses or an increase in the cardiac rate following atropine administration, the patient may benefit from oral anticholinergic agents or theophylline (blocks adenosine). A poor clinical response suggests the need for a temporary or permanent cardiac pacemaker.

   D. Congestive heart failure may also develop, in which case diuretics and vasodilators must be considered as the preferred treatment. Digitalis may exacerbate the sinus arrest in these cases, although it may be warranted if a demand pacemaker is utilized, and/or if the patient is carefully monitored.

Atrial Tachycardia

I. Location
   A. Impulses originate from an atrial site other than the sinus node.
   B. The atrium and AV junctional areas are also involved (a reentrant circuit that allows the impulse to restimulate the atrium as well as to pass to the ventricles). An abnormal automatic focus in the atrium may also be responsible for this arrhythmia.

II. Heart rate and rhythm
   A. The rate is above 160 to 180 in the dog; and above 240 bpm in the cat.
   B. The rhythm is usually regular, but may be slightly irregular.

III. P: QRS characteristics
   There is a P′ wave for each QRS complex, although the P wave is usually of different morphology than the sinus P wave. The PR interval is constant. The P wave may not be visualized as it may be fused with the T wave or occur simultaneously with the preceding QRS complex (Fig. 15-1D). The QRS complex may also be of different morphology due to aberrant conduction through the ventricular conduction system. An irregular R wave to R wave interval may be caused by concurrent AV block, or multifocal atrial tachycardia (P′ waves vary in shape; firing of two or more ectopic atrial foci).

IV. Differentials
   Sinus tachycardia, AV junctional tachycardia, and atrial flutter.

V. Significance
   A. Persistent (nonparoxysmal) atrial tachycardia supports severe myocardial or conduction system disease. This arrhythmia may also be secondary to digitalis toxicity or may occur under general anesthesia.
   B. Systemic disease that results in autonomic nervous systemic abnormalities may also be causative.
   C. In the cat, this arrhythmia is correlated with feline cardiomyopathy, hyperthyroidism, and other types of systemic disease.

VI. Treatment
   A. Sustained (nonparoxysmal atrial tachycardia) is often correlated with weakness, hypotension, and syncope and requires immediate therapy.
   B. If acute or chronic congestive heart failure is present, intense therapy including oxygen, cage rest, diuretics vasodilators, and digitalis is required. Intravenous fluid therapy and corticosteroids may be required for hypotension and shock.
   C. Vagal maneuver (mild ocular pressure or carotid sinus pressure) may effectively terminate a reentrant atrial tachycardia (see Fig. 15-3C). A vagal maneuver may also slow down the sinus rate and reveal sinus tachycardia or cause AV block and unmask atrial flutter (Fig. 15-3D), both differentials of atrial tachycardia.
   D. Intravenous digoxin may slow the ventricular response and improve the clinical status. If digoxin is not effective, intravenous propranolol or verapamil may convert atrial tachycardia to sinus rhythm or slow down the ventricular rate. The latter two drugs must be used with caution, as they may decrease cardiac contractility and exacerbate congestive heart failure. Intravenous adenosine has become the drug of choice in humans with

atrial tachycardia because AV nodal reentry is the predominant mechanism. It has very rapid excretions and limited side effects, which makes adenosine a favored choice, although its use is not established in our veterinary patients. Intramuscular quinidine gluconate has also been used to convert atrial tachycardia to normal sinus rhythm in dogs with refractory atrial tachycardia. Oral diltiazem may also be effective for arrhythmia termination in the dog and cat.

E. Electrophysiologic pacing methods such as overdrive suppression or premature atrial stimulation may also be effective in terminating atrial tachycardia, but should only be used by an experienced clinician. DC shock (cardioversion) should be reserved for refractory cases and only by a veterinarian experienced with this technique and possessing the proper equipment.

Atrial Fibrillation

I. Location

A high number of disorganized atrial impulses (multiple wavelets) bombarding the AV node is responsible for this arrhythmia. Many of these impulses approach the AV node in a refractory period (from concealed conduction of the previous impulses) and are not conducted to the ventricles.

II. Heart rate and rhythm

A. The rate is usually rapid, often above 180 bpm in the dog, and above 240 bpm in the cat.

B. The rhythm is very irregular and is correlated with an arterial pulse deficit.

III. P: QRS characteristics

No P waves are seen and there are normally shaped QRS complexes. Instead of P waves, small or large oscillations (f waves) are present. The interval between successive QRS complexes is very irregular because of intermittent AV block (Fig. 15-1E). There may be some variation and widening of the QRS complexes due to aberrant ventricular conduction or bundle branch block (Fig. 15-1F).

IV. Differentials

A. Frequent atrial premature complexes, AV junctional tachycardia with AV block, supraventricular tachycardia with AV block and atrial flutter with AV block are included.

B. Atrial flutter usually shows a regular RR interval and the atrial oscillations (F waves) are larger than f waves (Fig. 15-3D).

V. Significance

A. Atrial fibrillation is a severe arrhythmia and commonly occurs in patients with cardiomyopathy, advanced chronic valvular disease, and progressive congenital heart disease.

B. Other etiologies include severe ischemia or shock (gastric dilatation and after cardiac arrest), atrial tumor (hemangiosarcoma), or electrolyte disturbances (hyperkalemia).

C. Loss of atrial contraction decreases the stroke volume and cardiac output. The rapid ventricular rate also results in poor cardiac output. Slow atrial fibrillation (below 100 bpm) may signify concurrent AV block.

VI. Treatment
    A. Underlying congestive heart failure must be controlled. Digoxin is used
       to slow the ventricular response. Diuretics and vasodilator agents may be
       added as required. After approximately 5 to 7 days, if the ventricular rate
       is not controlled, propranolol may be added at a low dose. The propranolol
       dose is increased slowly until the ventricular rate is adequately controlled
       (<140 to 160 bpm). The lowest possible dose of propranolol will lessen
       the negative inotropic effects. Diltiazem may also be added to digoxin
       initially with rapid atrial fibrillation, as diltiazem does not reduce ventricu-
       lar contractility as does propranolol. Diltiazem is very useful in the treat-
       ment of atrial fibrillation in the cat.
    B. Although it is unusual to convert atrial fibrillation to normal sinus rhythm
       in dogs, the antiarrhythmic drug quinidine may be useful for this purpose.
       A normal-size heart and lack of congestive heart failure favors the use of
       quinidine. In certain cases, digitalis or diltiazem may also convert atrial
       fibrillation to normal sinus rhythm.
    C. Lidocaine should be avoided, as it may increase AV conduction velocity
       and lead to an even more rapid ventricular response.
    D. DC shock should be reserved for refractory cases without severe cardio-
       megaly. Experienced personnel and proper equipment are essential.

Atrioventricular Junctional Rhythm

  I. Location
     Impulses are generated in the AV junctional tissue and spread backward (ret-
     rograde) through the atrium and forward (antegrade) to the ventricles.
 II. Heart rate and rhythm
    A. The heart rate is variable (usually >60 bpm) depending on passive escape
       rhythm versus enhanced AV junctional rhythm (60 bpm, but <100 bpm
       in the dog).
    B. The rhythm is usually regular.
III. P: QRS characteristics
     The negative P' wave may occur before, during, or after the normal QRS
     complex. The P'R interval is constant, or RP' interval may be variable. The
     P'-wave location depends on the area of impulse generation, and relative
     speed of retrograde conduction through the atrium compared with antegrade
     conduction through the AV node, His bundle, and ventricular conduction
     system.
IV. Differentials
     Atrial standstill and slow atrial fibrillation are included.
 V. Significance
    A. Digitalis toxicity may cause an AV junctional rhythm. When abnormally
       rapid, this arrhythmia is difficult to distinguish from atrial tachycardia. If
       atrial fibrillation converts to an AV junctional rhythm in a patient taking
       digoxin, then digoxin toxicity is likely.
    B. An AV junctional escape rhythm may occur in patients with depressed
       sinus node function (e.g., the sick sinus syndrome).

VI. Treatment
   A. Usually no treatment is needed and the rhythm reverts spontaneously.
   B. If weakness or syncope is associated with a slow AV junctional rhythm, atropine, isoproterenol, or theophylline may be used in an attempt to accelerate the sinus node in order to help regain function as the primary pacemaker.
   C. Oral anticholinergic agents or theophylline may also be useful for chronic therapy. If congestive heart failure is present with an enhanced AV junctional rhythm, digitalis, diuretic, and vasodilator therapy may be needed.

VENTRICULAR ARRHYTHMIAS

Ventricular Premature Complexes

 I. Location
   Ectopic impulses are generated from a focus below the AV node and AV junction.
II. Heart rate and rhythm
   The rate is variable, depending on the frequency of VPCs; the rhythm is irregular. VPCs are usually related (coupled) to normal beats. If the VPCs are not coupled to a normal beat, the origination site is referred to as a parasystolic focus. There is usually a full compensatory pause (interval between the VPC and following sinus P wave) following a VPC as the ectopic beat does not usually conduct back to the atrium and affect the spontaneous sinus node discharge rate. Interpolated VPCs occur between normal beats and are not usually followed by a full compensatory pause.
III. P: QRS characteristics
   P waves that are seen are normal in shape, but are not associated with the QRS complex of the VPCs. The QRS complex is often wide and bizarre. If the major deflection of the QRS complex is negative in lead II, the ectopic focus is in the left ventricle (Fig. 15-2A); if the major deflection is positive in lead II, the ectopic focus is in the right ventricle (Fig. 15-2B).
IV. Differentials
   Atrial premature complexes with aberrant ventricular conduction and right or left bundle branch block are included.
 V. Significance
   A. Frequent VPCs, runs of VPCs, multifocal VPCs, or VPCs occurring during the QT interval of the previous beat may be dangerous. The ventricular arrhythmia may be due to cardiac disease (e.g., congestive heart failure, myocarditis, endocarditis).
   B. Secondary causes of VPCs include trauma, electrolyte disturbances, autonomic changes, hypoxia, and ischemia. Frequent VPC's may be hereditary in German shepherds. Frequent VPCs may lead to hypotension, shock, or congestive heart failure.
   C. Frequent VPCs or VPCs occurring during the preceding QT interval may be electrically unstable and may proceed to ventricular tachycardia and/or fibrillation and sudden death.

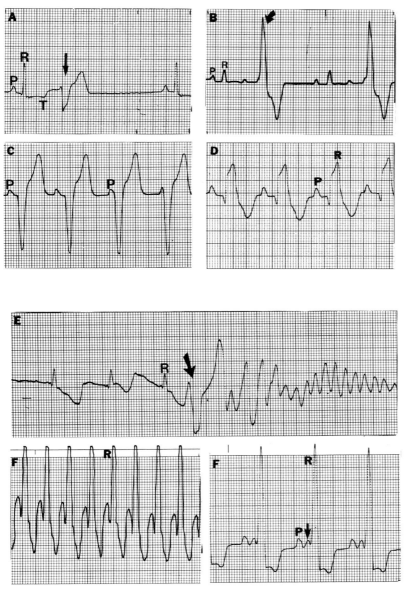

Fig. 15-2. Selected ventricular arrhythmias. Lead II rhythm strips, paper speed = 50 mm/ sec; 1 cm = 1 mV. **(A)** Left ventricular premature complex *(arrow)*, dog. **(B)** Right ventricular premature complex *(arrow)*, cat. **(C)** Ventricular tachycardia (P waves not related to QRS complexes), dog. **(D)** Left bundle branch block (can be confused with ventricular tachycardia, although note the constant PR interval), dog. **(E)** Ventricular fibrillation initiated by a forceful blow to the chest (during a QT interval) in a suspected cardiac arrest, dog. **(F)** *(left)* Supraventricular or ventricular tachycardia; *(right)* IV lidocaine interrupts the tachycardia and reveals ventricular preexcitation with a short PR interval and delta wave *(arrow)* supporting the Wolff-Parkinson-White syndrome.

VI. Treatment
    A. VPCs do not always require antiarrhythmic therapy. A medical data base including a thoracic radiograph, CBC and blood chemistry screen, and urinalysis is essential to rule out secondary causes of VPCs, which may require specific supportive therapy. Underlying congestive heart failure should be controlled with digitalis or other inotropic agents (e.g., dobutamine), diuretic, and vasodilator therapy.
    B. Antiarrhythmic therapy is advocated with frequent VPCs (greater than 20 to 30 per minute); repetitive complexes or runs of VPCs; multifocal QRS configurations; R-on-T phenomena (vulnerable period for development of ventricular fibrillation in animals with underlying heart disease; Fig. 15-2E), where the VPC occurs during the QT interval of the previous complex; and where clinical signs of poor cardiac output (e.g., weakness, dyspnea, and syncope) occur.
    C. Ventricular escape complexes that occur after a pause (similar to VPC configuration) should not be treated, as they represent a safety mechanism for maintaining cardiac output.
    D. Antiarrhythmic drugs commonly used to control VPCs include intravenous lidocaine and parenteral or oral procainamide, quinidine, propranolol and phenytoin (digitalis-induced VPCs). Newer antiarrhythmic agents that are being administered for VPCs include mexiletine, tocainide, and atenolol. Amiodarone, sotol, flecainide, and others are investigative antiarrhythmic drugs.

Ventricular Tachycardia

  I. Impulses are repetitively generated (greater than 3 VPCs in a row) from one or more ventricular foci. This arrhythmia may be paroxysmal or sustained.
 II. Heart rate and rhythm.
    A. The rate is usually above 100 bpm in the dog; and usually above 150 bpm in the cat.
    B. The rhythm is regular unless the arrhythmia is intermittent.
III. P: QRS characteristics
    The P waves that are seen are normal in shape but have no fixed relationship (AV dissociation) to wide and bizarre QRS complexes. The P waves occur before, during or after the QRS complexes, but have no fixed relationship (Fig. 15-2C).
IV. Differentials
    A. Sinus tachycardia, atrial tachycardia, or atrial fibrillation with a conduction disturbance (e.g., left or right bundle branch block) Figs. 15-1F, 15-2D, 15-3B) are included.
    B. A sustained ventricular rhythm slower than the above rates is termed an idioventricular rhythm.
 V. Significance
    A. Ventricular tachycardia is a life-threatening arrhythmia that, if sustained, may lead to hypotension, myocardial ischemia, syncope or seizures, shock, and death.

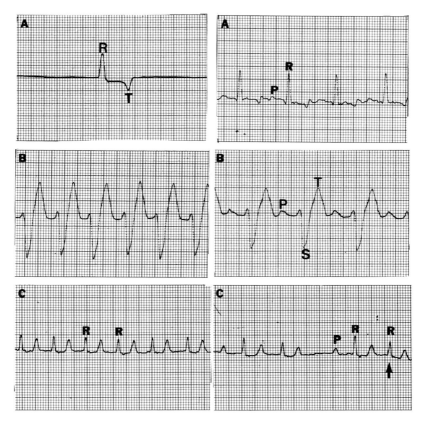

Fig. 15-3. Selected arrhythmias before and after treatment. Lead II rhythm strips, paper speed = 50 mm/sec; 1 cm = 1 mV. **(A)** *(left)* Atrial standstill; *(right)* Thirty minutes after IV normal saline and sodium bicarbonate, a conversion to normal sinus rhythm, dog. **(B)** *(left)* Suspected ventricular tachycardia; *(right)* IV lidocaine slows the cardiac rate and reveals right bundle branch block (prelidocaine ECG shows atrial tachycardia with right bundle branch block, a classic "quicksand of electrocardiography"), dog. **(C)** *(left)* Supraventricular tachycardia; *(right)* A vagal maneuver breaks the tachycardia abruptly (atrial premature complex, *arrow*), supporting an atrial tachycardia, dog. (*Figure continues.*)

  B. Some patients with ventricular tachycardia may show no clinical signs, especially if there is no underlying primary cardiac disease.

  C. This arrhythmia is electrically unstable and may lead to ventricular fibrillation and sudden death.

  D. All etiologies of VPCs (e.g., primary and secondary cardiac disease) may lead to a ventricular tachycardia. The arrhythmia may be hereditary in some young German shepherds.

 VI. Treatment

  A. Antiarrhythmic therapy is required in most patients with ventricular tachycardia. Exceptions include patients with complete heart block where the ventricular rhythm may be an escape mechanism, and severe acid-

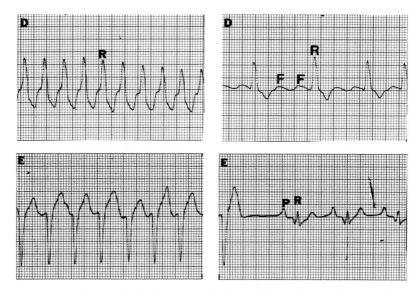

Fig. 15-3. (*Continued*). (**D**) (*left*) Supraventricular tachycardia; (*right*) a vagal maneuver results in varying degrees of AV block and atrial flutter, with flutter waves (**F**) and irregular RR intervals, dog. (**E**) (*left*) Ventricular tachycardia; (*right*) IV lidocaine converts ventricular tachycardia to normal sinus rhythm, dog.

     base or electrolyte disturbances, such as hypokalemia or hyperkalemia, which may respond to specific electrolyte or fluid therapy.

B. Lidocaine hydrochloride without epinephrine (2 to 3 mg/kg) via slow intravenous administration is the initial preferred treatment in the dog (Fig. 15-3E). This drug may also be used in the cat (0.5 mg/kg slow IV—beware of seizures). Seizures require intravenous diazepam. Hypotension may also occur if the bolus is administered too rapidly. The lidocaine bolus may have to be repeated several times at 10-minute intervals, although the higher dosages will increase the incidence of toxicity. A maximum total dose of 8 mg/kg is advised in the dog. Seizures will often occur before this dose is reached in the cat. Seizures may also occur in the dog at toxic doses.

C. The therapeutic effect of lidocaine is short termed and repeat boluses or constant-rate infusion may be required for a sustained antiarrhythmic effect (see antiarrhythmic drug section). If the ventricular arrhythmia is stable, intramuscular or oral therapy with procainamide or quinidine may be initiated and the lidocaine infusion slowly reduced over a 24- to 48-hour period. Hypokalemia and acidosis may cause therapeutic failure and must be treated.

D. When treatment with lidocaine is not indicated or practical, intramuscular quinidine or procainamide may be used to provide initial control of ventricular tachycardia. An initial loading dose of 12 to 20 mg/kg followed by repeat doses of 4 to 6 hour intervals at 6 to 12 mg/kg. Prolonged therapy may be continued with oral quinidine or procainamide at appropriate doses. Other antiarrhythmic drugs that may be useful include mexiletine, tocainide, propranolol, atenolol, and phenytoin.

E. DC shock should be reserved for the refractory arrhythmia and requires an experienced clinician and proper equipment.

F. The ECG should be monitored at frequent intervals. If the arrhythmia is poorly controlled, the advantage of increasing the drug dosage versus side effects must be considered. If the arrhythmia worsens, antiarrhythmic drug toxicity (i.e., proarrhythmia) must be considered as a cause of this abnormality. Multiform ventricular tachycardia due to procainamide or quinidine toxicity may be a life-threatening complication of antiarrhytymic medication (torsades de pointes).

G. Combinations of drugs (such as procainamide and quinidine, procainamide and propranolol, mexiletine and propranolol, or tocainide and propranolol) or added diazepam may be beneficial in refractory cases. The disadvantages of toxicity with combination therapy must be weighed against potential benefit.

H. If the arrhythmia is well controlled, it may be attempted to stop or slowly wean (controversial) the patient off the antiarrhythmic agent after a 2- to 3-week period. Attempting to stop the medication will avoid complications of long-term therapy and the great expense of antiarrhythmic drugs. The ECG must be evaluated before each decrease in dosage, and within 1 week after stopping the medication.

Ventricular Asystole

I. Location
No impulses are generated from atrial or ventricular pacemakers.

II. Heart rate and rhythm
There is no cardiac rate or ventricular rhythm.

III. P: QRS characteristics
P waves are of normal shape with complete AV block or are not present. No QRS complexes are seen.

IV. Differentials
Artifact (e.g., electrocardiograph is not on a proper lead or is connected improperly)

V. Significance
It is associated with cardiac arrest and no arterial pulses, and has a very grave prognosis.

VI. Treatment
A. Cardiopulmonary resuscitation must be undertaken immediately.
B. Pharmacologic intervention with intratracheal or intravenous epinephrine is mandatory.
C. An effective approach in human patients is to convert asystole to ventricular fibrillation followed by DC shock.

Ventricular Fibrillation

I. Location

Impulses are generated and propagated in the ventricles in a chaotic, asynchronous manner.

II. Heart rate and rhythm

A. The heart rate is rapid and disorganized.

B. The rhythm is irregular.

III. P: QRS characteristics

None are seen. There are no P waves present and there are no recognizable QRS complexes. There are continuous positive and negative oscillations that are chaotic and bizarre (Fig. 15-2E). The oscillations may be large (coarse) or small (fine).

IV. Differentials

Artifact (e.g., 60-cycle electrical interference or respiratory movement) is included

V. Significance

A. The most common arrhythmia associated with cardiac arrest is ventricular fibrillation.

B. There is no effective cardiac output, and no palpable atrial pulses are present.

C. Conditions such as myocardial ischemia, electrolyte imbalance, hypoxia, hypothermia, slow conduction, increased automaticity, autonomic nervous system dyssynergy, drugs, and unstable ventricular arrhythmias trigger ventricular fibrillation.

D. Ventricular fibrillation carries a very grave prognosis.

VI. Treatment

A. Cardiopulmonary resuscitation must be undertaken immediately.

B. Electrical defibrillation requires specialized equipment, but is mandatory.

C. Intratracheal lidocaine or propranolol may occasionally be successful in converting ventricular fibrillation to normal sinus rhythm.

D. Antifibrillatory agents such as bretylium have not been found very effective in animal patients.

E. Open-chest cardiac massage may be effective in converting ventricular fibrillation to normal sinus rhythm if no electrical cardioverter is available. External blows to the chest (thump-version) are less effective.

F. Sodium bicarbonate and calcium chloride are no longer routinely advocated. Sodium bicarbonate can be considered after 10 minutes of unsuccessful resuscitation efforts, or if significant acidosis is documented. Hypocalcemia is the only indication for calcium.

CONDUCTION DISTURBANCES

Atrial Standstill

I. Location

Impulses are not generated in the sinus node or are poorly conducted through the atrial tissues.

II. Heart rate and rhythm
   A. The rate is less than 60 bpm in the dog; less than 160 bpm in the cat.
   B. The rhythm is regular.
III. P: QRS characteristics
   No P waves are seen (Fig. 15-3A). The QRS complexes are normal or bizarre depending on the intraventricular conduction. The ST segment is elevated or depressed. The T wave may be tall due to shortened repolarization. The rhythm may be regular or irregular.
IV. Differentials
   AV junctional rhythm, idioventricular rhythm, and atrial fibrillation with complete heart block are included.
V. Significance
   A. Atrial standstill is a life-threatening abnormality associated with hyperkalemia (Addison's disease, acute renal failure, urinary obstruction, and diabetic ketoacidosis).
   B. Persistent atrial standstill is a disorder reported in English springer spaniels and other breeds, and select cats with dilated cardiomyopathy where there is degeneration and fibrosis of the atrial myocardial cells. There is often cardiac enlargement, although the blood electrolytes are normal. This abnormality may be correlated with a type of muscular dystrophy as seen in humans.
VI. Treatment
   A. If hyperkalemia is suspected, emergency therapy is undertaken if clinical history supports this possibility. The therapy is designed to transfer extracellular potassium into the body cells, thus restoring normokalemia.
   B. Initially, 2 mEq/kg of sodium bicarbonate is administered slowly intravenously coupled with normal saline, and may restore sinus rhythm within 15 to 30 minutes (beware of paradoxical cerebral acidosis) (Fig. 15-3A).
   C. Alternative therapy includes 0.5 U/kg of regular insulin coupled with 2 g of dextrose per unit of insulin by slow intravenous administration.
   D. Calcium gluconate (1 ml of a 10 percent solution/10 kg body weight) by slow intravenous administration.
   E. Intravenous normal saline with intravenous corticosteroids (e.g., 20 mg/kg hydrocortisone sodium succinate, 0.5 to 1 mg/kg dexamethasone, or 2 mg/kg of prednisolone).
   F. Intravenous 5 percent dextrose in water.

Incomplete AV Block (First- and Second-Degree AV Block)

I. Location
   The cardiac impulse is delayed or intermittently blocked in the region of the AV node or AV junction.
II. Heart rate and rhythm
   A. The rate is variable, depending on the rate of the sinus node pacemaker.
   B. The rate is usually regular in first-degree AV block, unless other arrhyth-

mias are present. The rhythm is usually irregular with second-degree AV block.

III. P: QRS characteristics
   A. First-degree AV block shows a prolonged, constant PR interval (AV conduction) with normal P wave and QRS complexes, at a 1:1 ratio.
   B. Second-degree AV block has normal P wave and QRS complexes with a constant PR interval, and with intermittent P waves not followed by QRS complexes. In Mobitz type I (Wenckebach) AV block, the PR interval gradually prolongs before a dropped ventricular beat occurs. The rhythm is regularly irregular. Mobitz-type II AV block, demonstrates a consistent PR interval prior to a dropped ventricular beat. The rhythm is often irregular.

IV. Differentials
   Complete AV block is included.

V. Significance
   A. First-degree AV block and Mobitz type I second-degree AF block are often caused by an increase in vagal tone (e.g., brachycephalic breeds, respiratory, gastrointestinal, or neurologic disease), digitalis, and sedatives (e.g., xylazine, acetylpromazine). Antiarrhythmic drugs (propranolol, quinidine, procainamide, and verapamil) and AV nodal disease are also associated with these types of AV block. Endogenous adenosine release may also be involved in AV block. Physiologic AV block may occur following ectopic beats or atrial tachyarrhythmias that occur during the AV node absolute or relative refractory periods (will slow down or block impulse).
   B. Mobitz type II AV block is a more advanced degree of block, and occurs in the AV junction, His bundle, or below. It may progress to complete heart block. Causes include idiopathic fibrosis (older dogs and cats), hereditary stenosis of the His bundle in the pug, hypertrophic cardiomyopathy in the dog and the cat, neoplastic infiltration secondary to metastatic neoplasia, and electrolyte disorders.
   C. Whether clinical signs develop (e.g., weakness, syncope, or congestive heart failure) may depend on the degree of AV block, ventricular rate, and ventricular function (i.e., contractility).

VI. Treatment
   A. For Mobitz type I AV block, treatment is usually not required. If related to drug toxicity, the drug should be stopped or dosage lowered.
   B. For Mobitz type II AV block, therapy depends on the clinical signs. If the cardiac rate is slow and weakness or syncope is evident, then atropine, theophylline (blocks adenosine), isoproterenol, or a temporary or permanent cardiac pacemaker is required.

Complete (Third-Degree) AV Block

I. Location
   The cardiac impulse is completely blocked in the region of the AV junction, and/or His bundle, and/or all bundle branches.

II. Heart rate and rhythm

The atrial rate (PP interval) is within normal limits, and there is a slow idioventricular escape rhythm. The rhythm is usually regular. An idioventricular escape rhythm is below 40 bpm, whereas a low AV junctional (idiojunctional) escape rhythm has a rate of 40 to 60 bpm in the dog. An enhanced AV junctional or idioventricular rhythm (AV dissociation) shows a more rapid rate, with the ventricular rate approaching the atrial rate.

III. P: QRS characteristics

A. No relationship; the P wave is completely dissociated from the QRS complex

B. The PR interval is variable, and there are usually many P waves versus few QRS complexes (Fig. 15-1H).

C. The morphology of the QRS complexes varies depending on the location of the ventricular escape rhythm.

IV. Differentials

Advanced second-degree AV block, atrial standstill, and ventricular tachycardia

V. Significance

A. Complete AV block is often associated with the clinical signs of weakness, syncope, or congestive heart failure.

B. Underlying conditions resulting in this abnormality include congenital defects (e.g., aortic stenosis, ventricular septal defect, isolated AV block), infiltrative cardiomyopathy (e.g., amyloidosis, neoplasia), idiopathic fibrosis, myocardial infarction, hypertrophic cardiomyopathy, bacterial endocarditis, Lyme carditis, and idiopathic fibrosis in geriatric dogs (e.g., cocker spaniel, German shepherd). Other reported causes include hypokalemia and hyperkalemia.

VI. Treatment

A. A permanent cardiac pacemaker is the only effective treatment in symptomatic patients.

B. Asymptomatic patients may not require therapy.

C. Drugs used for this abnormality include atropine, isoproterenol, theophylline, and corticosteroids (anti-inflammatory). An intravenous isoproterenol infusion may be useful in increasing the rate of the ventricular escape rhythm during nonelective surgical procedures.

ARRHYTHMIAS AND CONDUCTION
DISTURBANCES

Sick Sinus Syndrome (SSS)

I. Location

A. The cardiac impulses are generated in the sinus node at a slower than normal rate or are blocked exiting the sinus node.

B. The atria and AV node may also be involved, resulting in an atrial tachyarrhythmia (e.g., atrial tachycardia, flutter, or fibrillation).

II. Heart rate and rhythm

The rate is rapid or slow, and long pauses (Fig. 15-1G) may be present on the ECG. There may be a bradycardia-tachycardia syndrome with alternating periods of slow and rapid heart rates.

III. P: QRS characteristics

There is a normal P wave for each QRS complex. The PR interval is constant unless the bradycardia-tachycardia syndrome is present.

IV. Differentials

A. Sinus bradycardia, sinus block and/or arrest, atrial tachycardia; a poor (blunted) response to atropine (e.g., less than 50 percent increase in heart rate) may support SSS

V. Significance

A. The clinical signs of the sick sinus syndrome are variable.

B. A reduction in cardiac output may result in hypoperfusion of vital organs and show clinical signs of marked weakness and/or syncope, or seizures.

VI. Treatment

A. If the animal is asymptomatic or has mild clinical signs, no therapy is required.

B. If there are severe clinical signs, injectable atropine or other oral anticholinergic agents (e.g., probantheline) may alleviate these signs.

C. An artificial ventricular-demand pacemaker is required for long-term control of bradyarrhythmias, while digoxin or diltiazem may control the tachyarrhythmia.

Ventricular Preexcitation and the Wolff-Parkinson-White (WPW) Syndrome

I. Location

The cardiac impulses are generated in the sinus node but spread to the ventricle via an anomalous conduction pathway as well as the AV node.

II. Heart rate and rhythm

The cardiac rate and rhythm are normal in ventricular pre-excitation. The rate may be very rapid (e.g., 300 bpm) in the WPW syndrome.

III. P: QRS characteristics

The P waves are normal in ventricular pre-excitation or are unrecognizable in the WPW syndrome. The QRS complex is widened with notching of the R wave (delta wave) in ventricular pre-excitation. The QRS complex may be normal, wide, or bizarre in the WPW syndrome depending on the circuit the atrial tachycardia follows. The QRS complexes are wide when the cardiac impulse spreads antegrade via the anomalous pathway and retrograde via the AV node. The QRS complexes are narrow when the cardiac impulse spreads antegrade via the AV node and retrograde via the anomalous pathway. The PR interval is short in ventricular pre-excitation. In the WPW syndrome, there is often a P wave for every QRS complex (1:1 conduction). A short PR interval may be correlated with a normal QRS complex if the anomalous pathway bypasses the AV node to the area of the His bundle (Lown-Ganong-Levine syndrome, in humans).

IV. Differentials

AV junctional tachycardia, atrial tachycardia, and ventricular tachycardia are included.

V. Significance

Ventricular pre-excitation and WPW syndrome may be a congenital problem in the dog or cat occurring with or without other congenital heart defects (e.g., atrial septal defect, valvular dysplasia, or fibrosis).

VI. Treatment

A. Ventricular pre-excitation without tachycardia may not require therapy.

B. The WPW syndrome requires control and/or conversion of the tachycardia with a vagal maneuver (e.g., ocular or carotid sinus pressure) (Fig. 15-2F) digoxin, lidocaine, propranolol, quinidine, procainamide, verapamil, or DC shock). Digoxin is only indicated in narrow QRS complex WPW syndrome. In wide QRS complex WPW syndrome, digoxin may decrease the refractory period of the anomalous pathway and increase the rate of the tachycardia. Only lidocaine, procainamide, quinidine, mexiletine or tocainide should be used in this situation.

ANTIARRHYTHMIC THERAPY

Cardiac arrhythmias and conduction disturbances may have profound effects on cardiac output, coronary artery perfusion, arterial blood pressure, and vital organ perfusion. The clinical signs that result from specific arrhythmias have been previously described. Antiarrhythmic therapy may result in a control or abolishment of the arrhythmia and a return to normal hemodynamic function. It is important to have a thorough knowledge of the properties of the agents available to treat specific rhythm disturbances. Many of the available antiarrhythmic drugs are classified based on their electrophysiologic mechanisms (Table 15-3). The investigative agents are new drugs not available for routine clinical use. Antiarrhythmic drugs may decrease electrical instability (antifibrillatory) and lessen the possibility that an arrhythmia will result in ventricular fibrillation and sudden death. The antifibrillatory activity of an agent does not have to correlate with its antiectopic activity.

COMMONLY USED ANTIARRHYTHMIC DRUGS

Atropine Derivatives

I. Indications

Symptomatic sinus bradycardia, sinus block and/or arrest; incomplete AV block; sick sinus syndrome

II. Pertinent mechanisms

Parasympatholytic agent; decreases vagal tone to the sinus and AV nodes

III. How supplied

A. Atropine sulfate injection 0.4 mg/ml USP, and 0.4-mg tablet (Eli Lilly)

TABLE 15-3. CLASSIFICATION OF ANTIARRHYTHMIC AGENTS[a]

Type	Agent	General Mechanism
I	Quinidine Procainamide Lidocaine Disopyramide Phenytoin Aprindine* Encainide* Flecainide* Mexiletine Tocainide	Membrane-stabilizing agent (local anesthetic) Decreases the membrane conductance to sodium ions, depresses phase 4 depolarization (automaticity)
II	Propranolol Metoprolol Nadolol* Timolol* Atenolol Pindolol* Sotolol	Sympatholytic agent β-adrenergic blockade) Depresses phase 4 depolarization (automaticity)
III	Bretylium* Amiodarone* Bethanadine*	Prolongation of action potential duration Depresses phase 4 depolarization (automaticity) Antiadrenergic effects
IV	Verapamil Diltiazem Nifedipine*	Decreases the slow inward current, primarily the calcium ion Depresses phase 4 depolarization (automaticity) Depresses conduction in fibers with slow current.

[a] Asterisk (*): investigative agents, and/or not established for routine clinical use.

    B. Isopropamide (Darbid 5-mg tablet; Smith, Kline and French)
    C. Propantheline (Pro-Banthine, 7.5 or 15-mg tablet; Searle)
    D. Glycopyrrolate (Robinul 0.2 mg/ml, injection; Robbins)
  IV. Dosage
    A. Dog
      1. Atropine: 0.01 to 0.02 mg/kg IV, IM; 0.02 to 0.04 mg/kg SC q6–8h
      2. Isopropamide: 2.5 to 5.0 mg q8–12h
      3. Propantheline: 7.5 to 15 mg q8–12h
      4. Glycopyrrolate: 0.005 to 0.01 mg/kg IV, IM; 0.01 to 0.02 mg/kg SC q8–12h
    B. Cat
    Atropine: 0.02 to 0.04 mg/kg q4–6h; SC, IM, IV
   V. Side effects and toxicity
    A. Sinus tachycardia, ectopic beats, and ocular, gastrointestinal, and pulmonary effects
    B. Initial response may be parasympathomimetic (e.g., bradycardia), especially when administered IV

Digitalis Glycosides

  I. Indications
    A. Atrial premature complexes; atrial tachycardia; and atrial flutter or atrial fibrillation
    B. Sinus tachycardia due to congestive heart failure

II. Pertinent mechanisms
   A. Digitalis decreases the velocity of AV conduction by direct and parasym-
      pathomimetic effects.
   B. Cardiac contractility and cardiac output improve in congestive heart fail-
      ure, resulting in diminished sympathetic tone to the sinus and AV nodes.
   C. Parasympathomimetic (vagal) tone is increased and may result in a de-
      creased cardiac rate.
   D. The refractory period of atrial and ventricular cell transmembrane poten-
      tials is decreased and may result in ectopia.
   E. Improves baroreceptor function and autonomic nervous system influence
      on cardiac rhythm and conduction.
III. How supplied
   A. Digitoxin (crystodigin injection 0.2 mg/ml, 0.1- to 0.2-mg tablets, Eli Lilly).
   B. Digoxin (Lanoxin elixir 0.05 mg/ml; 0.125-, 0.25-, 0.5-mg tablet; Bur-
      roughs Wellcome); (Cardoxin elixir, 0.05, 0.15 mg/ml; Evsco).
IV. Dosage
   A. Dog
      1. Digitoxin
         a) Oral maintenance: 0.04 to 0.1 mg/kg divided q8h
         b) Rapid parenteral: 0.01 to 0.03 mg/kg, one-half of dose IV, wait 30
            to 60 minutes and give one-fourth of dose; wait 30 to 60 minutes
            and give remaining dose if required
      2. Digoxin
         a) Oral maintenance: 0.01 to 0.02 mg/kg divided BID
         b) Rapid oral: 0.02 to 0.06 mg/kg divided BID for the first day; then
            go to maintenance level
         c) Rapid parenteral: 0.01 to 0.02 mg/kg in divided doses as per Digi-
            toxin
   B. Cat
      1. Digitoxin: not routinely administered to cats
      2. Digoxin
         a) Oral maintenance: 0.22 mg/m^2 or 0.007 to 0.015 mg/kg SID to every
            other day (average cat, one-fourth of a 0.125-mg tablet every other
            day; elixir not well tolerated)
         b) Rapid IV: 0.005 mg/kg lean body weight divided between three
            doses or to effect; one-half the calculated dose IV, 60 minutes later,
            one-quarter of the calculated dose, and 60 minutes later the final
            one-quarter dose if necessary (stop if marked bradycardia, dimin-
            ished AV conduction, digoxin-related arrhythmias, or clinical signs
            are evident). Oral maintenance digoxin is started immediately after
            the last IV dose, in the dog and the cat.
V. Side effects and toxicity
   A. Gastrointestinal (anorexia, vomiting, diarrhea)
   B. Neurologic (lethargy, ataxia)
   C. Cardiac (e.g., AV block, AV junctional rhythm, ectopic beats from atrium
      or ventricle, ventricular tachycardia, and any other arrhythmia or conduc-
      tion disturbance)

Epinephrine

  I. Indications
     Ventricular standstill is the primary indication; high degree or complete AV block, until an artificial or permanent pacemaker is inserted; electromechanical dissociation
 II. Pertinent mechanisms
     It is a sympathomimetic (α- and β-receptor stimulation) agent. Epinephrine accelerates the atrial and ventricular rate in complete AV block (e.g., enhances automaticity).
III. How supplied
     Epinephrine hydrochloride 1:1,000 solution, 1 mg/ml injectable (Adrenalin, Parke-Davis)
 IV. Dosage
     Dog and cat: 0.2 mg/kg IV q3–5 ml of 1:1000 dilution IV; double dose for intratracheal administration
  V. Side effects and toxicity
     Cardiovascular (arterial hypertension, atrial and ventricular ectopia, and atrial or ventricular tachycardia and/or fibrillation)

Isoproterenol

  I. Indications
     Sinus bradycardia; sinus block and/or arrest; complete AV block; and to maintain an escape pacemaker during general anesthesia
 II. Pertinent mechanisms
     Sympathomimetic effects (e.g., stimulation of the cardiac and respiratory β-adrenergic receptors); cardiac effects are primarily on the sinus and AV nodes
III. How supplied
     A. Isuprel hydrochloride injection, 0.2 mg/ml, 1 and 5 ml ampule, 10-mg glossets (Breon)
     B. Proterenol 20-, 40-mg tablet (Key)
 IV. Dosage
     A. Dog
        1. Isuprel: 0.4 mg in 250 ml of 5% dextrose/water titrated to effect
        2. Proterenol: 10 to 20 mg q4–6h
        3. Isuprel glossets: 5 to 10 mg per rectum q4–6h
     B. Cat
        Isuprel: 0.4 mg per 250 ml of 5% dextrose/water titrated to effect
  V. Side effects and toxicity
     A. Gastrointestinal (vomiting)
     B. Neurologic (excitation)
     C. Cardiac (sinus tachycardia, ectopic complexes)

Lidocaine Hydrochloride

  I. Indications
     Frequent ventricular premature complexes; paroxysmal or persistent ventricular tachycardia; atrial tachyarrhythmias conducted over anomalous pathway in WPW syndrome

II. Pertinent mechanisms
   A. Depresses automaticity in ventricular myocardial cells; has minimal effects on atrial cells
   B. Lidocaine may decrease the refractory period of the AV node, causing an increase in the ventricular response in patients with atrial flutter or fibrillation.
III. How supplied
   Xylocaine (lidocaine), without epinephrine, 2 percent (20 mg/ml), (Astra)
IV. Dosage
   A. Dog
      1. 2 to 4 mg/kg slow IV, repeat every 10 minutes to a maximum of 8 mg/kg
      2. Constant-rate infusion (CRI) 25 to 75 μg/kg/min; approximately 2 mg/ml of 5 percent dextrose/water administered in a slow IV drip to effect. CRI equals body weight (kg) × dose × 0.36 = total dose in kg slow IV over 6 hours
   B. Cat
      0.5 mg/kg slow IV (cats are sensitive to this drug and may undergo seizures; control with diazepam)
V. Side effects and toxicity
   A. Gastrointestinal (emesis)
   B. Neurologic (tremors, seizures, excitation, control with diazepam)
   C. Cardiovascular (hypotension, increased AV conduction with atrial flutter or fibrillation)

Phenytoin

I. Indications
   Digitalis-induced atrial and ventricular tachyarrhythmias; digitalis-induced AV block; used in place of lidocaine or procainamide with refractory ventricular arrhythmias
II. Pertinent mechanisms
   A. Depresses diastolic depolarization and automaticity, shortens the duration of the action potential and the effect of refractory period
   B. Increases the conduction velocity in the atrium, and counteracts the depressant effect of AV conduction induced by digitalis or procainamide
III. How supplied
   30- and 100-mg capsule, 125 mg/5 ml syrup, 50 mg/ml injectable (Parke-Davis)
IV. Dosage
   A. Dog: 4 to 8 mg/kg PO divided q6–8h; 4 mg/kg slow IV
   B. Cat: not used; toxic
V. Side effects and toxicity
   A. Skin reactions (dermatoses)
   B. Neurologic (ataxia, tremors, depression)
   C. Cardiac (AV block)

Procainamide

  I. Indications
     Ventricular premature complexes; ventricular tachycardia; supraventricular
     tachycardia in WPW syndrome with wide QRS complexes; supraventricular
     tachyarrhythmias (not established in the dog).
 II. Pertinent mechanisms
     A. Prolongation of refractory period in the atria and the ventricles
     B. Slowing of electrical conduction, depression of automaticity, and prolon-
        gation of the refractory period of atrial and ventricular myocardial cells
     C. Indirect vagolytic effects (e.g., AV conduction may improve with low
        doses and decrease with higher doses)
III. How supplied
     A. Procan sustained-release (SR), 250-, 500-mg tablet (Parke-Davis)
     B. Pronestyl: 200, 500 mg tablet (Squibb)
     C. Pronestyl injection: 100, 500 mg/ml (Squibb)
 IV. Dosage
     A. Dogs
        1. Procan-SR: 8 to 20 mg/kg q6–8h
        2. Pronestyl tablets: 8 to 20 mg/kg q6h
        3. Pronestyl injection: 6 to 12 mg/kg IM q6–8h (the initial dose may be
           doubled), and 6 to 12 mg/kg IV over 5 minutes; CRI 25 to 40 μg/kg/
           min
     B. Cats: not routinely administered
  V. Side effects and toxicity
     A. Gastrointestinal (anorexia, vomiting, diarrhea)
     B. Cardiovascular (weakness, hypotension, decreased cardiac contractility;
        widening of the QRS complex and QT interval and AV block; multiform
        ventricular tachycardia)
     C. Systemic (fever, leukopenia; lupus erythematosus syndrome in humans,
        not established in the dog)

Propranolol Hydrochloride

  I. Indications
     A. Atrial premature complexes and tachyarrhythmias; atrial fibrillation in
        conjunction with digitalis; and ventricular premature contractions (second
        choice to quinidine or procainamide)
     B. Propranolol effective with digitalis induced atrial and ventricular tachyar-
        rhythmias.
     C. Atrial tachycardia secondary to Wolff-Parkinson-White syndrome with
        normal QRS complexes.
     D. Cats with hypertrophic cardiomyopathy
 II. Pertinent mechanisms
     A. Propranolol is a β-adrenergic receptor (β_1 and β_2) blocking agent that
        inhibits sympathetic stimulation to the heart.
     B. There is also a direct depressant action on the transmembrane potentials

of the cardiac cells, reducing automaticity and conduction. Propranolol may show antifibrillatory activity.

III. How supplied
  A. Inderal 10-, 20-, 40-, 80-mg tablet; 1-ml vial (1 mg/ml) (Ayerst)
  B. A selective β_1 blocking drug (less bronchoconstriction) atenolol is available in 25-, 50- and 100-mg tablets (Tenormin)

IV. Dosage
  A. Dog
    1. Propranolol: 0.04 to 0.06 mg/kg IV slowly; 0.2 to 1.0 mg/kg PO q8h
    2. Atenolol: 0.25 to 1.0 mg/kg PO SID–BID
  B. Cat
    1. Propranolol: 0.04 mg/kg IV slowly, 2.5 to 5.0 mg q8–12h
    2. Atenolol: 6.25 to 12.5 mg PO SID

V. Side effects and toxicity
  A. Respiratory (bronchoconstriction)
  B. Cardiac (decreased contractility, hypotension, bradycardia, and AV block)
  C. Systemic (hypoglycemia)

Quinidine

  I. Indications
    A. Ventricular premature complexes; ventricular tachycardia; acute atrial fibrillation; refractory supraventricular tachycardia; supraventricular arrhythmias with anomalous conduction in the WPW syndrome
 II. Pertinent mechanisms
    A. Inhibition of the fast sodium channel of the transmembrane potential
    B. Prolongation of the refractory period in the atria and ventricles
    C. Slows phase 0 of the action potential and depresses spontaneous diastolic depolarization (automaticity)
    D. An indirect vagolytic effect
III. How supplied
    A. Quinidine sulfate USP 200-mg tablet, 300 mg Extentab (Parke-Davis)
    B. Quinidine gluconate USP injection 80 mg/ml (Eli-Lilly); Quinaglute duratab 324 mg (Cooper)
    C. Quinidine polygalacturonate 275-mg tablet (Cardioquin, Purdue-Frederick)
IV. Dosage
    A. Dog
      1. Quinidine sulfate 6 to 16 mg/kg PO q6h (sulfate), q8h (Extentabs)
      2. Quinidine gluconate 6 to 20 mg/kg IM q6h, 8 to 20 mg/kg PO q6–8h (Quinaglute)
      3. Quinidine polygalacturonate 8 to 20 mg/kg q6–8h (Cardioquin)
    B. Cat: not routinely administered
 V. Side effects and toxicity
    A. Gastrointestinal (anorexia, vomiting, diarrhea)
    B. Cardiac (weakness, hypotension, decreased cardiac contractility, widen-

ing of the QRS complex and Q-T interval, AV block, and syncope due to
multiform ventricular tachycardia)
  C. Drug interaction (increases serum digoxin levels)

Tocainide and Mexiletine

  I. Indications
     Ventricular arrhythmias that are responsive to IV lidocaine
 II. Pertinent mechanisms
     Tocainide and mexiletine are synthetic analogs of lidocaine developed in an
     attempt to find an orally active lidocaine-type preparation. The electrophysio-
     logic mechanisms are similar to those of lidocaine.
III. How supplied
     A. Tocainide HCl 400-, 600-mg tablets (Tonocard, Merck)
     B. Mexiletine 150-, 200-, 250-mg capsules (Mexitil, Boehringer Ingelheim)
 IV. Dosage
     1 to 2 mg/kg/day divided BID–TID (tocainide and mexiletine); not established
     in small animals.
     A. Tocainide 20 mg/kg PO TID
     B. Mexiletine 6 mg/kg PO TID
  V. Side effects and toxicity
     Similar to lidocaine in humans; also blood dyscrasias and pulmonary fibrosis

LESS COMMONLY USED ANTIARRHYTHMIC DRUGS

Disopyramide

  I. Indications
     A. The prevention and treatment of ventricular tachyarrhythmias.
     B. Disopyramide has also been reported effective for supraventricular tachy-
        arrhythmias (atrial fibrillation or flutter) in humans, although it may be
        less effective for this purpose in the dog.
 II. Pertinent mechanisms
     A. Similar to quinidine and procainamide
     B. Decreases the slope of phase IV depolarization (automaticity)
     C. Anticholinergic effects
     D. A potent negative inotropic agent
III. How supplied
     100-mg, 150-mg capsule (Norpace, Searle)
 IV. Dosage
     Not well established, due to rapid excretion in the dog; not used in the cat
  V. Side effects and toxicity
     A. Should not be administered in patients in congestive heart failure or shock
        due to its negative inotropic effects
     B. Gastrointestinal (dry mouth, vomiting)

C. Cardiac (AV block, sinus node depression, multiform ventricular tachycardia)
D. Systemic (urinary retention, glaucoma, depression)

Diazepam

I. Indications
   A. Refractory supraventricular and ventricular tachyarrhythmias, combined with other antiarrhythmic drugs
   B. Arrhythmias induced by nervous systemic excitation or the autonomic nervous system
II. Pertinent mechanisms
   Sedative effect on the central nervous system that may be indirectly causing a cardiac arrhythmia
III. How supplied
   10-ml vials (5 mg/ml), 2-, 5-, 10-mg tablets (Valium, Roche)
IV. Dosage
   A. Dog
      2.5 to 20 mg IV, 0.1 to 0.2 mg/kg PO q8–12h
   B. Cat
      2.5 to 5 mg (5 mg/ml) IV, 0.1 to 0.2 mg/kg PO q12h
V. Side effects and toxicity
   Neurologic (marked sedation or coma)

Edrophonium Chloride

I. Indications
   Atrial tachycardia
II. Pertinent mechanisms
   Short-acting parasympathomimetic drug (increases vagal tone)
III. How supplied
   1-ml, 10-ml vials; 10 mg/ml (Tensilon, Roche)
IV. Dosage
   A. Dog
      1 to 2 mg slow IV over 30 seconds; if no response, give 3 to 5 mg additionally (atropine sulfate should be available if marked bradycardia occurs)
   B. Cat: not used in the cat
V. Side effects and toxicity
   A. Neurologic (excitation and seizures)
   B. Respiratory (dyspnea)
   C. Gastrointestinal (vomiting, diarrhea)
   D. Cardiac (bradycardia, hypotension)

Potassium Chloride

I. Indications
   Chemical ventricular defibrillator (dog and cat); digitalis-induced ventricular arrhythmias (dog)

II. Pertinent mechanisms
    A. Hyperkalemia decreases automaticity and conduction.
    B. Hypokalemia exacerbates digitalis-induced ventricular arrhythmias.
    C. Hypokalemia may result in tachyarrhythmias that are refractory to drug
       therapy.
III. How supplied
    10-ml ampules (2 mEq/ml) (Abbott)
IV. Dosage
    Monitor serum potassium and ECG
    A. Dog
       1. 0.5 to 2.0 mEq/kg/day slow IV (40 mEq diluted in 500 ml of 5% dex-
          trose/water), not to exceed 0.5 mEq/kg/hr (rate of infusion is critical)
       2. 1.0 mEq of potassium chloride/kg with 6.0 mg of acetylcholine/kg intra-
          cardiac (ventricular defibrillation only)
    B. Cat
       1. Should not exceed 0.5 mEq/kg/hr slow IV (e.g., hypokalemia)
       2. 0.25 to 0.75 mEq followed by calcium chloride IC (chemical defibril-
          lation)
V. Side effects and toxicity
    Cardiac arrest

Verapamil and Diltiazem

I. Indications
    A. Atrial tachyarrhythmias, particularly those generated by a re-entrant
       mechanism
    B. Reciprocating tachycardia with normal QRS complexes in the WPW syn-
       drome
    C. To decrease the ventricular rate by slowing AV conduction in atrial fibril-
       lation
II. Pertinent mechanisms
    A. Verapamil and diltiazem are calcium blocking agents, originally developed
       as antianginal drugs in humans, that block the influx of calcium and sodium
       ions at the slow channels of cardiac tissue.
    B. These agents slow the sinus node rate and prolong the absolute and rela-
       tive refractory period of AV nodal tissue.
III. How supplied
    A. Verapamil hydrochloride injectable 5 mg/2 ml; 80-, 120-mg tablets (Calan,
       Searle)
    B. 2-ml ampules, 2.5-mg/ml; and 80-, 120-mg tablets (Isoptin, Knoll)
    C. Diltiazem (Cardizem) 30-, 60-, 90-, and 120-mg tablets
IV. Dosage
    A. Dog
       1. Verapamil
          a) 0.05 to 0.15 mg/kg over 2 minutes, 5 mg total dose
          b) Oral dose not established at this time

    2. Diltiazem: 0.5 to 1.5 mg/kg PO TID
  B. Cat: Diltiazem, 1.0 to 2.5 mg/kg PO TID
V. Side effects and toxicity
  A. Gastrointestinal (constipation)
  B. Systemic problems (urinary retention)
  C. Cardiovascular (hypotension and shock, AV block, sinus bradycardia, and sinus block and/or arrest)
  D. For hypotension and shock, IV fluids, calcium chloride supplementation, and catecholamines (dobutamine, dopamine, or isoproterenol) may reverse these signs
  E. Drug interaction (verapamil may increase serum digoxin levels).
  F. Diltiazem causes less myocardial depression than verapamil

INVESTIGATIVE ANTIARRHYTHMIC AGENTS

Amiodarone

I. Indications
Acute and chronic atrial and ventricular tachyarrhythmias; atrial tachyarrhythmias correlated with the WPW with narrow or aberrant QRS complexes in humans
II. Pertinent mechanisms
  A. Amiodarone prolongs the duration of the action potential in the atria and the ventricles. This agent shows antifibrillatory effects in humans.
  B. The sympathetic nervous system is inhibited.
  C. The sinus node rate is slowed and the sinus node recovery time is prolonged.
  D. The absolute and relative refractory periods of the AV node and His-Purkinje system are prolonged.
  E. The absolute refractory period of the AV node and anomalous pathway is prolonged in the WPW syndrome.
III. How supplied
Not available for routine clinical usage
IV. Dosage
Not established in small animals
V. Side effects and toxicity (reported in humans)
  A. Gastrointestinal (vomiting)
  B. Systemic (hypothyroidism or hyperthyroidism, pulmonary fibrosis, and corneal deposits)

Aprindine

I. Indications
  A. Supraventricular tachyarrhythmias; ventricular premature contractions and incessant ventricular tachycardia; arrhythmias induced by digoxin

toxicity; and supraventricular tachycardias in the WPW syndrome with wide QRS complexes

    B. Ventricular arrhythmias that are refractory to quinidine or procainamide

II. Pertinent mechanisms

Mechanisms are similar to quinidine and procainamide; delays conduction in all levels of the heart; prolongs the effective refractory period of the atria, AV node, and His-Purkinje system

III. Dosage

    A. Dog

       0.5 to 2.0 mg/kg IV or PO, q8h

    B. Cat: not used

IV. How supplied

100-mg tablets (Eli Lilly)

V. Adverse effects not well documented in the dog

    A. Neurologic (tremors, ataxia)

    B. Systemic (agranolocytosis and cholestatic jaundice in humans)

    C. Cardiac (decreases contractility)

Bretylium

I. Indications

    A. Life-threatening, drug-resistant ventricular tachycardia, or ventricular fibrillation in humans.

    B. Limited clinical experience in the dog does not favor injectable bretylium as an antifibrillatory agent. This drug may actually worsen ventricular tachycardia and promote ventricular fibrillation, although this remains controversial and may depend on the dose administered.

II. Pertinent mechanisms

    A. Bretylium has direct membrane effects on the myocardium and indirect effects by blocking the sympathetic nervous system.

    B. Bretylium increases the action potential duration and absolute refractory period in isolated tissue.

III. How supplied

Bretylium tosylate injectable, 50 mg/ml (American Critical Care)

IV. Dosage

Not established in small animals

V. Side effects and toxicity (in humans)

    A. Gastrointestinal (vomiting)

    B. Cardiovascular (hypotension)

Note: The oral agent bethanadine may have a role as an antifibrillatory drug in the dog and cat.

NONPHARMACOLOGIC METHODS TO TREAT CARDIAC ARRHYTHMIAS

Vagal Maneuver

Increasing parasympathetic tone to the sinus and AV node via ocular or carotid sinus pressure

I. Indication

To provide a diagnostic aid in undefined atrial tachyarrhythmias and sus-pected sick sinus syndrome patients; terminate atrial tachycardia in some patients

II. Mechanisms

A. In sinus tachycardia, a vagal maneuver usually causes a slight slowing of the heart rate due to the effect on the sinus node.

B. With atrial tachycardia or flutter, physiologic AV block often occurs, and the RR intervals become irregular, showing an underlying atrial mecha-nism for the arrhythmia.

C. Supraventricular tachycardia that depends on circus (re-entrant) routes through AV junctional tissue may respond to a vagal maneuver by sudden termination of the tachycardia or speeding or slowing of the cardiac rate.

D. Although a tachycardia may be resolved only temporarily, it may aid in establishing the best choice of antiarrhythmic therapy if needed.

III. Contraindications and complications

A. Sick sinus syndrome (bradycardia-tachycardia syndrome): patients may show a marked symptomatic bradycardia

B. Breeds that are hypersensitive to a vagal maneuver (brachycephalic breeds) may show a marked symptomatic bradycardia

C. On termination of the tachycardia, a continued vagal maneuver may result in prolonged ventricular asystole; stop the vagal maneuver as soon as the tachycardia terminates.

Artificial Cardiac Pacing

I. Indications

A. Temporary pacing

1. Symptomatic and drug-resistant second- or third-degree AV block

2. Symptomatic and drug-resistant sinus bradycardia, sinus arrest and/or sinus block, and slow AV junctional rhythm (sick sinus syndrome)

3. Atrial or ventricular tachyarrhythmias unresponsive to drug therapy (use premature stimulation or overdrive suppression)

B. Permanent pacing

1. Symptomatic heart block

2. Symptomatic sinus block and/or arrest, bradycardia, AV block (sick sinus syndrome)

3. Symptomatic chronic second-degree AV block (Mobitz type II)

4. Recurrent drug-resistant tachyarrhythmias benefited by short-term pacing

5. Symptomatic bilateral bundle branch block

II. Mechanisms and types of pacemakers

A. Functions as natural pacemaker by initiating electrical impulses via a bat-tery. The electrical impulse travels through small wires to the heart

B. An atrial pacemaker is required to suppress atrial arrhythmias.

C. A ventricular pacemaker is satisfactory for complete AV block, although the lack of sequential atrioventricular pumping will result in less than maximal cardiac output.

D. Bifocal pacing (AV sequential pacing) is commonly used in humans.

E. A demand pacemaker (functions only when the heart rate is below a critical level) avoids a major complication of fixed pacemakers, competition between the natural rhythm and pacemaker-induced rhythm.

III. Complications and malfunctions

A. Malfunctioning pacemakers (slowing, irregularity, sensing failure, loss of capture, promoting arrhythmias)

1. Requires replacement of the malfunctioning unit with a new pacemaker
2. Loss of capture may be due to malposition or fracturing of the electrodes or wires.
3. Improper sensing of atrial ventricular rhythm (AV sequential pacemaker) resulting in a pacemaker induced tachycardia.

B. Ventricular fibrillation
The most common cause is competition of the regular rhythm with a fixed-rate pacemaker and R-on-T phenomenon.

C. Infection at surgical sites or along wire tracts; surgical drainage or removal of the infected sites may be required.

D. Arrhythmias related to underlying heart disease.

Cardioversion and Defibrillation

I. Indications
Electroshock therapy is used as an emergency procedure during ventricular fibrillation and also for the conversion of selected tachyarrhythmias (e.g., atrial fibrillation in which underlying cause has been corrected; atrial tachycardia, atrial flutter, and ventricular tachycardia unresponsive to drugs and correlated with clinical signs).

II. Mechanism
Cardioversion electrically converts arrhythmias to a sinus rhythm by a synchronized discharge of current during the depolarization (QRS complex) part of the electrical cycle. Defibrillation does not require a synchronized delivery of current.

III. Contraindications for cardioversion

A. Digitalis toxicity and/or hypokalemia
B. Severe mitral insufficiency and/or marked left atrial enlargement
C. Chronic atrial fibrillation
D. Atrial fibrillation or atrial flutter with AV block
E. Sick sinus syndrome
F. A cardioverter that is not synchronized to the QRS complex

SUGGESTED READINGS

Anderson JL: Antifibrillatory versus antiectopic therapy. Am J Cardiol 54(2): 7A, 1984
Bolton GR: Handbook of Canine Electrocardiography. WB Saunders, Philadelphia, 1975
Bonagura J: Therapy of cardiac arrhythmias. p. 360. In Kirk RW (ed): Current Veterinary Therapy VIII. WB Saunders, Philadelphia, 1983

Bonagura JD: Cardiac dysrhythmias diagnosis and treatment. Scientific Proceedings of the American Animal Hospital Association 87, 1980

Bonagura JD, Muir WW: Antiarrhythmic therapy. In Tilley LP (ed): Essentials of Canine and Feline Electrocardiography. 3rd Ed. Lea & Febiger, Philadelphia, 1992

Chung EK: Principles of Cardiac Arrhythmias. 3rd Ed. Williams & Wilkins, Baltimore, 1983

Fenster PE: Use of antidysrhythmic drugs. p. 117. In Hurst JW (ed): Clinical Essays on the Heart. Vol. I. McGraw-Hill, New York, 1983

Jenkins WL, Clark DR: A review of drugs affecting the heart. J Am Vet Med Assoc 171(1): 85, 1977

Mandel WJ: Cardiac Arrhythmias. JB Lippincott, Philadelphia, 1980

Miller MS: Quicksands of Electrocardiography. p. 707. Ann Proc ACVIM, 1991

Miller MS: Electrocardiographic Waveform Patterns Associated with Heart Disease. p. 247. In August JR (ed): Consultations in Feline Internal Medicine. 2nd Ed. WB Saunders, Philadelphia, 1994

Miller MS, Calvert CA: Special tests to diagnose arrhythmias. p. 289. In Tilley LP (ed): Essentials of Canine and Feline Electrocardiography. 3rd Ed. Lea & Febiger, Philadelphia, 1992

Miller MS, Smith FWK, Tilley LP: Disorders of cardiac rhythm. p. 421. In Birchard SJ, Scherding RG (eds): Small Animal Practice. WB Saunders, Philadelphia, 1994

Miller MS, Tilley LP: Electrocardiography. p. 43. In Fox PR (ed): Canine and Feline Cardiology. Churchill Livingstone, New York, 1988

Miller MS, Tilley LP: Cardiac Electrophysiology. p. 105. In Swenson M, Reece W (eds): Dukes Physiology of Domestic Animals. 11th Ed. Cornell University Press, 1993

Opie LH (ed): Drugs for the Heart. American Edition. Grune & Stratton, Orlando, FL, 1984

Selzer A: Drug therapy. p. 117. Principles and Practice of Clinical Cardiology. 2nd Ed. WB Saunders, Philadelphia, 1983

Tilley LP: Essentials of Canine and Feline Electrocardiography, Interpretation and Treatment. 3rd Ed. Lea & Febiger, Philadelphia, 1992

Tilley LP, Miller MS: Treatment of Cardiac Arrhythmias and Conduction Disturbances. p. 346. In Kirk RW (ed): Current Veterinary Therapy IX. WB Saunders, Philadelphia, 1986

Tilley LP, Miller MS, Smith FWK: Canine and Feline Cardiac Arrhythmias. Lea & Febiger, Philadelphia, 1993

16

Key Treatment Principles for Cor Pulmonale

Philip A. Padrid

INTRODUCTION

Cor pulmonale refers to a change in the structure and/or function of the right ventricle that results from a change in the structure and/or function of the respiratory apparatus, including the airways, lung parenchyma, and lung vasculature. For purposes of this chapter, cor pulmonale is defined as "right-heart enlargement secondary to disease(s) of the respiratory apparatus." In the absence of right-heart failure, cor pulmonale might be considered a syndrome without clinical relevance. However, although frank heart failure in the setting of cor pulmonale is exceedingly uncommon in dogs and cats, structural changes in the right ventricle may be the first indication of the severity of underlying pulmonary disease. Thus, cor pulmonale can suggest to the veterinary practitioner the need to frequently evaluate the patient to detect progression of the respiratory disorder(s). Cor pulmonale as a result of heartworm infestation is discussed in Chapter 10 and will be mentioned here only briefly.

PATHOGENESIS

Central to the development of cor pulmonale is an elevated pulmonary artery pressure against which the right ventricle must empty. Pulmonary hypertension and right-heart failure due to, for example, mitral stenosis or congenital left-to-right shunt is not cor pulmonale. This distinction is important, because it places a primary focus of interest on the lung rather than the heart. Thus, consideration of therapeutic strategies to alleviate the signs and progression of cor pulmonale begins with a review of the factors that underlie its development.

ACUTE ONSET COR PULMONALE

I. Pulmonary Embolus
   A. Pulmonary embolus is an example of an acute disorder of the lung vasculature, in which a sudden rise in impedance to right ventricular outflow can lead to acute right ventricular failure (acute cor pulmonale).
   B. More common in veterinary patients is the presence of heartworm infesta-

tion, which causes pulmonary hypertension in about one-third of cases in which pressures are measured. This syndrome is characterized by a sudden increase in pulmonary artery pressure, which results from embolic "showers" induced by heartworm death. In severe cases, heart failure may result in death of the patient.

C. Somewhat less well-characterized pulmonary embolus can occur spontaneously, in the setting of hyperadrenocorticism, hypothyroidism, renal amyloidosis, glomerulonephritis, and postoperatively. As a direct result of vessel occlusion, or indirectly as a result of release of vasoactive mediators, total pulmonary resistance rises, leading to the development of pulmonary hypertension. Regardless of cause, the primary symptom of acute pulmonary embolus is dyspnea.

CHRONIC COR PULMONALE

I. Increased pulmonary artery pressure can develop as a result of three basic mechanisms.

A. Elevated left atrial pressure: By definition, cor pulmonale refers to right ventricular enlargement secondary to pulmonary disease; therefore, elevated left atrial pressure is not considered a cause of cor pulmonale.

B. Elevated pulmonary arterial blood flow: Elevated pulmonary arterial blood flow most commonly occurs in the presence of congenital heart defects with left-to-right shunt, such as patent ductus arteriosus.

C. Elevated pulmonary vascular resistance: Elevated pulmonary vascular resistance can occur as a result of three basic mechanisms.

1. Vasoconstriction of the pulmonary vascular bed

a) Vasoconstriction of the pulmonary vascular bed is generally a consequence of alveolar hypoxemia and/or secretion or release of vasoconstrictive mediators, such as leukotrienes, or serotonin (from platelets or mast cells).

b) Additionally, chronic hypoxemia may stimulate the secretion of a growth factor for connective tissue from pulmonary vascular smooth muscle. Thus, the small pulmonary arteries may be rendered less distensible.

c) The most common cause of chronic hypoxemia-induced cor pulmonale in humans is chronic bronchitis with or without emphysema.

d) Although chronic bronchitis is a well recognized syndrome in older dogs (and cats), there is reason to believe that chronic bronchitis in dogs does not routinely result in cor pulmonale and almost never progresses to right-heart failure.

(1) The canine pulmonary vasculature is particularly resistant to the effects of chronic hypoxemia relative to other species.

(2) Dogs with chronic bronchitis do not routinely develop severe hypoxemia (Pao_2 < 60 mmHg), and only rarely retain carbon dioxide.

(3) With the increased availability and use of color flow Doppler, pulmonary hypertension and tricuspid insufficiency are now

being recognized in dogs with chronic respiratory disease. Yet right ventricular failure remains a very uncommon finding in this setting.

(4) Therefore, even though the dog suffers naturally occurring bronchitis, the resulting derangements in gas exchange are relatively mild in many cases. The canine pulmonary vasculature seems to respond minimally to a chronic environment of low-oxygen tensions, and when pulmonary hypertension develops it rarely leads to frank right-heart failure.

e) The existence, development, and natural progression of hypoxemia in cats with bronchitis or severe chronic asthma is unknown.

(1) The primary mediator released from feline airway mast cells may be serotonin, and this mediator may cause smooth-muscle constriction and have profound effects on the feline pulmonary vasculature. Therefore, in chronic feline bronchitis or severe asthma, cor pulmonale could theoretically develop as a consequence of hypoxemia, and/or release of serotonin.

(2) Postmortem examination of the respiratory tract from affected cats may reveal medial hypertrophy of the small pulmonary arteries. In any other species this would be strong evidence for the existence of hypoxic vasoconstriction during life. However, medial hypertrophy of the pulmonary arterioles is a common finding in cats with no signs of heart or lung disease.

(3) It should be emphasized that the existence of pulmonary hypertension secondary to chronic feline lung disease has not been documented in clinical cases.

2. Obstruction of the pulmonary vascular bed

a) The most common cause of obstruction of the pulmonary vascular bed in veterinary medicine is probably heartworm disease.

(1) Lesions within the vascular wall, especially the smaller pulmonary arteries of the caudal lung lobes, result in blood flow obstruction.

(2) This may progress to total obstruction of blood flow in the caudal lobes, a condition that has been confirmed by arteriogram and lung scan.

(3) Vascular obstruction results in pulmonary hypertension and leads to right ventricular dilatation.

(4) This leads to increased stretch of the ventricular free wall and increased wall tension (Laplace law). This in turn leads to increase right ventricular output (Starling principle).

(5) In advanced cases, the ventricle dilates and ultimately fails, leading to signs of right-heart failure, including ascites, hydrothorax, and hydropericardium.

(6) Less commonly reported, pulmonary embolus can cause massive acute right-heart failure. This is discussed in the section on acute cor pulmonale.

3. Obliteration of the pulmonary vascular bed

a) Obliteration of the pulmonary vascular bed is a common finding in people with emphysema (most commonly due to chronic inhalation of cigarette smoke) or a congenital lack of enzyme alpha-1 antitrypsin.

b) Diffuse emphysema in dogs with or without chronic bronchitis is extremely uncommon. Although anecdotal evidence (hyperinflation on chest radiographs) and occasional case reports have supported the clinical impression of emphysema, the documented incidence of diffuse emphysematous change in feline lungs is very low.

c) Diffuse fibrosis of the interstitium of the lung may also lead to destruction of a significant portion of pulmonary vasculature.

    (1) Interstitial fibrosis is often suspected in dogs with or without coexisting bronchitis. Significant interstitial fibrosis has been documented in older dogs, and it is reasonable to conclude that the combination of hypoxemia due to ventilation/perfusion inequalities, and mechanical obstruction of small pulmonary arterioles from inflammation could result in pulmonary hypertension.

    (2) If should be noted, however, that a dilated or hypertrophied right heart in the presence of interstitial fibrosis has rarely been well documented in dogs or cats.

II. Primary pulmonary hypertension

This is a relative uncommon disorder recognized in humans. It is a diagnosis of exclusion, made when pulmonary hypertension is found in individuals free of other heart, lung, or circulatory ailments. The syndrome of primary pulmonary hypertension in dogs or cats is rarely suspected on clinical grounds and is very poorly documented.

TREATMENT

TREATMENT OF ACUTE COR PULMONALE

Acute right-heart failure secondary to primary respiratory disease is almost always the result of heartworm infestation. Therefore, treatment of acute cor pulmonale may be found in Chapter 10.

TREATMENT OF CHRONIC COR PULMONALE

I. Treatment of right-heart failure

Right-heart failure is exceedingly uncommon in dogs and cats with cor pulmonale. Treatment for right-heart failure should be based upon consultation with or direct supervision of a veterinary cardiologist. Listed below are general approaches only.

A. As has been reviewed, pulmonary arterial hypertension is not a disease, but rather the potential result of a number of different pathologic processes, including chronic bronchitis, chronic thromboembolism, and pulmonary fibrosis. Regardless of etiology, sustained increases in right ventricular afterload may theoretically progress to right ventricular failure.

B. In humans, prognosis of patients with cor pulmonale due to bronchitis, pulmonary fibrosis, etc., is linked causally with the ability of the right heart to sustain cardiac output. Therefore, rational therapeutic strategies should be designed in part to reduce right ventricular afterload and improve right ventricular function.

1. Cage rest

2. Low sodium diet

3. Diuretics

   a) Diuretic therapy is rational when there is a component of passive pulmonary hypertension. This has been documented in cor pulmonale in humans.

   b) In the setting of right-heart failure due to pulmonary disease, diuretic therapy will lower central volume and may lower cardiac output. In clinical veterinary practice, this does not seem to adversely affect the patient's clinical status unless the animal becomes clinically dehydrated.

   c) Diuretics should be used for patients with cor pulmonale in conjunction with serious attempts to improve underlying respiratory dysfunction, and only when peripheral edema or ascites is causing significant patient discomfort.

4. Digitalis

   a) The primary indication for digitalis in cor pulmonale is to control superventricular tachycardia when the increased heart rate is contributing to heart failure.

   b) New-onset superventricular tachycardia should alert the clinician to the possibility of worsening hypoxemia as a result of worsening of the underlying lung disease or worsening of the right-heart function.

   c) As a positive inotrope, digitalis increases cardiac output and lowers right ventricular diastolic pressure in some humans with cor pulmonale. However, this results in an increase in output to the restricted pulmonary vascular bed, and increases pulmonary artery pressure.

   d) Patients with chronic respiratory disease may be more susceptible to the toxic effects of digitalis, and may suffer an increased incidence of arrhythmias while taking digitalis.

   e) Digitalis is not recommended for the treatment of cor pulmonale unless superventricular tachyarrhythmias develop that compromise the animal's hemodynamic status.

5. Phlebotomy

   a) Chronic hypoxemia may theoretically lead to increased production of red blood cell mass, and polycythemia. Hematocrits of greater than 55 mmHg are associated with increased ventricular work in humans, and small, frequent phlebotomy to gradually reduce hematocrit to less than 50 mmHg have been advocated as a way to decrease pulmonary artery pressure in humans with cor pulmonale.

   b) Polycythemia due to chronic lung disease in dogs and cats is poorly described, and mild when documented. There is no information available on the need or appropriateness of phlebotomy in these cases.

6. Vasodilators
   a) The theoretic application of vasodilators in the treatment of cor pulmonale is based upon the premise that vasoconstriction plays a role in the genesis and sustenance of pulmonary hypertension.
      (1) Experiments in rats and dogs exposed to acute or chronic hypoxic ventilation and vasoconstricting drugs have shown that vasodilators have a beneficial effect of decreasing pulmonary pressure in these research settings.
      (2) Histologic study of pulmonary vasculature demonstrates medial hypertrophy of the pulmonary artery in dogs and especially in cats.
      (3) Humans with chronic obstructive lung disease have such changes seen postmortem, although the changes are mild. However, humans with chronic thrombotic disease and pulmonary fibrosis do not display changes suggestive of a chronic vasoconstrictive process.
   b) Anecdotal experience using vasodilators in humans with cor pulmonale is confusing about the benefits of vasodilators. Reports demonstrating that vasodilators reduce pulmonary artery pressures, increase cardiac output, and reduce clinical signs are tempered by other reports demonstrating no effect or serious adverse effects associated with vasodilator therapy.
   c) The efficacy of vasodilatory therapy for pulmonary hypertension is based almost exclusively on studies of patients with primary pulmonary hypertension, a syndrome which may or may not exist in veterinary medicine, and which may or may not respond to vasodilators in the same way as other causes of pulmonary hypertension.
   d) Increased ventricular output without decreased pulmonary arterial pressure, as occurs in humans with primary pulmonary hypertension on vasodilator therapy, has the theoretic problem of increasing flow without decreasing pressure, therefore increasing right ventricular work.
   e) There are no currently available vasodilators with selective actions on the pulmonary vascular bed. In humans, high-dose calcium channel blockers seem to be most beneficial in patients with primary pulmonary hypertension who demonstrate an initial beneficial response to acute administration of these drugs.
   f) An approach used in humans with cor pulmonale is to evaluate the hemodynamic response to acute administration of a potent and short-acting vasodilator. The drug of choice in this setting seems to be intravenous titratable prostacyclin. It appears that humans who respond favorably to acute administration of prostacyclin have the greatest chance of responding favorably to any other vasodilators in the long term.
   g) Pulmonary artery pressure of veterinary patients may be estimated using color flow Doppler. This information may be useful in estimat-

TABLE 16-1. RECOMMENDED DRUGS FOR TREATMENT OF CHRONIC
LOWER AIRWAY DISEASE

Feline Bronchial Disease
Acute drug therapy
   Bronchodilator
   1. Terbutaline 0.01 mg/kg IV, IM, SQ
   Anti-inflammatory
   1. Prednisone sodium succinate 5 mg/kg IV
   2. Dexamethasone 1 mg/kg IV, IM, SQ
Chronic drug therapy
   Bronchodilator
   1. Terbutaline 0.05–0.1mg/kg orally twice daily *as needed*
   Anti-inflammatory
   1. Prednisone 1 mg/kg orally twice daily for 5 days, then 0.5 mg/kg orally twice daily for 5
      days, then 0.25 mg/kg orally twice daily every other day (or lowest effective dose to control
      clinical signs)
   Antibiotic
   1. Amoxicillin 10 mg/kg orally 2–3 times daily for 7–10 days
   2. Oxytetracycline 10 mg/kg orally 3 times daily for 10–14 days (as tolerated)
   3. Chloramphenicol 25 mg/kg orally 3 times daily for 10–14 days (as tolerated)

Canine Bronchial Disease
Chronic drug therapy
   Bronchodilator
   1. Albuterol syrup 0.02–0.04 mg/kg orally 2–3 times daily *as needed*
   Anti-inflammatory
   1. Prednisone 1 mg/kg orally twice daily for 5 days, then 0.5 mg/kg orally twice daily for 5
      days, then 0.1–0.25 mg/kg orally twice every other day (or lowest effective dose to control
      coughing)
   Antibiotic
   1. Chloramphenicol 50 mg/kg orally 3 times daily for 7–10 days

---

ing acute changes associated with intravenous vasodilator therapy
in the setting of cor pulmonale with right-heart failure. If a beneficial
clinical response is noted, long-acting oral agents may be used on a
trial basis.

    h) Clinical evaluation of right-heart function should be followed closely
by individuals familiar with subtle changes in these signs and
findings.

II. Treatment of underlying respiratory disease (Table 16-1)
    A. Treatment of cor pulmonale directed toward the primary respiratory disor-
der(s) should result in improvement in airflow and alveolar ventilation.
    B. This approach results in clinical improvement in humans, even though
objective changes in hemodynamic parameters are minimal.
    C. The most common etiology of cor pulmonale in dogs and cats is probably
chronic bronchial disease (including asthma in cats).
    D. Although the etiology of chronic bronchitis and asthma is unknown, a
common feature of these obstructive airway diseases is inflammation of
airway mucosa and submucosa, with variable degrees of airway edema,
mucus hypersecretion, and bronchoconstriction.
    E. The degree of pulmonary hypertension that may develop as a result of
these syndromes is not known, but treatment of these disorders should
improve gas exchange. As a result, pulmonary hypertension that may develop in response to chronic hypoxemia might be ameliorated as well.

1. Oxygen therapy
    a) The only therapeutic intervention proven effective in cor pulmonale secondary to chronic bronchitis or emphysema in humans is oxygen therapy. Although oxygen is frequently prescribed for a wide variety of medical ailments, indiscriminate use of oxygen can result in great harm to the patient.
    b) Oxygen therapy is not meant to cure the underlying problem, but may have profound beneficial short-term effects until other therapies that address the underlying pathological process(es) causing the hypoxemia take effect.
    c) Humans with cor pulmonale often benefit from daily oxygen, usually given during most of their waking hours and during sleep. Unfortunately, this is not practical for the treatment of dogs and cats.
    d) Oxygen can be effectively delivered to dogs or cats by either mask or nasal cannula; 100 percent oxygen can be delivered through a mask, in which case approximately 60 to 80 percent FiO_2 is delivered to the patient. Oxygen can be delivered at a variable flow rate (0.5 to 4 L/min) through a nasal cannula to deliver 30 to 50 percent FiO_2 to the patient, depending upon patient size. The method of delivery should be empirically tested in each case, and the least stressful method should be used.
    e) Oxygen therapy for the veterinary patient with cor pulmonale is most likely to have a beneficial effect in the following circumstances.
        (1) Acute dyspnea from bronchoconstriction in feline chronic asthma
        (2) Acute dyspnea in canine and feline chronic bronchitis
        (3) Acute dyspnea during exacerbation of canine chronic tracheal collapse or chronic layngeal paralysis
        (4) Acute dyspnea from pneumothorax (oxygen reduces the amount of nitrogen in alveoli, driving gas out of tissue and blood, and allows more inspired oxygen into tissue and blood)
        (5) Acute dyspnea from aelurostrongylus infestation in cats
2. Bronchodilators
    a) Beta adrenoreceptor agonists such as terbutaline and albuterol are the bronchodilator drugs of choice in dogs and cats.
    b) A small but consistent number of dogs with chronic bronchitis that are exercise limited by their disease and/or have crackles and wheezes on chest auscultation may benefit from these drugs when given as needed.
    c) A significant number of cats with chronic bronchial disease have a reversible bronchoconstriction that will respond favorably to acute and long-term administration of these drugs.
3. Glucocorticoids
    a) Chronic bronchitis and asthma are chronic inflammatory diseases of the airways. Therapy for these diseases must address the underlying inflammatory changes in airway structure that lead to pathologic changes in gas exchange and airway function.
    b) Glucocorticoids have been shown both clinically and experimentally,

to be the single most effective class of drugs for the treatment of chronic bronchitis and asthma in humans.

c) They are the most effective drugs to minimize clinical signs of chronic bronchitis and asthma in dogs and cats.

d) Glucocorticoids are not indicated solely for the treatment of cor pulmonale. However, for dogs and cats with chronic moderate-to-severe bronchial disease, glucocorticoids should be considered the mainstay of therapy whether or not cor pulmonale is suspected.

4. Antibiotics

a) Aerobic bacteria may be recovered from both the healthy canine and feline lower airways.

b) Although exacerbations of chronic lung disease in humans are commonly due to bacterial infection, there is as yet no objective evidence that bacterial infections play an important role in the perturbation of canine or feline chronic airway or lung disease.

c) Antibiotics are specifically indicated for dogs or cats with cor pulmonale when there is evidence of genuine airway infection by bacteria. This can be reasonably assumed by growth of material taken from airway swabs or washings on a primary culture plate. Choice of antibiotics is then based on culture and sensitivity data.

d) Empiric use of antibiotics should be avoided. If antibiotics are given on this basis, the preferred drug for use in dogs is chloramphenicol, due to high bioavailability and absorption into bronchial tissue.

e) Mycoplasma is recovered from the lower airway of approximately 25 percent of cats with signs of lower airway disease. This organism can produce H_2O_2, and may cause damage to airway epithelium which can take months to heal.

f) Tetracycline may be given to cats with chronic symptoms of bronchial disease—even if culture results are unavailable or negative—due to the high potential number of false-negative mycoplasma culture results obtained in clinical and academic veterinary practice.

PROGNOSIS

I. The prognosis for dogs and cats with cor pulmonale is dependent upon
   A. the presence or absence of right ventricular failure
   B. the response to cardiovascular therapy
   C. the severity of the underlying respiratory disease
   D. the response to respiratory therapy

II. In general, right-heart enlargement secondary to chronic disease (without heartworm infection) probably occurs in less than 50 percent of cases, *documented* right-heart enlargement secondary to chronic lung disease probably occurs in less than 10 percent of cases, and right ventricular *failure* secondary to chronic lung disease probably occurs in less than 1 percent of cases. Therefore, while the development of right ventricular failure carries a poor prognosis, the great majority of heartworm-free dogs with cor pulmonale do not suffer cardiovascular compromise and are limited primarily by their underlying pulmonary disorder.

ACKNOWLEDGMENT

I thank Drs. Mark Kifflesen, Neil Harpster, Joel Edwards, Paul Pion, and Frank Smith for their clinical experience and contributions to key treatment principals for Cor Pulmonale.

SUGGESTED READINGS

Atkins CE: The role of noncardiac disease in the development and precipitation of heart failure. p. 1035. In: Hamlin RL (ed): Veterinary Clinics of North America, Small Animal Practice 21:5. WB Saunders, Philadelphia, 1991

Barer GR, Shaw PH: Stimulus-response curves for the pulmonary vascular bed to hypoxia and hypercapnia. J Physiol 211:139, 1970

Bishop MJ, Kennard S, Artman LD, Cheney FW: Hydralazine does not inhibit canine hypoxic pulmonary vasoconstriction. Am Rev Respir Dis 128:998, 1983

Brewster RD, Benjamin SA, Thomassen RW: Spontaneous cor pulmonale in laboratory beagles. Lab Animal Sci 33:299, 1983

Chapleau MW, Fish RE, Levitzky MG: Regional hypoxic pulmonary vasoconstriction in dogs with asymptomatic dirofilariasis. Am J Vet Res 46:1341, 1985

Daley WJ: Pathogenesis and treatment of cor pulmonale. p. 117. In: Brashear RE, Rhodes ML (eds): Chronic Obstructive Lung Disease, Clinical Treatment and Management. CV Mosby, St. Louis, 1978

Fishman AP: Pulmonary hypertension and cor pulmonale. p. 999. In: Fishman AP (ed): Pulmonary Diseases and Disorders. Vol. 2. McGraw-Hill, New York, 1988

Fishman AP: Pulmonary hypertension. p. 269. In: Wyngaarden JB, Smith LH, Jr, Bennett JC (eds): Textbook of Medicine. 19th Ed. WB Saunders, Philadelphia, 1992

Flenley DC, Picken J, Welchel L et al: Blood gas transfer after small airway obstruction in the dog and minipig. Respir Physiol 15:39, 1972

Hollinger MA: Inhalation therapy. p. 83. In: Tallarida RJ (ed): Respiratory Pharmacology and Toxicology. WB Saunders, Philadelphia, 1985

Kuriyama T, Wagner WW, Jr: Collateral ventilation may protect against high-altitude pulmonary hypertension. J Appl Physiol 51:1251, 1981

Leffler CW, Passmore JC: Contribution of prostaglandins to the regulation of pulmonary vascular resistance in adult cats and dogs. Prostaglandins and Medicine 3:343, 1979

Marshall BE, Marshall C, Benumof J et al: Hypoxic pulmonary vasoconstriction in dogs: Effects of lung segment size and oxygen tension. J Appl Physiol 51:1543, 1981

Marshall BE, Marshall C: Pulmonary hypertension. p. 1177. In: The Lung: Scientific Foundation. Vol. 1. Raven Press, New York, 1991

Mecham RP, Whitehouse LA, Wrenn DS, Parks WC et al. Smooth muscle mediates connective tissue reproduction in pulmonary hypertension. Science 237:423, 1987

Padrid P: Chronic lower airway disease in the dog and cat. p. 320. In: Spaulding GL (ed): Problems in Veterinary Medicine. Vol. 4, No. 2. JB Lippincott, Philadelphia, 1992

Padrid P, Ndukwu IM, Leff AR, Mitchell RW. Schultz-Dale contraction of airway smooth muscle from immune sensitized cats is attenuated by cyptroheptadine. J Vet Int Med 7: 120A, 1993

Paraskos JA: Pulmonary heart disease including pulmonary embolism. p. 1. In: Parmley WW, Chatterjee K: Cardiology. Vol. 2. JB Lippincott, Philadelphia, 1988

Peake MD, Harabin AL, Brennan NJ et al: Steady-state vascular responses to graded hypoxia in isolated lungs of five species. J Appl Physiol 51:1214, 1981

Rawlings CA: Heartworm Disease in Dogs and Cats. WB Saunders, Philadelphia, 1986

Reeves JT, Grover EB, Grover RF: Circulatory responses to high altitude in the cat and rabbit. J Appl Physiol 18:575, 1963

Tucker A, McMurtry IF, Reeves JT, et al: Lung vascular smooth muscle as a determinant of pulmonary hypertension at high altitude. Am J Physiol 228:762, 1975

Weir EK: Acute vasodilator testing and pharmacologic treatment of primary pulmonary hypertension. p. 485. In: Fishman AP (ed): The Pulmonary Circulation: Normal and Abnormal, Mechanisms, Management, and the National Registry. University of Pennsylvania Press, Philadelphia, 1990

17

Cardiopulmonary Arrest and Resuscitation

Andrew W. Beardow
Nishi Dhupa

INTRODUCTION

The goal of this chapter is to present the currently accepted techniques for cardiopulmonary resuscitation (CPR). Many of these techniques are undergoing constant revision as contradictory evidence often exists for the efficacy of a given intervention. The reader is directed to the suggested readings for detailed discussion.

DEFINITION OF CPR

CPR represents the attempt to restore normal respiratory and circulatory function with minimal damage to essential organs such as the lungs, heart, and brain. The recognition of the importance of "cerebral resuscitation" in order to preserve normal neurologic function after cardiopulmonary resuscitation has led to the development of modifications in the traditional CPR (now often termed cardiopulmonary cerebral resuscitation CPCR) protocol. CPR is initiated in any circumstance where ventilation becomes ineffective or ceases, and systemic perfusion or circulation fails, that is, in a situation of cardiopulmonary arrest (CPA). CPR provides artificial ventilation and circulation (basic life support) until therapeutic interventions directed at the underlying arrhythmias can be instituted (advanced cardiac life support) and spontaneous cardiopulmonary function restored.

RECOGNITION OF CARDIOPULMONARY ARREST

The diagnosis of CPA should be established before initiating CPR, as CPR is associated with complications including trauma to the heart and lungs.

  I. Absence of ventilation (apnea) is determined by
      A. Visual assessment of chest excursions
      B. Auscultation
      C. Feeling for the movement of air from the mouth or nostrils. Agonal gasping may occur and should not be confused with effective ventilation.
 II. Absence of a palpable femoral pulse or heart sounds on auscultation

425

III. Lack of response to sensory stimulation
IV. Dilation of the pupils
 V. Electrocardiographic (ECG) evidence of asystole or ventricular flutter/fibrillation

GOALS

 I. CPR is used to institute artificial cardiovascular and respiratory support
 II. To identify arrhythmias causing hemodynamic compromise, and institute immediate and appropriate therapy
III. To provide continuous support to stabilize cardiovascular function and to minimize damage to vital organs.

PRACTICAL ASPECTS

From a practical point of view, CPR should be considered in three phases.
 I. Anticipation
 II. Prevention
III. Organization

Anticipation

Most human and animal studies suggest that CPR will only be effective in a very small number of cases. The figure is higher for well patients and significantly lower for the severely ill patient with pre-existing multi-organ dysfunction. Resuscitation is only 100 percent effective when CPA is anticipated and prevented.

 I. CPA should be anticipated in the following clinical scenarios
   A. Primary cardiovascular disease states
   B. Respiratory pathology resulting in hypoxemia or hypercapnia
   C. Polysystemic trauma, particularly thoracic trauma or trauma associated with blood loss
   D. The use of anesthetic or antiarrhythmic drug therapy
   E. Severe acid-base disturbances
   F. Electrolyte abnormalities, particularly hyperkalemia and hypocalemia
   G. Overwhelming septicemia or endotoxemia
   H. Pre-existing cardiac arrhythmias: Certain arrhythmias are more likely to degenerate into ventricular fibrillation (VF).
      1. Ventricular tachycardia (exhibiting the R-on-T phenomenon) (Fig. 17-1).
      2. Ventricular flutter
      3. Frequent and multiform ventricular premature contractions (Fig. 17-2)
   I. Increases in parasympathetic tone related to vomiting, intratracheal intubation, and laryngeal, pharyngeal, ocular or abdominal surgery
   J. Prolonged seizures

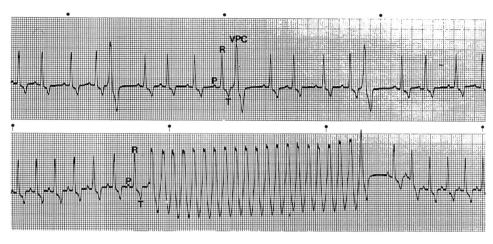

Fig. 17-1. Two separate strips 1 hour apart in a dog with episodes of fainting. A reveals VPCs that represent the R-on-T phenomenon. The R wave of the VPC is near the peak of the preceding T wave, the vulnerable period. The R-on-T phenomenon is not always a critical determinant of ventricular tachyarrhythmias, VPCs during the vulnerable period may result in ventricular tachycardia (as observed later on in strip B) or ventricular fibrillation, as well as in deteriorating hemodynamic status. Paper speed, 25 min/sec. (From Tilley LP: Essentials of Canine and Feline Electrocardiography. 3rd Ed. Lea & Febiger, Philadelphia, 1992, with permission.)

K. Electric shock

L. Cardiovascular surgery, angiocardiography, or pericardiocentesis:

In veterinary patients, hypoxemia and anesthesia represent the two greatest risk factors for CPA, with life-threatening arrhythmias occurring secondary to respiratory compromise or dysfunction. These arrhythmias include ventricular flutter or fibrillation, asystole, or electromechanical dissociation (EMD). Many patients become bradycardic before CPA ensues.

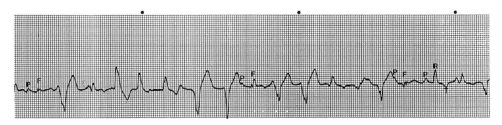

Fig. 17-2. Multiform ventricular tachycardia at an average rate of 220/min in a dog with severe digitalis toxicity. The rhythm is interrupted toward the end of the strip by a conducted sinus complex, which captures the ventricle. Numerous ventricular fusion complexes (F) also are present, a simultaneous activation of the ventricle. (From Tilley LP: Essentials of Canine and Feline Electrocardiography. 3rd Ed. Lea & Febiger, Philadelphia, 1992, with permission.)

II. Code Status

Current understanding and techniques allow resuscitative efforts to be instituted in all cases of CPA. When faced with this situation the clinician now has to decide not only how to resuscitate the patient but also whether to resuscitate the patient. Anticipation, therefore, not only demands recognition of patients at greatest risk for CPA, but also prior discussion with the owner to determine the extent of the resuscitative efforts (code status) to institute should CPA occur.

A. A *do not resuscitate* (DNR) request by the owner allows no interference once CPA ensues. In terminally ill cases, the owner should be encouraged to select this code status.

B. A *positive* code status requires the veterinarian to institute basic life support with artificial ventilation and manual external cardiac compression, and to support vital organ function.

C. A *full* code status allows the veterinarian to institute internal cardiac compression following an emergency thoracotomy, in addition to other basic life support measures.

Prevention

I. Hypoxemia

Hypoxemia is the commonest antecedent to CPA in the veterinary patient. Steps should therefore be taken to alleviate hypoxemia as soon as it is recognized.

A. Associated with hypoventilation during anesthesia
1. Switch off inhalant anesthetic gas
2. Ventilate patient with 100 percent oxygen (O_2)

B. Associated with pulmonary edema
1. Institute diuretic and vasodilator therapy.
2. Provide supplemental oxygen (100 percent O_2 initially) using intranasal delivery, O_2 mask or cage, and ventilatory support if necessary.

C. Associated with chronic respiratory disease
1. Provide supplemental O_2 and ventilatory support if necessary.
2. Treat the underlying disease process (e.g., with bronchodilators in the case of chronic obstructive bronchial disease; with steroids and bronchodilator in cases of allergic or asthmatic reactions).

D. Associated with thoracic effusions
1. Immediate thoracocentesis to alleviate respiratory compromise
2. Provide supplemental O_2 and ventilatory support if necessary.

E. Associated with thoracic trauma
1. Immediate thoracocentesis for pneumothorax or hemothorax
2. Provide supplemental O_2 and ventilatory support if necessary.

If these initial interventions fail to sustain adequate oxygenation and ventilation (defined as $Pao_2 > 60$; $Sao_2 > 85$, $Paco_2 < 40$; recognized clinically by sustained cyanosis and dyspnea), intratracheal intubation and mechanical ventilation (with sedation if needed) may be required to prevent CPA.

II. Bradycardia

Bradycardia frequently precedes CPA in debilitated or critically ill patients. If recognized

  A. Ensure adequate oxygenation by providing supplemental O_2 if necessary.
  B. Correct intravascular volume deficits, acid-base disturbances, and electrolyte abnormalities.
  C. Use atropine (0.02 mg/kg IM or IV) or glycopyrrolate (0.01 mg/kg) to increase heart rate.
  D. If atropine is ineffective, positive chronotropic agents such as dobutamine (5 to 15 μg/kg/min), dopamine (5 to 10 μg/kg/min) or epinephrine (0.045 to 0.2 mg/kg bolus or 0.1 to 1.5 μg/kg/min continuous rate infusion) may be required.

III. Ventricular arrhythmias

Ventricular tachycardia—particularly if it is multiform, exhibits the R-on-T phenomenon, or renders the patient hemodynamically unstable—may progress to a pulseless ventricular arrhythmia (pulseless ventricular tachycardia, ventricular flutter, ventricular fibrillation)

  A. Use lidocaine at 2 mg/kg slow intravenous bolus. Dose may be repeated three times, up to a total of 8 mg/kg. Conversion to a stable rhythm may be followed by institution of a continuous rate infusion (CRI) of lidocaine at 50 μg/kg/min. As lidocaine has a very short half-life (2 minutes), there should be minimal delay between administering the bolus and starting the infusion.
  B. Alternatively, procainamide can be used. The dose is 6 to 8 mg/kg IV over 5 minutes, followed by a CRI of 25 to 40 μg/kg/min. If given intramuscularly instead, the dose is 6 to 20 mg/kg q 4–6 h. If given orally, the dose is 6 to 20 mg/kg q 6–8 h.

Organization

Organization is the key to effective CPR following documented CPA. Training of all personnel should include

  I. The ability to recognize signs of impending CPA, and to initiate appropriate preventative or therapeutic measures
 II. The ability to implement mouth-to-nose resuscitation, the use of a face mask, intratracheal intubation, and basic CPR
III. If resuscitative efforts in the practice involve several people, they should be organized into a team with a team leader. This team follows a previously approved and practical set of guidelines for CPR. The team leader (a veterinarian) directs the effort and keeps a chronologic record of events during the resuscitative effort. Other personnel perform the basic CPR skills of ventilation and closed-chest compressions, the attachment of the ECG oscilloscope, the establishment of intravenous access, the drawing up of drugs, and their administration when ordered by the veterinarian.
IV. The designation of an area within the clinic for CPR: Facilities should include O_2 supplementation, good lighting, access to a surgical set, laryngoscope and

endotracheal tubes, ability to provide suction, an ECG monitor, an anesthetic machine or ventilator, an emergency drug-dosage charge, intravenous fluids and administration equipment, and an electrical defibrillator. This area should be checked and stocked regularly.

V. A *crash kit* should be readily available and should contain the following drugs: epinephrine, atropine, sulphate, lidocaine hydrochloride, dexamethasone, sodium bicarbonate, calcium gluconate and procainamide.

VI. A *defibrillator* should be available as defibrillation results in the most consistent success in resuscitation. A defibrillator may occasionally be purchased from a local hospital, and should provide direct current countershock.

CARDIAC LIFE SUPPORT

CPR has traditionally been organized into basic cardiac life support (BCLS) and advanced cardiac life support (ACLS). BCLS is the provision of traditional CPR, involving mouth-to-mouth or mouth-to-nose breathing, or intubation and artificial ventilation (via self-inflating resuscitation [Ambu] bag or mechanical ventilator) and manual chest compressions (The ABC of CPR). ACLS includes the identification and rectification of life-threatening arrhythmias, such as ventricular fibrillation, pulseless ventricular tachycardia, or EMD. The most recent CPR guidelines in human medicine have moved defibrillation to the initial phases of CPR. Hence, arrhythmia recognition and management has been used during the earliest stages of CPR, and the traditional division between BCLS and ACLS no longer exists. ACLS has now been expanded to include multi-organ support, and in particular directed toward cerebral resuscitation. Traditional cardiac compression techniques have also been modified to maximize cerebral and coronary blood flow.

The ABCDs of CPR

A. Airway management
B. Breathing/ventilatory management
C. Circulation
D. Drugs/defibrillation

These are the vital components of any CPR protocol or algorithm.

I. A: Airway management
The airway can be visualized by extending the patient's head and neck and pulling the tongue forward. The airway should be cleared of any secretions, vomit, or foreign material, and a patent airway secured by orotracheal intubation. If a complete obstruction exists, an alternative airway can be created with an emergency tracheostomy.

II. B: Breathing/ventilatory management
If spontaneous breathing movements are not seen once the patency of the airway is ensured, artificial ventilation should be initiated.
A. Techniques for artificial ventilation
1. Mouth-to-mouth or mouth-to-nose ventilation uses exhaled air to provide 16 percent O_2. If mouth-to-nose resuscitation is attempted, the

patient's mouth should be held closed and the resuscitator's mouth placed over both nostrils to form an air-tight seal with the lips.

2. A face mask, with ventilation provided by an Ambu bag
3. The preferred technique is endotracheal intubation and ventilation with an Ambu bag, the reservoir bag on an anesthesia machine, or a mechanical ventilator. The use of 100 percent O_2 delivered at a flow rate of 150 ml/kg/min is recommended at this stage.

B. As hypoxemia precipitates many CPA events, adequate ventilation and oxygenation may be the only intervention necessary to restore cardiovascular and respiratory function. Following the administration of a few breaths, the patient should be carefully assessed for the return of effective circulation (increase in heart rate, palpable pulse, improvement in mucous membrane color and perfusion). If spontaneous improvement does not occur, the CPR protocol is continued.

III. C: Circulation

A. Manual compression of the chest has been shown to provide, at best, only 30 percent of normal cardiac output. Open-chest CPR is consistently two to three times more effective in generating cerebral blood flow. The primary goal of cardiac compression is to maintain basal perfusion of the heart and brain. Perfusion of the coronary arteries occurs predominantly during diastole and is determined by the difference between aortic and right atrial pressures. Perfusion of the brain occurs during systole and is determined by the difference in systolic carotid pressure and cerebral venous or intracranial pressure. The aim of cardiac compression is therefore;

1. To maximize peak systolic arterial pressures
2. To increase diastolic aortic pressures
3. To decrease diastolic right atrial pressures (The administration of large volumes of shock intravenous fluids and the use of shock trousers may be contraindicated in previously normovolemic patients, as these techniques will result in an increase in right atrial pressure.)

B. Hemodynamic studies in animal models have provided evidence to suggest that several different mechanisms exist for the generation of blood flow (artificial systole) during chest compression. The creation of artificial systole is now known to result from the combination of direct compression of the ventricles (cardiac pump) and indirect fluctuations in thoracic intravascular pressures as a result of the phasic fluctuations in intrathoracic pressure (thoracic pump) generated during manual chest compression.

1. Cardiac pump mechanism
Compression of the chest wall during closed-chest CPR causes indirect compression of the cardiac chambers and generates artificial systole. However, in animals larger than 15 kg, this mechanism is thought to play only a minor role in the forward flow of blood.

2. Thoracic pump mechanism
External chest compression is thought to augment circulation in large part due to the creation of significant cyclic changes in intrathoracic pressure. Sudden forcible compression of the chest wall generates a positive intrathoracic pressure, generating a significant forward blood flow in the major arteries. Retrograde flow in the veins is prevented

by intraluminal one-way valves. In animals greater than 15 kg, this mechanism is thought to play the major role in effective CPR.
C. Compression techniques
   1. Chest compressions should be rapid in order to increase and decrease intrathoracic pressure rapidly. The chest wall should be displaced approximately 30 percent.
   2. In patients weighing 5 to 15 kg, the cardiac pump effect can be maximized by placing the patient in left lateral recumbency and using the heel of the palm on the lower one-third of the chest at the level of the fifth intercostal space. If this proves ineffective, the heel should be moved to the mid-third of the chest in order to maximize the thoracic pump effect.
   3. In large patients (> 15 kg), the thoracic pump is maximized when the patient is placed in dorsal recumbency and the heel of the hand is placed over the caudal one-third of the sternum. This position requires stabilization of the patient with a V-shaped trough made of wood or plastic. Lateral recumbency can also be used, and may be easier in large, narrow-chested dogs.
   4. The chest should be compressed at least *60 to 80* times per minute, with total release between compressions to maximize the diastolic component of the resuscitation cycle. The systolic compressions should take up 40 percent of the cycle time.
D. Compression and ventilation techniques
   Changes in intrathoracic pressure form the basis of the thoracic pump, and it has been suggested that synchronizing chest compression with manual ventilation may potentiate this mechanism. Simultaneous ventilation compression (SCV) is only possible if the patient is intubated. The recommendations for the coordination of compression with ventilation therefore vary depending on the resuscitative methods used.
   1. If mouth-to-mouth or mouth-to-nose ventilation or a face mask are used, ventilation should be interposed with compressions (one ventilation for every five compressions) in order to maximize the efficacy of both.
   2. For intubated patients
      a) Ventilate without compression twice, in order to ensure lung expansion and to assess the need for cardiac compression.
      b) Ventilate *simultaneously* with every second or third compression, in order to augment the thoracic pump mechanism.
      c) Do not maintain residual positive pressure in the airways between ventilations, as this may impair venous return and therefore cardiac output.
      d) Interpose abdominal compression between chest compressions. This has been shown to increase cerebral and coronary blood flow (by increasing aortic diastolic pressure) in dogs.
E. Open-Chest CPR
   Direct cardiac massage requires opening the thorax and pericardium. It is indicated if external chest compressions are ineffective in producing a palpable femoral pulse. This failure may result from an inability to gener-

ate high intrathoracic pressures or low systemic arterial and venous pressures. A decision to open the chest should not be delayed more than 2 minutes after the onset of CPA. Cerebral perfusion and the chances of neurologic recovery are optimized by direct cardiac massage.

1. Indications
   a) Dogs larger than 20 to 30 kg
   b) Flail chest
   c) Severe obesity
   d) Pleural space disease: pneumothorax, hemothorax, diaphragmatic hernia
   e) Pericardial effusion
   f) Severe hypovolemia: shock, hemorrhage, gastric dilatation, and volvulus
2. Technique
   This requires an emergency left-sided thoracotomy, together with a pericardiotomy.
   a) Use clippers in heavily coated long-haired dogs in order to facilitate incision of the skin.
   b) Use a scalpel blade to incise the skin on the left lateral chest wall, just behind the elbow (½-inch caudal for every 5 kg of body weight), and extending dorsally from the origin of the ribs down to near the sternum.
   c) Push the tips of curved Mayo scissors into the fifth or sixth intercostal space near the costochondral junction, and use them to penetrate the pleural space. Spread the tips to enlarge the opening, and then use them to extend the incision both dorsally and ventrally along the cranial edge of the caudal rib.
   d) Use a Balfour abdominal retractor or Finochietto rib spreader to provide good exposure and visualization of the heart and pericardium.
   e) Open the pericardium near its apex, using the index finger to hook the pericardial-diaphragmatic ligament, elevate it toward the thoracic opening, and cut through it using the Mayo scissors. Enlarge the cut with scissors and spread it open further with fingers. Lift the heart out of the pericardial sac prior to initiating cardiac massage.
   f) Following successful return of spontaneous cardiac systole, irrigation of the thoracic cavity is followed by aseptic closure of the chest wall.
3. Direct cardiac massage
   a) Use the palmar surfaces of the fingers and thumb to compress the right and left ventricles. Initiate compressions at the apex and extend to the base in order to empty the ventricles. The rate (60 to 100 compressions/minute) is dictated by the rate of ventricular filling. Care should be taken not to tip the apex upward (laterally) as this kinks the base of the heart. Avoid rotation and digital pressure at the heart base.
   b) If ventricular filling is impaired, the massage rate should be lowered while venous return is improved by the use of intravenous fluids, epinephrine, or interposed abdominal compressions.

    c) Cranial perfusion can be maximized by temporarily occluding the descending aorta with a finger.

IV. D: Drugs/Defibrillation

An ECG monitor should be attached to the animal as soon as possible. Water-based ECG coupling cream should be used. Alcohol-based and ultrasound coupling gel should *NOT* be used, as alcohol will ignite during defibrillation.

A. Arrhythmia recognition
1. Asystole
   a) This is defined as the absence of electrocardiographic activity.
   b) Ventricular fibrillation can masquerade as asystole if the fibrillatory waves are perpendicular to the ECG lead. Therefore, a diagnosis of asystole should always be confirmed by checking the perpendicular lead.
   c) When present, asystole implies significant myocardial ischemia.
   d) Treatment involves the initiation of BCLS CPR, followed by administration of either epinephrine, atropine, or sodium bicarbonate, as indicated.
   e) A precordial thump may also be useful (see next section).
   f) Transvenous or transvenous pacing has also been described (see Suggested Readings).
   g) Reversible abnormalities, such as severe acidosis, electrolyte imbalances (particularly hyperkalemia), or high vagal tone, should be addressed immediately.
2. Electromechanical dissociation
   a) In electromechanical dissociation (EMD), the ECG trace may be fairly normal, but there is ineffective circulation due to the presence of severe inotropic depression of the myocardium.
   b) Electrical activity is uncoupled from contraction.
   c) Pulseless idioventricular rhythms are examples of EMD.
   d) Hypovolemia, tension pneumothorax, and pericardial tamponade may cause "apparent" EMD. These situations should be corrected once identified.
   e) Treatment guidelines advise the use of basic CPR and high-dose epinephrine. Methoxamine (an alpha adrenergic agonist) has also been used.
   f) Calcium administration is recommended only in cases of wide QRS complex arrhythmias.
   g) Sodium bicarbonate and high-dose corticosteroids are not currently recommended.
3. Ventricular fibrillation (Fig. 17-3)
   a) This is defined as chaotic depolarization of the ventricular myocardium.
   b) Ventricular fibrillation is described as either coarse or fine. Fine fibrillation carries the poorer prognosis.
   c) If DC defibrillation is available, it should be carried out as soon as the arrhythmia is recognized (see section on defibrillation).
   d) Epinephrine can be used in an attempt to coarsen the fibrillation, both before electrical defibrillation or if a defibrillator is not available. This is not always successful.

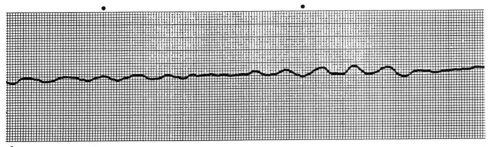

A

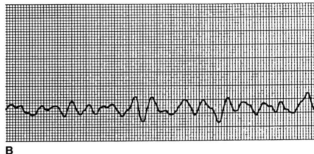

Fig. 17-3. (A) Fine ventricular fibrillation. **(B)** Coarse ventricular fibrillation. (From Tilley LP: Essentials of Canine and Feline Electrocardiography. 3rd Ed. Lea & Febiger, Philadelphia, 1992, with permission.)

B

e) The use of a precordial thump has also been advocated. This is performed by using the heel of the palm to deliver a thump to the chest wall. The transfer of energy to the heart may convert ventricular fibrillation into a sinus rhythm, although in practice this is rarely successful.

f) Nonlethal arrhythmias may degenerate into ventricular fibrillaion following a precordial thump, and therefore the procedure should be considered only when there is ECG confirmation of ventricular fibrillation.

B. Arrhythmia management

1. Defibrillation

Studies in human medicine have shown that defibrillation is the best method of managing ventricular fibrillation and that it is most effective if administered in the first few minutes of CPR. Ventricular fibrillation is recognized in approximately 40 percent of veterinary cardiac arrests. In general, the success of the defibrillation is inversely proportional to the duration of fibrillation as well as the health, perfusion, and viability of the myocardium. Defibrillation can be achieved chemically or electrically. The former is rarely effective, and therefore direct current (DC) defibrillation should be carried out as soon as ventricular fibrillation is recognized.

2. DC defibrillation

a) Defibrillators are dangerous in unskilled hands.

b) Only direct current (DC) defibrillators should be used. Older model alternating current (AC)–based defibrillators should not be used.

c) To maximize the efficacy of defibrillation, the paddles should be

positioned to ensure a maximum amount of electrical energy
through the myocardium.

   d) If the animal is in dorsal recumbency, the paddles are placed on
either side of the chest in the precordial region.

   e) If in lateral recumbency, a flat electrode can be substituted for the
conventional paddle to allow maximum patient stability.

   f) A water-based coupling solution should be used. *Alcohol will ignite.* The paddles should be completely covered with the coupling
gel and enough pressure applied to maximize skin contact. Poor
contact will result in arcing and burns.

   g) "Clear": It is the responsibility of the team leader or person controlling the electrical discharge (usually the person holding the paddles) to ensure that no personnel are in contact with the patient,
table, or any equipment attached to the patient. If the ECG device
being used in not protected from defibrillation, it should be discon-
nected temporarily (disconnect the cable instead of unclipping the
patient). If the defibrillator requires activation from the main unit
rather than the paddles, the operator should not initiate a discharge
until all personnel are clear.

   h) The energy of the discharge is dependent on the animal's weight.

   i) For external defibrillation, the initial setting should be

      (1) 2 J/kg (animals under 7 kg body weight)

      (2) 5 J/kg (8 to 40 kg body weight)

      (3) 5 to 10 J/kg (over 40 kg body weight)

        Note: If the internal paddles are applied directly to the heart
during open-chest CPR, energy settings should start at 0.2 J/
kg. Do not exceed 50 J with internal defibrillation.

   j) If the first discharge is ineffective, a second should be given immediately, using the same amount of energy. Conductivity will *increase* with successive discharges, resulting in a greater current
with successive shocks.

   k) If the second discharge is ineffective, repeat a third time at one
and a half times the preceding energy.

   l) After each discharge

      (1) Check the ECG monitor

      (2) Check for a pulse

      (3) If a flat line is seen on the ECG monitor, select another lead
(lead AVF in lead II was previously used)

      (4) Check patient position and restabilize if necessary

  m) If three discharges are ineffective, resume CPR, and administer
epinephrine.

3. Chemical defibrillation

   a) Can be tried if DC cardioversion is unavailable

   b) Success rates are very low. This should be considered a technique
of last resort.

   c) Technique for chemical defibrillation

      (1) Conversion of ventricular fibrillation to asystole

        This is achieved by raising intracellular potassium concentrations, which halts fibrillation in the myofibrils. Use a combination of potassium chloride (1.0 mEq/kg) and acetylcholine chloride (6.0 mg/kg). Acetylcholine is believed to increase potassium flux across the cell membrane. Prior administration of atropine may negate this effect, rendering the technique ineffective. Acetylcholine is expensive and has a short shelf life.

(2) Conversion of asystole to sinus rhythm
This is achieved using a combination of calcium gluconate and epinephrine.

(3) Bretyllium tosylate has also been used alone for chemical defibrillation, although results have been inconsistent in clinical practice.

C. Chemical adjuncts to CPR (Table 17-1)
1. Epinephrine
a) The cornerstone of ACLS
b) Epinephrine's major beneficial effects during CPR are related to its alpha adrenergic receptor–stimulating properties, which cause peripheral vasoconstriction and therefore maintain arterial pressure.
c) The alpha adrenergic effects also increase myocardial blood flow (by increasing aortic diastolic pressure) and cerebral blood flow during CPR.
d) The beta adrenergic effects may increase myocardial oxygen demand and cause an increased incidence of arrhythmias after return

TABLE 17-1. CPR DRUG AND DEFIBRILLATION DOSAGES

Drug	Dose	Dose (ml)								
		2 kg	5 kg	10 kg	15 kg	20 kg	25 kg	30 kg	40 kg	50 kg
Epinephrine (1:1000)	0.2 mg/kg (high)	0.5	1.0	2.0	3.0	4.0	5.0	6.0	8.0	10.0
	0.05 mg/kg (low)	0.125	0.25	0.5	0.75	1.0	1.25	1.5	2.0	2.5
Atropine (0.5 mg/ml)	0.05 mg/kg	0.25	0.5	1.0	1.5	2.0	2.5	3.0	4.0	5.0
Lidocaine (2%—20 mg/ml)	2.0 mg/kg	0.25	0.5	1.0	1.5	2.0	2.5	3.0	4.0	5.0
Dexamethasone SP (4 mg/mL)	4.0 mg/kg	2.5	5.0	10.0	15.0	20.0	25.0	30.0	40.0	50.0
Sodium Bicarbonate (1 mEq/ml)	1.0 mEq/kg	2.5	5.0	10.0	15.0	20.0	25.0	30.0	40.0	50.0
Calcium Gluconate (100 mg/ml)	10 mg/kg	0.25	0.5	1.0	1.5	2.0	2.5	3.0	4.0	5.0

DC Countershock		Energy in watt seconds								
External	0.5–5 ws/kg	25	50	100	150	200	250	300	400	500
Internal	0.05–0.5 ws/kg	2.5	5.0	10.0	15.0	20.0	25.0	30.0	40.0	50.0

of spontaneous circulation. However, positive effects include cerebral microvascular dilation.

e) The success of resuscitation in canine models correlates with epinephrine administration and alpha adrenergic stimulation.

f) The effects may be antagonized by acidosis.

g) The dose-response curve suggests that epinephrine produces its response in the range 0.045 to 0.2 mg/kg. High-dose epinephrine (0.2 mg/kg) has recently been advocated, although its use in all CPR attempts remains controversial. High-dose epinephrine may be particularly useful in clinical cases refractory to standard doses.

h) If the ventricles have been fibrillating for more than four minutes, administration of epinephrine is recommended prior to electrical defibrillation.

i) Epinephrine may be of value in treating asystole via activation of pacemaker β_1-adrenergic receptors, thereby increasing cardiac automaticity.

2. Lidocaine

a) This is a class 1B, membrane-stabilizing antiarrhythmic drug. It acts by blocking the movement of sodium into myocardial cells.

b) Lidocaine may have a role after CPR in the management of recurrent malignant arrhythmias.

c) Several studies have indicated that prior administration of lidocaine increased the electrical energy required for defibrillation; therefore, it is better avoided in early CPR.

3. Bretylium tosylate

a) This is a class 3 antiarrhythmic drug.

b) Its actions are inconsistent, but it may be useful for treatment of refractory ventricular fibrillation.

c) Unlike lidocaine, bretyllium does not appear to increase the defibrillation threshold.

d) The recommended dose is 25 to 50 mg/kg IV.

4. Atropine

a) Used for the treatment of bradycardia

b) Counters excessive parasympathetic neural tone that may contribute to suppression of sinoatrial automaticity

5. Sodium bicarbonate

a) Its use is indicated in animals with metabolic acidosis prior to cardiac arrest.

b) In animals with normal acid-base status before CPA, acidosis may be controlled with adequate ventilation and cardiac compression.

c) Adverse effects of bicarbonate administration include hypernatremia, hyperosmolality, paradoxical CNS acidosis, decreased plasma concentration of ionized calcium and a shift in the oxyhemoglobin dissociation curve (with decreased oxygen delivery to tissues).

d) Paradoxical CNS acidosis may be a result of the dissociation of carbonic acid (H_2CO_3) formed by the bicarbonate into highly diffusible H^+, which freely crosses the blood-brain barrier.

    e) Administration of bicarbonate should be guided by measurement of blood pH.

    f) Bicarbonate administration may be indicated if CPR efforts are continuing beyond 15 to 20 minutes without the return of spontaneous cardiac function.

    g) Bicarbonate administration may also be indicated if the patient appears to be refractory to the administration of epinephrine.

6. Calcium

    a) The routine use of calcium during CPR protocols is now considered to be contraindicated except in special circumstances.

    b) Calcium entry into cells has been implicated in re-oxygenation-reperfusion injury after resuscitation, particularly in the myocardium and the brain.

    c) The use of calcium during CPR is recommended only in known cases of hypocalcemia, hyperkalemia, or hypermagnesemia.

7. Fluid therapy

    a) This should be guided by the patients status before CPA.

    b) Volume loading during CPR causes increases in both right atrial and intracranial pressures and subsequent decreases in coronary and cerebral blood flows.

    c) Hypovolemic patients need to receive crystalloid or colloid solutions (or, if indicated, blood transfusions) rapidly.

    d) Avoid glucose-containing fluids, as glucose has been associated with progressive neuronal injury, possibly due to the provision of a substrate for production of neuronal lactic acid.

D. Routes of drug administration

1. Endotracheal

    a) If an endotracheal tube is in place before an indwelling intravenous line is established, epinephrine should be administered into the patients tracheobronchial tree.

    b) Endotracheal delivery of the drug can be improved by doubling the dose, dilution with saline (1:10), using a long catheter to deposit the drug below the endotracheal tube, and by forceful ventilation following administration in order to help dispersion.

    c) Epinephrine, atropine, calcium, and lidocaine can be administered intratracheally.

    d) Sodium bicarbonate should not be administered intratracheally, as it inactivates surfactant.

2. Intravenous

    a) Intravenous administration is the preferred route.

    b) With intravenous administration of drugs during CPR, central vein injections are preferred over peripheral vein injections.

3. Intraosseous

    a) This involves intramedullary administration into the humerus, femur, or tibia, via an intramedullary cannula.

    b) Rapid delivery of drugs to the central circulation is accomplished via the abundant endosteal medullary blood supply.

4. Intralingual
   a) Small volumes of drugs (1 to 15 ml) are injected into the abundant submucosal vessels just under the dorsal mucosal surface of the tongue. These vessels remain patent and functioning during CPR.
   b) This route provides rapid uptake into the central circulation.
5. Intracardiac
   a) This route should be used only if other sites are unavailable, unless the chest is open.
   b) Risks associated with this method of injection include hemorrhage, coronary artery laceration, cardiac tamponade, and pneumothorax.

POSTRESUSCITATIVE CARE

Animal studies have demonstrated that specific steps taken early in the postresuscitation phase can influence outcome. Postresuscitation life-support protocols to preserve cerebral integrity have been established in humans.

Processes known to exacerbate neuronal dysfunction after successful CPR include central nervous system edema, hypercapnia (due to hypoventilation), hypocapnia (hyperventilation), hypoperfusion, and intracellular dysfunction and cell membrane instability related to re-oxygenation-reperfusion. Cardiac, pulmonary, and renal function must also be supported. Complications of CPR, including fractured ribs or sternebrae, pneumothorax, pulmonary contusions, and pulmonary edema, should be addressed.

I. Postresuscitative treatment
   A. Ventilatory support, if necessary, to ensure a Pa_{CO_2} level of 25 to 35 mmHg. Hypercapnia induces vasodilation and may exacerbate cerebral edema.
   B. Blood pressure support using inotropic agents or vasopressors such as dobutamine (5 to 15 μg/kg/min) and dopamine (5 to 10 μg/kg/min). The aim is to maintain diastolic blood pressure above 60 mmHg. These agents will also provide chronotropic support. Atropine can be used, if necessary, for severe bradycardias. It should not be assumed that atropine will invariably control bradyarrhythmias in the periresuscitative period. If atropine proves ineffective, the drugs listed above or epinephrine should be used.
   C. Supplemental oxygen, if the patient is ventilating adequately, can be administered by nasal catheter supplying 40 percent oxygen.
   D. Neuroprotective and anti-edema therapeutic interventions include the use of corticosteroids (rapid-acting dexamethasone sodium phosphate at 0.5 mg/kg IV), mannitol (1 to 2 g/kg IV) and furosemide (1 to 2 mg/kg IV). The use of agents such as dimethylsulfoxide, desferoxamine, and lidoflazine for their free-radical scavenging, iron-chelating, and calcium channel blocking effects, respectively, is still controversial. The reader is referred to the Suggested Readings.
   E. Metabolic support involving the supply of fluids, electrolytes, and nutrition
   F. Antiarrhythmic management with lidocaine at a continual rate infusion (50 μg/kg/min), particularly if the arrest rhythm was ventricular fibrillation
   G. Diuretics and morphine may be indicated in the presence of pulmonary edema. Central venous pressure monitoring may be useful.

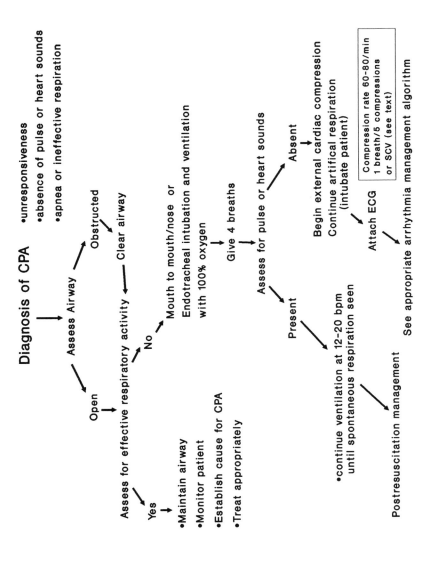

Fig. 17-4. Diagnosis of CPA. This general algorithm should be followed in all cases of CPA. These principles should be adhered to throughout the resuscitation attempt, including during interventions for arrhythmia management. Please refer to the relevant section of the text for a more detailed discussion.

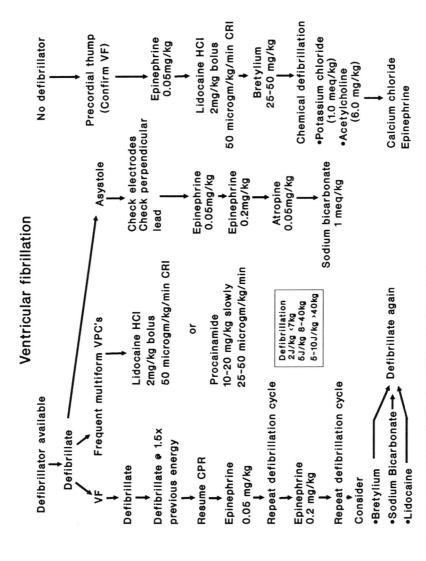

Ventricular fibrillation

No defibrillator → Precordial thump (Confirm VF) → Epinephrine 0.05mg/kg → Lidocaine HCl 2mg/kg bolus 50 microgm/kg/min CRI → Bretylium 25–50 mg/kg → Chemical defibrillation
•Potassium chloride (1.0 meq/kg)
•Acetylcholine (6.0 mg/kg) → Calcium chloride Epinephrine

Asystole → Check electrodes Check perpendicular lead → Epinephrine 0.05mg/kg
Epinephrine 0.2mg/kg → Atropine 0.05mg/kg → Sodium bicarbonate 1 meq/kg

Defibrillator available

Defibrillate → Frequent multiform VPC's → Lidocaine HCl 2mg/kg bolus 50 microgm/kg/min CRI
or
Procainamide 10–20 mg/kg slowly 25–50 microgm/kg/min

VF → Defibrillate → Defibrillate @ 1.5x previous energy → Resume CPR → Epinephrine 0.05 mg/kg → Repeat defibrillation cycle → Epinephrine 0.2 mg/kg → Repeat defibrillation cycle → Consider
•Bretylium
•Sodium Bicarbonate → Defibrillate again
•Lidocaine

Defibrillation
2 J/kg <7kg
5 J/kg 8–40kg
5–10 J/kg >40kg

Fig. 17-5. Ventricular fibrillation. This algorithm for the management of ventricular fibrillation is divided according to the availability of a defibrillator. After each intervention the ECG should be re-evaluated and the next step initiated if VF is still seen. If a new arrhythmia develops the appropriate algorithm should be selected. If sinus rhythm is seen postresuscitation management should be instituted (see text). Please note the increasing dose for epinephrine as we progress through the algorithm.

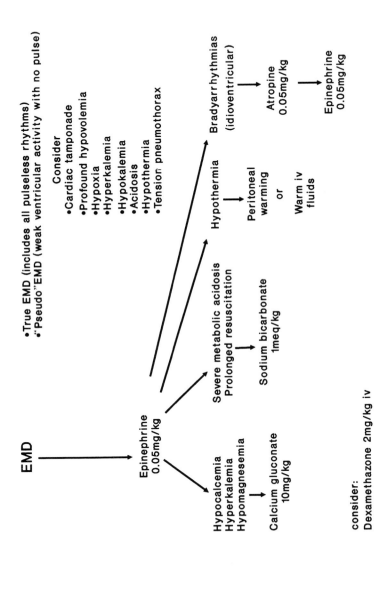

Fig. 17-6. Electromechanical Dissociation (EMD). The EMD algorithm covers all rhythms where the ECG shows organized complexes but no clinically appreciable circulation is present. EMD is divided into "true" EMD, where no mechanical ventricular activity is seen, or "pseudo" EMD, where weak mechanical ventricular activity is seen. Each of the many different factors that contribute to the development of EMD should be considered and managed (if recognized) when EMD is diagnosed.

443

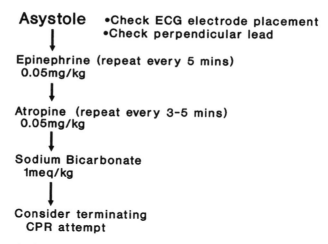

Fig. 17-7. Asystole. No electrical or mechanical activity is seen during asystole. Electrode placement should always be checked if no electrical activity is recorded. A perpendicular lead should be checked (Lead aVL for lead II) to ensure isoelectric ventricular fibrillation is absent.

    H. Renal function and urine output should be monitored (preferably by catheterization). If urine production is inadequate, intravenous fluids, and furosemide, mannitol, and dopamine (1 to 2 μg/kg/min) should be used.

  II. Prediction of outcome

After cardiac arrest, the rapid recovery of upper airway and ocular reflexes is a good prognostic sign. If the absence of oculocephalic (doll's eye) or oculo-vestibules (caloric) reflexes, the nonreactivity of the pupils, and continuing unconsciousness persist 6 to 12 hours after arrest, the prognosis is poor. Progressive deterioration of reflexes after initial recovery may indicate progressive cerebral insult due to the damaging effects of ischemic anoxia on the brain.

CPR ALGORITHMS

These algorithms (Figs. 17-4 to 17-7) are designed to help in the decision making process during a resuscitation attempt. The general algorithm applies in all cases and the arrhythmia-specific algorithms are used once that rhythm is recognized. As the rhythm changes, switch to the appropriate algorithm.

SUGGESTED READINGS

American Heart Association: Guidelines for cardiopulmonary resuscitation and emergency cardiac care. JAMA 268:16, 1992

Haskins SC: Internal cardiac compression. J Am Vet Med Assoc 200:1945, 1992

Henik RA: Basic life support and external cardiac compression in dogs and cats. J Am Vet Med Assoc 200:1925, 1992

Kass PH, Haskins SC: Survival following cardiopulmonary resuscitation in dogs and cats. Vet Emer Crit Care 2:57, 1992

Moses BL: Cardiopulmonary resuscitation. p. 508. In: Murtaugh RJ, Kaplan PM (eds): Veterinary Emergency and Critical Care Medicine. CV Mosby, St. Louis, 1992

Robello CD, Crowe DT: Cardio-pulmonary resuscitation: Current recommendation. Vet Clin N Amer Critical Care 19:1127, 1989

Van Pelt DR, Wingfield WE: Controversial issues in drug treatment during cardiopulmonary resuscitation. J Am Vet Med Assoc 200:1938, 1992

Van Pelt DR, Wingfield WE: Neurologic management following cardiac arrest and resuscitation. p. 112. In: Kirk RW, Bonagura JD (eds): Current Veterinary Therapy XI. WB Saunders, Philadelphia, 1992.

18

Emergency Management and Critical Care

Andrew W. Beardow

INTRODUCTION

On presentation, an animal in severe congestive or low-output heart failure is often hemodynamically unstable, rendering even the simplest of diagnostic tests potentially fatal. The patient must therefore be managed symptomatically to allow stabilization before proceeding with tests such as radiographs, echocardiography, and so on.

Heart failure is associated with a number of syndromes, depending on the side of the heart primarily affected and the nature of the precipitating heart disease. These syndromes represent the final common pathway in the pathogenesis of heart failure associated with most cardiac diseases. Therefore, the first section will briefly describe the etiopathogenesis and management of these syndromes, and then a review of the heart diseases associated with them will be presented.

Although each of the syndromes will be described separately, it is clear that neither ventricle operates in isolation; consequently, these syndromes will often occur concurrently.

SYNDROMES ASSOCIATED WITH CARDIAC FAILURE

   I. Left-sided congestive (or backward) heart failure
  II. Right-sided congestive heart failure
 III. Biventricular failure
 IV. Low-output or "forward" failure

LEFT-SIDED CONGESTIVE HEART FAILURE

   I. Cardinal sign
     A. Pulmonary edema
  II. Pathophysiology
     Left-sided cardiac pathology and the activation of the body's compensatory mechanisms (sympathetic nervous system, renin-angiotensin-aldosterone

447

system, atrial naturetic peptide) result in the following physiologic responses.

   A. Tachycardia, increased sodium and water retention, and peripheral vasoconstriction (venous vasoconstriction increases preload, and arterial vasoconstriction increases afterload)

   B. An increase in left atrial or left ventricular filling pressure

   C. An increase in pulmonary venous pressure, which leads to a greater tendency for extravasation of fluid into the lung parenchyma

   D. Accumulation of this fluid in the interstitium and alveoli as pulmonary edema, leading to compromised respiratory gaseous diffusion, a reduction in the surface area of tissue available for gaseous exchange, narrowed airways, and decreased lung compliance. Hypoxia, tachypnea, and—when the animal becomes distressed—dyspnea develop as a result. Fluid accumulation within the airways causes coughing, which may become productive. If so, the animal coughs up frothy serosanguinous fluid.

  III. Clinical signs

   A. Tachypnea and dyspnea

     1. May be occur suddenly (especially in cats) or have developed over a period of time

     2. If severe, the animal will adopt a classic "air-hungry" stance, with its neck extended and forelimbs abducted

     3. Patients are often unable to lie down, as this may hamper the effort to breathe or increase venous return. Many patients sleep for protracted periods once the pulmonary edema is controlled.

   B. Coughing

    Usually a cough softer than the harsh, honking cough seen with tracheobronchial disease occurs. However, left atrial enlargement may compress the left mainstem bronchus, leading to tracheobronchial irritation and a honking cough.

   C. Tachycardia

    Usually accompanied by a loss of sinus arrhythmia. When atrial and ventricular myocardial disease occur in an environment of tissue hypoxia and increased sympathetic tone, atrial and ventricular tachyarrhythmias may develop.

  IV. Therapeutic goals in the management of left-heart failure

   A. Decrease left atrial and pulmonary venous pressures, hence decreasing pulmonary edema

   B. Provide respiratory support until pulmonary edema is under control

   C. Facilitate the clearance of pulmonary edema through systemic volume contraction

  V. Methods

   A. Decreased preload to minimize left ventricular and left atrial filling pressures.

     1. Diuretics (e.g., furosemide, bumetanide)

     2. Venodilators (e.g., nitroglycerin; IV furosemide has been shown to induce vasodilation and this effect may precede the diuretic effect)

     3. An animal in congestive heart failure may require elevated left atrial

pressures to maintain left ventricular filling and left ventricular end-diastolic volume, thus maximizing the benefits from the Frank-Starling relationship. An excessive fall in left atrial filling pressure may therefore lead to a decrease in stroke volume and, as a result, cardiac output. Thus, when venodilators or high doses of diuretics are used, monitor the patient for signs of compromised cardiac output including
   a) Cooling of the periphery
   b) Prolongation of the capillary refill time
   c) Increase in weakness or dyspnea
   d) Decreasing urine output
   e) Progressive tachycardia
   4. These changes are most noticeable in patients with
      a) Primary myocardial failure (i.e., dilated cardiomyopathy)
      b) Diastolic dysfunction (i.e., hypertrophic cardiomyopathy)
B. Decrease afterload
   1. Decreasing afterload (i.e., the force against which the heart has to pump) increases stroke volume and cardiac output. This tends to decrease left atrial pressure, especially in cases of mitral regurgitation (MR).
   Arterial dilators (e.g., hydralazine)
   2. Excessive afterload reduction can lead to hypotension and tachycardia. Hydralazine, in particular, has been associated with these changes. Where cardiac output is compromised, this can lead to
      a) Increased myocardial oxygen demand and consequent myocardial damage
      b) Weakness
      c) Collapse
C. Decrease both preload and afterload with balanced vasodilators
   1. Angiotensin converting enzyme (ACE) inhibitors (enalapril, captopril, lisinopril)
   2. Sodium nitroprusside
D. Oxygen for respiratory support
   1. Oxygen cage: normally using a 40 percent concentration (FIO_2), but increasing up to 100 percent for short periods (up to 18 to 24 hours) if necessary. Prolonged exposure to 100 percent oxygen can lead to lung damage, which compromises gaseous diffusion and oxygenation.
   2. A closely fitted face mask if the animal will tolerate it without struggling.
   3. Intranasal catheter
      a) An excellent technique for delivering oxygen in mid-sized to larger dogs
      b) Technique for intranasal oxygen delivery
         (1) Use a red rubber Tomcat catheter
         (2) From the tip of the catheter, measure a length equivalent to the distance from the tip of the dog's nose to the medial canthus of the eye.
         (3) Form a butterfly attachment at that point with zinc oxide tape.
         (4) Instill 2 to 3 drops of 2 percent lidocaine into the nostril to be intubated, or apply lidocaine gel to the catheter tip.

       (5) Advance the catheter into the nostril, directing it ventrally and caudally to the level of the tape butterfly.

       (6) Secure the butterfly to the skin of the lateral portion of the nose caudal to the nostril. A second butterfly can be used to secure the distal end of the catheter to the patient's forehead.

       (7) Use an appropriately sized anesthetic machine adaptor or a 3-cc syringe with the plunger removed to allow connection to an oxygen supply.

       (8) Deliver humidified oxygen at 50 to 100 ml/kg/min. The oxygen supply can be humidified by passage through a water bubbler (Bubble Humidifier, Becton and Dickinson, Lincoln Park, NJ).

VI. Therapeutic approach
   A. Recognition of left-heart failure
      1. Signalment
         a) Age
         b) Breed
         c) Sex
      2. History
         a) Previous history of heart disease
         b) Familial history of heart disease
         c) History of major clinical signs associated with heart disease or heart failure
            (1) Cough
            (2) Weakness
            (3) Syncope
            (4) Hyperpnea/dyspnea, tachypnea
      3. Physical examination
         a) Auscultation
         b) Presence of moist rales
         c) Presence of a murmur
         d) Presence of gallop rhythms
            (1) S_3 or protodiastolic gallops are usually associated with myocardial failure seen with dilated cardiomyopathy in the dog and cat.
            (2) S_4 gallops are associated with hypertrophic cardiomyopathy or diastolic dysfunction in cats.
         e) Presence of an arrhythmia
      4. Body temperature
      Body temperature is often normal to subnormal, but low-grade fevers have been associated with peripheral vasoconstriction and loss of thermal regulation in humans. In dogs, where thermal regulation is mainly through the respiratory tract, this may not be appreciated.
      5. Pulses
         a) Weak or snapping (short duration) pulses
         b) Pulse deficits

TABLE 18-1. A GUIDE TO THE THERAPEUTIC MANAGEMENT OF DOGS IN
CONGESTIVE HEART FAILURE

| Severity Grade | Initial Management | | Intensive Care |
| | Extensive Care | | |
	Outpatient	Inpatient	
I	*Diuretic*—Lasix: 1–2 mg/kg PO B–TID *Balanced vasodilator:* *Enacard:* 0.25–0.5 mg/kg S–BID *Capoten:* 0.5–2.0 mg/kg B–TID Digoxin if SVT, AFib		As for extensive
II	As above	*Lasix:* 1–2 mg/kg PO; IM: IV *Nitroglycerin:* up to 1″ q 6hr for 48hrs[a] *ACE inhibitor:* (as grade I)[b] *Digoxin:* if SVT Afib	As extensive inpatient
III	*Lasix:* 2–4 mg/kg PO initially *Nitroglycerin:* up to 1″ 16h for 48hr[a] *ACE inhibitor:* (as grade I) *Digoxin:* BID <15 kg 0.005 mg/kg, >15 kg 0.22 mg/m^2, for SVT, AFib, cardiomegaly, or LOCHF	*Lasix:* IV, IM *Nitroglycerin:* up to 1″ q6h for 48hr[a] *Oxygen* cage: intranasal tube 40% *Digoxin:* BID as outpatient *ACE inhibitor:* (as grade I)[b]	*Lasix:* 2–4 mg/kg IV or IM *Dobutamine:* 1–10 g/kg/min for low-output failure *Dopamine:* 1–5 (10) g/kg/min if no arrhythmia, but oliguria *Nitroprusside:* 1–10 g/kg/min *Oxygen:* may need 100% initially *Morphine:* 0.1 mg/kg IM, IV
IV	Should be hospitalized	As Class III consider rapid digitalization	As Class III may require mechanical ventilation

LOCHF, Low-output congestive heart failure
[a] Nitroglycerin dose range .125–1″ depending on body size
[b] Hydralazine may be substituted for ACE inhibitors in CHF secondary to chronic valve disease

   6. Mucous membranes
       a) Prolonged capillary refill time (CRT), pale/cyanotic
       b) Peripheral vasoconstriction causes blanching of the mucous membranes.
       c) In cyanotic patients, the membranes appear to be gray rather than white.
   B. Emergency management
       Decisions regarding therapeutic management are made according to the clinical signs, physical findings, and results of a minimum cardiac database according to the principles previously discussed (Table 18-1).
       1. Minimize stress to the patient; avoid interventions or procedures that cause the patient to struggle or result in an increase in heart or respiratory rates.
       2. Assess the severity. Severity may be graded to allow appropriate, but not excessive, interventions.

3. Institute appropriate therapeutic interventions.
   a) Severity grade I
      (1) Comfortable in room air, able to move about without inducing respiratory distress or cyanosis
      (2) Auscultable crackles, but localized
      (3) Tachycardia, but with pink mucous membranes and a Capillary Refill Time less than 2 seconds
      (4) Normal body temperature
   b) Severity grade II
      (1) Comfortable at rest in room air but distressed and/or cyanotic with effort
      (2) Auscultation reveals crackles in all fields
      (3) Pale mucous membranes (exacerbated with effort) with normal or prolonged CRT
   c) Severity grade III
      (1) Distressed when breathing room air
      (2) Auscultation reveals crackles in all fields; may be coughing up serosanguinous fluid; weak or snapping pulses
      (3) Pale or gray mucous membranes with slow capillary refill time
      (4) Low normal to hypothermic body temperature
   d) Severity grade IV
      (1) Collapsed, severely dyspneic
      (2) Crackles and bubbling in all fields, and coughing up serosanguinous fluids, which may flow from the nose and mouth with little effort
      (3) Pale or gray mucous membranes, with very slow capillary refill times
      (4) Weak to almost imperceptible pulses with a very short duration
      (5) Hypothermia, cold periphery

Class I and class II

These patients may be able to undergo further diagnostics to complete a cardiac database without further interventions. A minimum cardiac database in these patients should include a physical examination, chest radiographs, and an ECG.

Throughout each procedure, the patient must be carefully monitored and the procedure aborted at the first signs of respiratory or cardiovascular compromise. Should these occur, the patient should be rested and managed therapeutically as discussed in the following section, and the planned techniques should be reviewed before proceeding.

Class III and IV

These patients may be placed at increased risk by radiology or electrocardiography. Symptomatic therapy is initiated to stabilize the patient. All aspects of the signalment, history, and physical examination should be reviewed to ensure that left-heart failure is the most likely diagnosis. Diuretics and venodilators may compromise respiratory and hemodynamic function in patients with diseases that mimic congestive heart failure.

The therapeutic approach will depend on the facilities and personnel available at the hospital. For the purposes of this chapter, emergency management has been divided into *extensive* or *intensive* care, depending on the personnel and facilities available. Extensive care is provided by the equipment and facilities commonly available to the general practitioner. The availability of specialized equipment, including infusion pumps, blood pressure monitoring devices, and the facility to provide continuous 24-hour monitoring, allows a more intensive approach to be adopted.

C. Extensive care

In both dogs and cats these initial measures are used until the patient is stable enough for further diagnostics and formulation of a long-term management plan.

1. Dogs
    a) Furosemide: 1 to 4 mg/kg every 4 to 8 hours
        (1) Some breeds, for example, Doberman pinchers, require lower doses.
        (2) Dobermans are dosed at 50 to 75 percent of the conventional dose.
    b) Vasodilators
        (1) Nitroglycerin
            i) Used percutaneously as paste, patch, or spray. Sublingual spray gives rapid onset within minutes. Paste and patches may take one to several hours for maximal effect, depending on the surface area covered (venodilator).
            ii) Dose
                (A) 2 percent paste (1 inch = 14 mg): 3.125 mg to 15 mg (0.25 to 1 inch), depending on size
                (B) 2.5 mg patch: Apply 0.25 to 1 patch for 24 hours. The paste should be rubbed into the hairless area in the axilla or groin, and its location noted to prevent accidental exposure by anyone handling the animal. Nitrate tolerance (see later notes) develops with prolonged exposure.
        (2) Balanced vasodilators
            i) Enalapril (Enacard): 0.5 mg/kg SID to BID
            ii) Captopril (Capoten): 0.5 to 2.0 mg/kg BID to TID
        (3) Arterial vasodilators
            i) Hydralazine (Apresoline): 0.5 mg/kg BID, titrating up to 2 mg/kg if necessary
            ii) Some authors prefer these agents in patients with left-heart failure secondary to mitral valve disease, because the onset of action occurs more rapidly than that of ACE inhibitors. Once the patient stabilizes, it is switched to an ACE inhibitor.
    c) Oxygen
        (1) 40 percent (cage, intranasal)
        (2) 100 percent for short periods (requires an oxygen cage)

      d) Digoxin
        (1) Indicated in dogs with supraventricular tachyarrhythmias (paroxysmal atrial tachycardia, atrial fibrillation) and myocardial failure (dilated cardiomyopathy, end-stage valvular disease). Myocardial failure is often difficult to define superficially. In general, it exists in patients with primary dilative myocardial disease and those in the later stages of chronic valvular and congenital disease where significant cardiomegaly is seen. Even when echocardiographic data is available, the point at which the heart muscle starts to fail (i.e., shows a decrease in contractility) cannot be defined definitively. This has lead to controversy among authorities about the appropriate time to introduce digoxin. If digoxin administration is required and the oral route is not available, IV administration can be used.
        (2) Technique for IV digitalization
          i) The dose is calculated at 0.01 to 0.02 mg/kg.
          ii) The calculated dose is divided into 4 aliquots to be administered at *hourly* intervals by slow (over 10 to 15 minutes) IV injection.
          iii) The patient is monitored for either the desired effect or the onset of signs associated with toxicosis; when either is seen the injections are terminated.
             Note: IV digitalization may cause gastrointestinal signs, vomiting, and arrhythmias, which may further complicate the congestive failure. Rapid IV injection has been associated with vasoconstriction (increased afterload).
      e) Cage rest
      f) Morphine
        (1) Can be used in patients that are distressed.
        (2) May cause peripheral vasodilation, shunting blood away from the pulmonary circulation, and thus enhancing the management of the pulmonary edema.
        (3) Dose: 0.1 mg/kg IM, IV (up to 0.5 mg/kg IM)
  2. Cats
    a) Lasix
      (1) Cats require lower Lasix doses. Cats with hypertrophic cardiomyopathy have poor ventricular compliance and require higher than normal ventricular filling pressures. Therefore, when Lasix is used, watch for signs of worsening cardiac output.
      (2) Dose: 1.0 to 2.0 mg/kg SID or BID
    b) Nitroglycerin: 0.125 inch to 0.25 inch TID or QID
    c) ACE inhibitors: Enalapril (Enacard) 0.25 mg/kg daily
    d) Digoxin
      (1) Indicated in cats with DCM. Has a variable half life and its pharmacokinetics are affected by concurrent drug administrations. Cats therefore must be carefully monitored for signs of toxicity.

        (2) Dose: 0.007 mg/kg q 24 to 48 hours

    e) Diltiazam

        (1) Indicated for cats with diastolic dysfunction (e.g., hypertrophic cardiomyopathy) and supraventricular tachyarrthymias

        (2) Dose: 7.5 mg TID

    f) Beta blocker

        (1) Indications as for diltiazem.

        (2) Dose

           i) Inderal: 2.5 to 5.0 mg TID

           ii) Atenolol: 6.25 to 12.5 mg SID

D. Intensive care

In the intensive care setting, continuously administered intravenous agents can be used. In some patients in late severity grade III and class IV, especially dogs with severe myocardial failure (e.g., Dobermans with dilated cardiomyopathy), the previously discussed protocol may not be effective. In that case, acute intravenous inotropic and vasodilator support become necessary.

1. Positive inotropes

    a) Dobutamine (Dobutrex)

        (1) A synthetic β_1-adrenergic agonist. It has more potent inotropic effects than chronotropic effects. It causes modest peripheral vasodilation (probably by indirect effects on sympathetic tone as the patient stabilizes). Administration may lead to tachycardia, increasing ventricular arrhythmias (although this effect is more often seen with dopamine), or increased ventricular response rate in patients with atrial fibrillation. Therefore, patients in atrial fibrillation should be digitalized, intravenously if necessary.

        (2) Dose

           i) Dogs: 1 to 10 µg/kg/min. Start at 1 µg/kg/min and increase in 1 µg/kg/min increments every half hour to effect

           ii) Cats: 1 to 5 µg/kg/min. It is important to start at the lower dose and titrate carefully. May induce arrhythmias, seizures (focal fascial, petit or grand mal), and has been reported to be associated with sudden death. If seizures are seen, discontinue the infusion. If necessary, reintroduce at half the infusion rate.

    b) Dopamine

        (1) A norepinephrine precursor that acts to release norepinephrine from neural stores. It is more arrhythmogenic than dobutamine. It acts peripherally at presynaptic dopamine receptors to induce vasodilation. At low doses (<5 µg/kg/min) it induces increased blood flow in the renal, coronary, cerebral, and mesenteric vascular beds. At higher doses, it causes alpha stimulation and potentially detrimental peripheral vasoconstriction (5 to 10 µg/kg/min).

        (2) Dose: 1 to 10 µg/kg/min. As for dobutamine but monitor carefully for arrhythmias.

2. Vasodilators
   a) Sodium nitroprusside (Nipride)
      (1) A potent, balanced vasodilator, useful in the acute management of severe cardiogenic pulmonary edema. Sodium nitroprusside may induce severe hypotension. The hypotensive effects are balanced by improved cardiac output principally due to the drug's effects on afterload. Hemodynamic response shows rapid onset and offset.
      (2) Sodium nitroprusside is metabolized to cyanmethemoglobin and free cyanide in red blood cells. The cyanide is then converted to thiocyanate in the liver and undergoes renal excretion.
      (3) The use of nitroprusside requires constant monitoring of blood pressure due to its potent hypotensive effects.
      (4) Requires fresh preparation and protection from light during an infusion.
      (5) May induce lactic acidosis due to cyanide accumulation, and excess thiocyanate may induce toxicity characterized by depression and nausea. Rapid infusion and overdosage may induce cyanide intoxication.
      (6) Dose: 1 to 10 μg/kg/min (most patients require 5 to 7 μg/kg/min)
   b) Nitroglycerin
      (1) Mainly a preload reducer
      (2) Available for percutaneous or intravenous use by constant rate infusion.
      (3) Dose: 1 to 5 μg/kg/min. Start at the low end and titrate up by 1 μg/kg/min every 30 minutes.
      (4) Nitrate tolerance
          Nitrates induce vasodilation by providing an exogenous source for endogenous nitric oxide (NO) production. NO has been shown to be a potent endogenous vasodilator working at the muscular level. For activity, nitrates require free sulphydryl groups to be present. Chronic exposure to nitrates leads to oxidation of these groups and loss of their potency—that is, tolerance develops. Therefore, after 24 to 48 hours of exposure of nitrates, a nitrate-free interval of 12 hours must be incorporated. This applies to all nitrates, whether cutaneously, intravenously, or orally (isosorbide dinitrate) administered.
3. Agents with both inotropic and vasodilating properties
   a) Milrinone (Primacor)
      (1) A positive inotrope and a balanced vasodilator
      (2) May induce ventricular arrhythmias
   b) Amrinone (Inocor)
      A positive inotrope and vasodilator
   c) Both amrinone and milrinone are available for intravenous short-term support, but are not available for long-term oral use.

       (1) Amrinone dose: 1 to 3 mg/kg IV bolus (slow), followed by constant rate infusion of 10 to 100 µg/kg/min

       (2) Milrinone dose: 1 to 10 µg/kg/min

  4. Intravenous fluid administration

Diuretic use, increased insensible fluid losses due to increased respiratory efforts and adipsia may all contribute to excessive volume depletion, which may prove detrimental to maintaining effective cardiac output and renal function. A patient's fluid status must be carefully monitored and, if necessary, supplemented with judicious intravenous fluids. Half-strength saline or D5W are appropriate fluids, and are normally administered at 0.5 to 0.75 of the calculated maintenance fluid rate. It may appear paradoxical to have a patient on both parenteral fluids and diuretics, but a balance of fluid into and out of the patient is essential. One could look upon it as replacing the sodium-rich urine with sodium-depleted fluid, thus decreasing total body sodium. Indeed hyponatremia may result. It is impossible to overemphasize the need for continual monitoring of a patient in heart failure during the administration of parenteral fluids. If possible, urine production should be measured and central venous pressure assessed to prevent fluid overload. The lungs should be frequently ausculated, the patient's respiratory efforts monitored, and the patient's girth measured if ascites is present.

VII. Patient monitoring

During the critical phases of the management of congestive heart failure, monitoring the patient and its response to therapy is essential. As the therapy becomes more aggressive, the need for greater and ever more sensitive monitoring increases. Two broad groups of monitoring exist, noninvasive and invasive.

  A. Noninvasive monitoring techniques

    1. Physical examination

      a) Mucous membranes

        (1) Color: pale? cyanotic?

        (2) Moist or dry?

      b) Capillary refill time: prolonged?

      c) Pulse rate

        (1) Should fall with effective treatment

        (2) Increases with hypotension, tachyarrhythmias, stress

        (3) Quality of pulses should increase in strength and duration

        (4) Duration should increase

        (5) Regularity: dropped beats?

      d) Auscultation

        (1) Gallops may resolve as the patient improves

        (2) Resolution of crackles

        (3) Heart rate and rhythm: intensity of sound should increase if pleural effusion is resolving

      e) Palpation: Apex beat should strengthen (except in cats with HC)

      f) Percussion: To assess pleural effusion

      g) Temperature: should normalize

      h) Body weight: should decrease as volume contraction occurs.

2. Assessment of blood pressure

Many patients will sustain systolic blood pressure within the normal range until the terminal stages of heart failure. Despite this, monitoring arterial blood pressure is still useful in the critical patient for a number of reasons.

a) Assessing the response to vasodilators e.g., nitroglycerin

b) Assessing the response in hypotensive patients given positive inotropes (dobutamine, dopamine, milrinone, amrinone).

c) Noninvasive techniques

Several techniques are described for noninvasive assessment of blood pressure. They are broadly divided into two main groups: oscillometric (e.g., Dinamap) and Doppler. Both techniques use an air-filled cuff to occlude arterial blood flow. The pressures are determined by deflating the cuff and measuring the changes in blood flow in the artery distal to the cuff. It is the method used to detect this flow that distinguishes these two techniques.

Both techniques may be unreliable if cardiac output is low or if arrhythmias are present (especially the oscillometric). Both tend to give reasonably accurate assessment of systolic blood pressure, provided careful attention is paid to technique. They are particularly useful in assessing trends. Doppler techniques may be more accurate in smaller animals with an irregular heart rate.

3. Serial thoracic radiography

Serial thoracic radiographs help assess resolution of pulmonary edema, pleural effusion, and are often necessary if effusions obscure the cardiac silhouette. In that situation, tracheal position relative to the vertebrae and sternum give an indication of cardiomegaly.

4. Electrocardiography

A continuous ECG should be recorded if possible. Alternatively, intermittent ECG can be recorded, but in this circumstance, frequent auscultation is recommended and an ECG should be run if changes in the heart rate or rhythm are heard. Bradycardia may indicate impending problems, and is often seen as a prelude to cardiopulmonary arrest. Arrhythmias may be present or develop during the course of management of CHF, especially with agents such as dopamine or dobutamine.

5. Pulse oximetry

Pulse oximetry is used to assess the saturation of hemoglobin in peripheral blood. It can be used to assess trends in oxygen saturation, which should increase as the patient improves.

B. Invasive monitoring techniques

1. Biochemistry screen

a) BUN and creatinine

Elevations may suggest poor renal perfusion (especially if urine specific gravity is elevated).

b) Sodium and potassium levels

(1) Hypokalemia will complicate the management of congestive heart failure, predispose to arrhythmias, and predispose to

digoxin intoxication. It is common in debilitated patients in congestive failure, particularly cats. Appropriate potassium supplementation should be used.

    (2) Profound hyponatremia can lead to weakness and collapse. Dilutional hyponatremia occurs in patients with congestive heart failure, due to the failure of free water excretion associated with increased vasopressin and antidiuretic hormone levels. The use of furosemide, ACE inhibitors and sodium-depleted diets (or sodium-depleted fluids) can exacerbate hyponatremia.

2. Arterial or venous blood gases

An arterial partial pressure of oxygen (Pao_2) less than 65 mmHg is an indication for oxygen supplementation. If the Pao_2 decrease is sustained, or $Paco_2$ climbs to greater than 50 mmHg, this is an indication for mechanical ventilation. In venous blood, the Pvo_2 is used as an index of peripheral perfusion. As peripheral perfusion decreases, the tissues extract more oxygen, and therefore Pvo_2 decreases. However, a higher than normal Pvo_2 may be seen, suggesting shunting of blood away from tissues or lack of peripheral perfusion.

3. Central venous pressure

    a) A measurement used as an indicator of right atrial pressure, and hence peripheral venous congestion.

    b) Prone to errors due to technique, positioning, and maintenance of catheter patency.

    c) Useful for assessing *trends* in right atrial filling pressures

        (1) Upwards: Can be used to monitor excessive increases (usually greater than 5 cm of water above baseline) in central venous pressure due to fluid therapy.

        (2) Downwards: May indicate excessive volume reduction and potential compromise of cardiac output, or the need for judicious IV fluid supplementation (as a guide, optimal preload is usually obtained with a CVP of 10 cm H_2O)

    d) The measurement of CVP may therefore be useful in patients where concurrent diseases warrant a careful balance of volume expansion and depletion (e.g., concurrent renal and cardiac disease.

    e) Technique

        (1) Aseptic technique should be used.

        (2) Clip and scrub the skin over the right jugular vein.

        (3) Use a "through the needle" catheter of appropriate length (when placed, the tip of the catheter should lie in the cranial vena cava and not the right atria, where there is potential for rupture, occlusion, or arrhythmogenesis).

        (4) The fluid-filled catheter should be attached by fluid-filled, non-distensible tubing to a water-filled manometer (available in disposable form).

        (5) The manometer is held in a clamp and the base should be secured at the level of the right atrium.

        i) When the animal is in *lateral* recumbency, the level of the tip of the thoracic vertebral spinous process can be used as a guide.

        ii) When the animal is in *sternal* recumbency, a level half to two-thirds of the way up the chest can be used.

    (6) A three-way tap is inserted between the catheter and the manometer. The three-way tap is opened and the level of the fluid in the manometer given 30 seconds to equilibrate with the CVP.

  f) The normal value for CVP is variable and a baseline (usually less than 10 cm of water) should be estimated for each patient. Serial measurements of CVP should be used to assess trends in CVP, especially if IV fluids or diuretics are being used.

4. Cardiac catheterization

  a) Specialized catheters exist to measure a number of hemodynamic parameters

    (1) Cardiac output

    (2) Wedge or occlusive pressure

    (3) Right atrial pressure

    (4) Pulmonary arterial pressure

  b) For use in the clinical setting, a cooperative (or sedated) patient and an intensive care environment with constant patient monitoring are required.

    (1) Cardiac-output measurement requires a cardiac-output computer. The thermodilution technique normally is used to assess cardiac output, but special catheters exist that have built-in flow probes.

    (2) Wedge or occlusive pressure

    A balloon-tipped (Swan-Ganz) catheter is placed, via the jugular vein, through the right side of the heart into the pulmonary artery. The measuring tip of the catheter is distal to the balloon. When inflated, the balloon protects the tip of the catheter from the pulmonary arterial pressure and the catheter measures the wedge or occlusive pressure. As the pulmonary capillary and venous systems show poor compliance, the occlusive pressure is a reflection of pulmonary venous, and hence left atrial, pressure. It is left atrial pressure that is critical in the formation of pulmonary edema, and thus occlusive pressure can be used not only to assess the magnitude of elevation of left atrial pressure, but its response to therapeutic intervention. These catheters also have a measuring port positioned to lie in the right atrium to give continuous measurement of right atrial pressure. This technique requires special catheters and intensive monitoring, but can be used to fine tune and direct therapy in the critical patient.

VIII. Prolonged in-hospital management

The desirability of a prolonged hospital stay and the management decisions made will depend on many factors.

    A. Methods used for initial stabilization
    B. Presumptive diagnosis
    C. Level of staffing, equipment, and expertise available
    D. Cost factors and owner commitment
    E. Realistic long-term prognosis
    F. After 12 to 24 hours, many patients in left congestive heart failure will have responded to initial emergency interventions and can be switched to a medication protocol and discharged to the owner. This usually includes oral equivalents of those medications already used. ACE inhibitors usually substitute for nitroglycerin for long-term management to circumvent the effects of nitrate tolerance.
    G. For patients requiring longer hospital stays for continued intervention and monitoring, the approach includes addressing the following questions.
       1. Diagnosis
         a) Is it correct?
         b) Are other diseases present to compromise therapy, (e.g., pneumonia)?
       2. Therapy
         a) Is it appropriate? Completion of a cardiac database may dictate your approach.
         b) Is it adequate? Can we push harder (e.g., increase dose frequency or amount) or move to a more intensive approach?
       3. Severity
        Is there a realistic hope for stabilization and discharge?

RIGHT-SIDED CONGESTIVE HEART FAILURE

  I. Cardinal signs
    A. Ascites
    B. Pleural effusion
    C. Jugular venous distension
 II. Pathophysiology
    Cardiac pathology and activation of the body's compensatory mechanisms result in
    A. An increase in right ventricular and right atrial pressures
    B. Engorgement of the splanchnic tissues and consequent hepatosplenomegaly
    C. Raised systemic venous pressure, with disruption of Starling's forces across the capillary bed, leading to a net efflux of fluid into the interstitium
    D. Overload of systemic lymphatic system, which initially removes this excessive extracellular fluid
    E. Accumulation of this fluid in the pleural (pleural effusion), peritoneal (ascites), and subcutaneous spaces (peripheral edema).
III. Clinical signs
    A. Abdominal distension, jugular venous distension, dyspnea, peripheral edema
    B. Cardiogenic edema of the gastrointestinal tract may lead to diarrhea and vomiting, weight loss

C. Clinical signs depend mainly on the site of fluid accumulation (e.g., pleural, peritoneal, subcutaneous or GI)
IV. Therapeutic goals
  A. Remove the fluid either pharmacologically or mechanically
  B. Decrease right atrial pressure
V. Methods
  A. Decreasing right atrial pressure
    1. Decrease preload
       In right-heart failure, diuretics are the safest means of reducing preload. Venodilators can also be used, but may depress right ventricular filling pressure below a critical level. In a failing right ventricle, these critical levels occur at a higher venous pressure. Therefore, right-heart failure may be exacerbated by venodilators. Dehydration will also decrease right atrial pressure and have a similar detrimental effect on right ventricular filling. ACE inhibitors are useful in this setting. Their primary beneficial effect results from minimizing RAAS-mediated sodium retention. Some authors do report limited pulmonary vasodilating properties.
    2. Increasing cardiac output
       An increased output from the right ventricle will also decrease right atrial pressure. Pulmonary arterial dilators with an efficacy comparable to those used peripherally are not available, and thus positive inotropes are used to increase cardiac output from the right side (e.g., digoxin). Dobutamine, dopamine, amrinone, and milrinone can be considered, but are often unnecessary in pure right-sided failure.
VI. Approach
  A. Recognition of right-heart failure
    1. Appearance of the cardinal signs, in association with clinical and physical signs, consistent with underlying right-heart disease.
    2. These diseases are divided into
       a) Congenital: Tricuspid dysplasia, pulmonic stenosis, pulmonary hypertension
       b) Acquired: Tricuspid endocardiosis with concurrent pulmonary hypertension, pericardial effusion, heartworm disease, chagas disease. Pericardial effusion is prevalent in mid- to large breed dogs in middle to late age.
  B. Emergency management
    1. Abdominocentesis or pleurocentesis are recommended for immediate alleviation of signs associated with excessive fluid accumulation in these cavities.
    2. Moderate dose of diuretics (furosemide 1 to 2 mg/kg BID to TID).
    3. ACE inhibitors may prove a useful adjunct to therapy (see Left heart failure)
    4. Digoxin. Rapid digitalization is rarely necessary, slow digitalization using a conventional oral dose is usually adequate.
  C. Identification of the underlying cause
     Heartworm disease and pericardial effusion should be considered.

D. In-hospital care in the critical stage
Usually involves repeated pleural or abdominocentesis, continued diuretic use and monitoring. The measurement of central venous pressure may be particularly useful in patients in right heart failure.
E. Chronic client care

BIVENTRICULAR FAILURE

A. Biventricular failure often occurs in the later stages of cardiac disease, especially in cases of dilated cardiomyopathy or end-stage chronic valvular disease in dogs. In cats, biventricular failure may be seen with all types of cardiomyopathy but particularly with dilative restrictive disease.
B. Patients often have a history of left-heart failure, but not invariably.
C. Prognosis is guarded to grave at this stage.
D. Cardinal signs of left (e.g., pulmonary edema) and right (e.g., pleural effusion or ascites) congestive failure are seen
E. Biventricular failure is managed by a combination of medications used for left and right congestive failure.

LOW-OUTPUT CARDIAC FAILURE

I. Cardiac clinical signs
A. Weakness
B. Poor perfusion
C. Cold extremities
D. Hypothermia
II. Pathophysiology
A. Two main causes
1. Pump failure; represents systolic dysfunction and is associated with
a) Primary myocardial disease
b) Chronic ventricular volume overload (e.g., mitral valve disease)
2. Decreased cardiac filling; represents diastolic dysfunction and is associated with
a) Extracardiac compression
b) Pericardial effusion
c) Compromise of the ventricular chamber
d) Hypertrophied muscle
e) Space-occupying lesion (e.g., tumor)
3. Systolic and diastolic dysfunction lead to a decrease in stroke volume and cardiac output.
III. Clinical signs
A. Exercise intolerance due to poor muscle perfusion
B. Blanched mucous membranes, slow CRT
C. Cold extremities
D. Concurrent signs of congestive heart failure if present (see above comments)

      1. Right congestive failure in patients with pericardial effusion
      2. Left congestive failure with systolic dysfunction or diastolic dysfunction due to chamber compromise (e.g., hypertrophic cardiomyopathy).

IV. Therapeutic goals
  A. Increase cardiac output
    1. Systolic dysfunction
      a) Positive inotropes
        (1) Dobutamine or dopamine for short-term acute support
        (2) Digoxin, long-term oral or acute parenteral support
      b) Afterload reducers
        (1) Sodium nitroprusside
        (2) ACE inhibitors
      c) Decrease peripheral systemic resistance allowing increased stroke volume (remember stroke volume equals systolic pressure divided by peripheral vascular resistance)
    2. Diastolic dysfunction
      a) Extracardiac causes (e.g., pericardial effusion)
      Pericardiocentesis animals require high filling pressures to force blood into the compromised ventricle. Preload reducers (e.g., diuretics) should be used with extreme caution as they significantly decrease filling pressure. Once the external pressure is relieved, these agents can be used, but are often unnecessary.
      b) Cardiac causes (e.g., ventricular hypertrophy, HC in cats)
      Where excessive hypertrophy is causing compromise of diastolic filling and hence stroke volume, negative inotropes such as diltiazem and beta blockers are indicated. Diltiazam has positive lusitropic properties; it actively enhances ventricular relaxation.
      As it is the diastolic phase of the cardiac cycle that shortens during tachycardia, further exacerbating diastolic dysfunction, negative chronotropes, again diltiazem or beta blockers, are also indicated.
  B. Treat signs of congestive heart failure (see above)

V. Approach
  A. Recognition of low-output heart failure
  Recognition of the cardinal signs of low-output failure associated with clinical and physical signs consistent with heart disease.
  B. Emergency management of systolic dysfunction
    1. Acute inotropic management
      a) IV dopamine or dobutamine
      b) Rapid IV digitalization
      c) Intravenous amrinone or milrinone
    2. Diuretics
    Furosemide
    3. Acute vasodilation
      a) Intravenous sodium nitroprusside
      b) Nitroglycerin intravenously, percutaneously, or sublingually
      c) Many of these drugs are continued through the critical phase while the animal is hospitalized, and some, for example, percutaneous nitroglycerin, can be dispensed for chronic client administered care.

d) As a general rule all parenteral vasodilating agents should be weaned over 2 to 3 hours rather than abruptly discontinued.

C. The identification of the underlying cause

D. In-hospital care during the critical stages

E. Chronic client administered care.

SYNDROMES ASSOCIATED WITH CARDIAC DISEASES COMMONLY SEEN IN THE EMERGENCY ROOM

CHRONIC VALVE DISEASE

As the mitral valve is most adversely affected, left congestive heart failure is usually seen. As the disease progresses low-output failure becomes superimposed on the congestive changes due to myocardial failure. If chordae tendineae rupture occurs, low-output failure may occur acutely as a result of a sudden increase in the volume of regurgitation back into the left atrium accompanied by a consequential fall in cardiac output. Left atrial pressure rises rapidly as a result of this sudden change and peracute left CHF is also seen.

DILATED CARDIOMYOPATHY (Fig. 18-1)

A primary pump failure leading to both low-output failure and left LCHF. As the disease progresses, biventricular failure is seen.

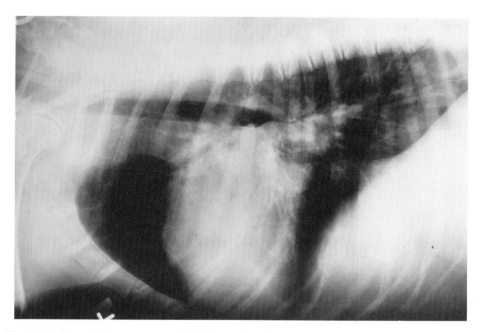

Fig. 18-1. Lateral chest radiograph of the patient showing cardiomegaly, pulmonary venous distension, and pulmonary edema.

A. Canine: Usually present in left LCHF and low-output failure. Atrial fibrillation is often seen in protracted or severe disease, biventricular failure is seen in end stages.

B. Feline: Usually present in low-output and biventricular failure (which manifests as a life-threatening pleural effusion).

Hypertrophic Cardiomyopathy (Figs. 18-2 and 18-3)

Rarely seen in dogs. Cats present with signs of left CHF due to diastolic compromise. May also show signs of biventricular failure. Dogs with secondary hypertrophy (i.e., due to subaortic stenosis) usually present with ventricular arrhythmias.

Pericardial Effusion

Patients present with signs of right CHF (the right ventricle is thinner and more susceptible to raised intrapericardial pressure) and low-output failure due to extra-cardiac compression.

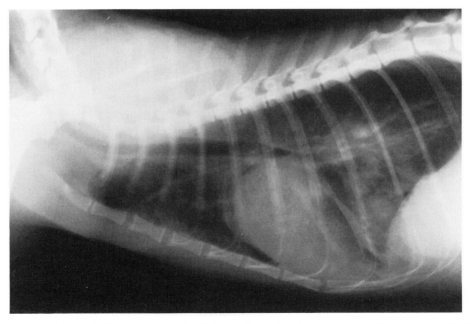

Fig. 18-2. Lateral chest radiograph of the patient showing cardiomegaly, particularly the atria, and pulmonary edema.

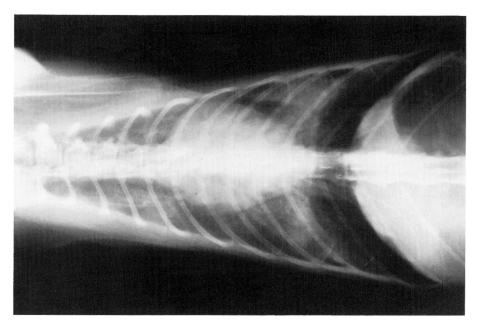

Fig. 18-3. Ventrodorsal radiograph of the patient showing the classic "valentine" shape that results from concentric hypertrophy of the ventricle and bi-atrial enlargement. Pulmonary edema is also seen.

SUGGESTED READINGS

Fox PR: Critical care cardiology. Vet Clin N Amer 19:1095, 1989

Harpster N: Pulmonary edema. p. 385. In Kirk RW (ed): Current Veterinary Therapy X. WB Saunders, Philadelphia, 1989

Opie LH: Drugs for the Heart. 3rd Ed. WB Saunders, Philadelphia, 1991

Rush JE: Emergency therapy and monitoring of heart failure. p. 713. In Kirk RW, Bonagura JD (eds): Current Veterinary Therapy XI. WB Saunders, Philadelphia, 1992

Wall RE, Rush JE: Cardiac emergencies. p. 213. In Murtaugh RJ, Kaplan PM (eds): Veterinary Emergency and Critical Care Medicine. Mosby-Year Book, St. Louis, 1992

Ware WA, Bonagura JD: Pulmonary edema. p. 205. In Fox PR (ed): Canine and Feline Cardiology. Churchill Livingstone, New York, 1988

Appendix 1
Recommendations for the Diagnosis of Heart Disease and the Treatment of Heart Failure in Small Animals

This document was created by the International Small Animal Cardiac Health Council, starting in May of 1992, to provide guidelines for diagnosing common cardiac diseases in small animals and for treating the heart failure that occurs secondary to these diseases. The International Small Animal Cardiac Health Council is comprised of eminent veterinary clinical cardiologists from around the world.

The International Small Animal Cardiac health Council has included the following members:

Dr. John Bonagura
Dr. Claudio Bussadori
Dr. David Church
Dr. Peter Darke
Dr. Steven Ettinger
Dr. Philip Fox
Dr. Robert Hamlin
Dr. Bruce Keene
Dr. Mark Kittleson
Dr. Chris Lombard

Dr. Jordi Manubens
Dr. Takeo Minami
Dr. Sydney Moise
Dr. Michael O'Grady
Dr. Paul Pion
Dr. Jean Louis Pouchelon
Dr. David Sisson
Dr. William Thomas
Dr. Larry Tilley
Dr. Yoshihisa Yamane

GENERAL PATHOPHYSIOLOGY OF HEART DISEASE LEADING TO HEART FAILURE

Heart disease and heart failure are defined differently. If any cardiac finding is outside accepted limits of normality (e.g., a systolic murmur or systolic click heard on auscultation, tall R waves or a bundle branch block on the electrocardiogram, or reduced wall motion on the echocardiogram), then by definition heart disease is present. Diverse examples of heart disease include mitral regurgitation, dilated cardiomyopathy, pulmonic stenosis, and anomalous coronary arteries. Heart failure occurs when heart disease becomes severe enough to overwhelm the compensatory mechanisms of the cardiovascular system. Heart failure is not a disease. Heart failure is present when a mechanical inadequacy of the heart results in elevated venous pressures leading to congestion and edema formation in the tissues (congestive or backward heart failure) and/or results in inadequate cardiac output (forward or low-output heart failure). It is important to remember that the presence of identifiable heart disease does not in any way imply that heart failure is present or ever will manifest as a clinical problem. Conversely, if heart failure is present, then by definition the patient must have heart disease.

Myocardial failure is defined as a decrease in myocardial contractility. Many types of heart disease result in myocardial failure. Although patients with myocardial failure commonly develop signs of heart failure, myocardial failure may be present when heart failure is not. As an example, taurine deficiency in cats may produce myocardial failure. Prior to recognition of the connection between taurine deficiency and myocardial failure and prior to adequate supplementation of most cat foods, cats with taurine-deficiency induced myocardial failure most commonly presented to veterinarians because they were manifesting signs of heart failure. However, experimental taurine deficiency commonly results in myocardial failure which may be detected for years by echocardiography without any evidence of heart failure.

Conversely, myocardial failure does not have to be present for heart failure to be present. There are several examples of cardiac disease in veterinary medicine where myocardial systolic function is believed to be normal, yet heart failure is present. Examples include hypertrophic cardiomyopathy, mitral regurgitation in small dogs, and chronic pericardial tamponade.

The cardiovascular system has three functions: (1) to maintain normal systemic arterial blood pressure, (2) to maintain normal blood flow (cardiac output), and (3) to maintain normal venous and capillary pressures. When cardiac disease becomes severe, the ability of the cardiovascular system to maintain these functions deteriorates. Consequently, heart failure may be manifested as high capillary pressure (edema), low cardiac output (hypoperfusion), and low blood pressure (hypotension). Generally in acute heart failure, hypoperfusion and hypotension prevail because chronic compensatory mechanisms have not had time to become effective. Acute heart failure can be severe enough to lead to cardiogenic shock. In chronic heart failure the body has time to compensate for the heart disease. Compensation commonly takes the form of renal sodium and water retention, which produces an increase in circulating blood volume. As venous return increases, the myocardium in the affected ventricle is stretched, stimulating it to grow into a larger chamber (volume overload or eccentric hypertrophy). The increase in end-diastolic volume provided by volume overload hypertrophy allows the affected ventricle to pump more blood for any given amount of myocardial shortening (shortening fraction).

Renal sodium and water retention is produced via a number of different mechanisms, but all are stimulated by a decrease in systemic (and therefore renal) blood flow or circulating blood volume. The renin-angiotensin-aldosterone system is one of the most important mechanisms for stimulation of salt and water retention. When the ability of the ventricle to enlarge becomes overwhelmed (reaches a maximum), the kidneys continue to retain salt and water because of the continued suboptimal cardiac output and renal perfusion. At this stage, the salt and water retention increases diastolic ventricular pressure to a clinically significant level. This increased diastolic pressure "backs up" into the atrium, veins, and capillaries behind the affected ventricle and causes edema. Signs of heart failure referable to edema formation are called congestive heart failure. Congestion and edema formation are the most common manifestations of chronic heart failure, so the term congestive heart failure is commonly used synonymously with heart failure. Diseases of the left heart result in left-heart failure, which is most commonly manifested as pulmonary edema. Diseases of the right heart result in right-heart failure. Manifestations of congestive heart failure secondary to right-heart disease are species dependant but in small animal medicine these manifestations are usually those of ascites and occasionally subcutaneous edema. Right and left congestive heart failure together commonly produce pleural effusion. Chronic heart failure patients can also have clinical signs referable to poor perfusion (low-output failure) but these signs are less common and generally occur later in the course of the disease. It is unusual for chronic heart failure patients to become clinically hypotensive.

It is useful to think of heart disease and failure as a continuum that may progress from heart disease to the preclinical phase to a phase with overt clinical signs.

HEART DISEASE

Heart disease includes numerous anatomic and physiologic abnormalities of diverse etiology which may become or may never be clinically significant to the patient.

THE PRECLINICAL PHASE

At this stage, cardiac structural abnormalities are identifiable using readily available diagnostic modalities (e.g., radiography, electrocardiography, echocardiography) but are not apparent to the owner because they are balanced by compensatory mechanisms that inhibit development of clinical signs of heart failure.

THE PHASE WITH OVERT CLINICAL SIGNS

At this stage, clinical signs of heart failure are observable by the client and clinician.

DEFINITION OF HEART FAILURE

Developing a precise definition of heart failure has provoked countless hours of debate. Although there are many proposed definitions, not one is universally accepted. One difficulty lies in the fact that heart disease may or may not lead to heart failure.

We present four currently employed definitions for your information.

DEFINITION 1 (PARMLEY)

"An inability of the heart to deliver enough blood to the peripheral tissues to meet metabolic tissue demands. A decreased cardiac output and a rise in atrial pressures are the hallmarks of the syndrome. In mild forms of heart failure, cardiac output falls and atrial pressures rise in response to physical exertion. As the heart failure syndrome worsens, clinical signs are detectable at lower levels of exertion and finally are apparent at rest." (Parmley WW, Chatterjee K: Principles in the management of congestive heart failure. p. 1. In Cardiology, JB Lippincott, Philadelphia, 1988.)

DEFINITION 2 (BRAUNWALD)

"Pathophysiologic state in which an abnormality of cardiac function is responsible for failure of the heart to pump blood at rate commensurate with the requirements of the metabolizing tissues or do so only at an elevated filling pressure." (Braunwald E: Diseases of the Heart. 4th Ed. p. 393. WB Saunders, Philadelphia, 1992.)

DEFINITION 3 (HAMLIN)

"When the cardiovascular system fails to circulate sufficient blood to meet the metabolic demands of the body for nutrients or when the blood backs up within a venous or capillary bed, the patient manifests a complex of clinical signs. These clinical signs resulting from cardiac dysfunction translate into a reduced quality of life and/or longevity."

DEFINITION 4 (KITTLESON)

"Heart failure is a pathophysiologic condition that becomes clinically apparent when heart disease causes systolic and/or diastolic cardiac dysfunction severe enough to produce clinical signs referable to congestion/edema and/or peripheral hypoperfusion at rest or with exercise."

FUNCTIONAL CLASSES OF HEART FAILURE

The current approach to heart failure classification in human patients employs a functional classification scheme that relates to the signs and symptoms of human patients at rest and during exercise (New York Heart Association (NYHA) functional classes 1 through 4).

This scheme often does not conveniently or appropriately apply to veterinary patients with heart failure primarily because many veterinary patients do not exercise vigorously. The members of the International Small Animal Cardiac Health Council unanimously concluded that this scheme did not serve the profession well and that the therapy of heart failure would be best approached by the use of a system emphasizing anatomic diagnosis and the severity of clinical signs at rest. Consequently, a new classification scheme that the Council believes is more applicable to the veterinary situation was developed.

INTERNATIONAL SMALL ANIMAL CARDIAC HEALTH COUNCIL SYSTEM OF HEART FAILURE CLASSIFICATION

I. The asymptomatic patient (heart disease associated with no clinical signs)
   Heart disease is detectable (e.g., cardiac murmur, arrhythmia, or cardiac chamber enlargement that is detected by radiography or echocardiography); however, the patient is not overtly affected and does not demonstrate clinical signs of heart failure. The need for treatment at this stage is arguable but not justifiable with currently available data. This stage can be subdivided as follows
   A. Signs of heart disease are present but no signs of compensation (volume or pressure overload ventricular hypertrophy) are evident (Class IA)
   B. Signs of heart disease are present and signs of compensation (volume or pressure overload ventricular hypertrophy) are detected radiographically or echocardiographically (Class IB).
II. Mild-to-moderate heart failure
   A. Clinical signs of heart failure are evident at rest or with mild exercise, and adversely affect the quality of life. Typical signs of heart failure include exercise intolerance, cough, tachypnea, mild respiratory distress (dyspnea), and mild to moderate ascites. Hypoperfusion at rest is generally not present (Class II).
   B. Home treatment is often indicated at this stage.
III. Advanced heart failure
   A. Clinical signs of advanced congestive heart failure are immediately obvious. These clinical signs could include respiratory distress (dyspnea), marked ascites, profound exercise intolerance, or hypoperfusion at rest. In the most severe cases, the patient is moribund and suffers from cardiogenic shock. Death or severe debilitation is likely without therapy.
   B. Patients with advanced heart failure are divided into two subcategories:
      1. Home care is possible (Class 3A)
      2. Hospitalization is mandatory (cardiogenic shock, life-threatening pulmonary edema, or a large pleural effusion is present) (Class 3B)

SYSTEMATIC APPROACH TO THE DOG OR CAT WITH CARDIAC DISEASE

HISTORY AND PHYSICAL EXAMINATION

I. Signalment
   Determining age, breed, and sex of the patient are important in formulating a rule-out list and in helping determine prognosis.

II. History

Current and pre-existing diseases should be noted. Current drugs or medications and clinical response to these medicaments are important points to be recorded. Presenting clinical signs, and duration and progression of the illness should be recorded.

III. Physical examination

In addition to a complete physical exam, a thorough cardiovascular examination should be performed and should include all of the following

   A. Auscultation
      1. Determine the heart rate
      2. Identify the presence or absence of the following
         a) Heart murmur (PMI, radiation, loudness, timing, character)
         b) Gallop sounds
         c) Other abnormal heart sounds (e.g., split S_1 or S_2, clicks, snaps, rubs)
         d) Arrhythmias
         e) Abnormal lung sounds
   B. Femoral pulse palpation (character, rate, rhythm, pulse deficits)
   C. Capillary refill time/mucous membrane color evaluation
   D. Jugular vein observation (distention and pulsation)
   E. Precordial palpation (apical impulse, presence of thrills)
   F. Thoracic percussion
   G. Abdominal palpation to assess organomegaly and detect ascites

CLINICAL TESTS

   I. Electrocardiography

   Assess the rate, rhythm, and axis; evaluate the P-QRS-T complex morphology.

   II. Thoracic radiography

   Evaluate cardiac size and shape for evidence of heart disease (cardiomegaly, specific chamber enlargement, pulmonary vascularity) and evaluate for presence or absence of heart failure (pulmonary edema, pleural effusion).

   III. Echocardiography

   Assess cardiac structure and function to determine the type and severity of the cardiac disease present; detect fluid accumulation; discover noncardiogenic causes of current clinical signs.

   IV. Clinical pathology
      A. CBC
      B. Serum biochemical profile
      C. Serum electrolyte concentrations (potassium, sodium, chloride, calcium)
      D. Acid-base status (blood pH, P_{CO_2}, bicarbonate)
      E. Blood gases (arterial and venous oxygen tensions)
      F. Serum thyroxine concentration
      G. Cytologic evaluation of effusions
      H. Heartworm antigen serology/microfilaria detection
      I. Other tests when appropriate (e.g. blood culture, leukemia virus tests,

FIV serology, plasma and whole blood taurine concentration, plasma carnitine concentration, plasma lactate concentration)

CLINICAL FINDINGS IN HEART DISEASE AND HEART FAILURE

I. Client complaints
   A. Dyspnea, orthopnea (pulmonary edema, pleural effusion)
   B. Cough (pulmonary edema, compression of bronchus by left atrium)
   C. Tachypnea (pulmonary edema, pleural effusion)
   D. Exercise intolerance (low cardiac output, pulmonary edema)
   E. Abdominal distention (ascites)
   F. Weakness (low cardiac output)
   G. Syncope (episodic cessation of cerebral blood flow due to arrhythmias)
   H. Weight loss
   I. Anorexia
   J. Depression
II. Physical examination (general)
   A. Respiratory signs (i.e., tachypnea, dyspnea)
   B. Ascites
   C. Distended and possibly pulsating jugular veins
   D. Abnormal femoral pulses (hypokinetic, hyperkinetic)
   E. Precordial thrills
   F. Palpable rhythm irregularities
   G. Hepatosplenomegaly
   H. Pale mucous membranes
   I. Prolonged capillary refill time (>2 sec)
III. Auscultation
   A. Murmurs
   B. Rate and rhythm irregularities
   C. Abnormal intensity of heart sounds
   D. Gallop sounds
   E. Crackles and wheezes (most commonly due to chronic bronchial disease)
   F. Muffled heart or lung sounds
IV. Radiography
   A. Cardiomegaly (generalized or specific chambers)
   B. Aortic root or main pulmonary artery bulges
   C. Pulmonary edema
   D. Pleural effusion
   E. Bronchial compression from atrial enlargement
   F. Pulmonary vascular patterns (e.g., pulmonary venous congestion, pulmonary arterial enlargement, pulmonary arterial blunting)
   G. Lung lobe collapse or torsion
   H. Pulmonary infiltrates (e.g., "inflammatory infiltrates", metastatic lesions)
V. Electrocardiography
   A. Increased or decreased heart rate

   B. Abnormal cardiac rhythm
   C. Abnormal mean electrical axis
   D. Morphologic abnormalities of P or QRS complexes
   E. ST segment or T-wave changes
  VI. Echocardiography
   A. Anatomic cardiac lesion (e.g., atrial or ventricular septal defect, atrial enlargement, intra- or extracardiac tumors or thrombi, valvular lesions)
   B. Cardiac hypertrophy patterns
      1. Eccentric hypertrophy: volume overload ventricular hypertrophy (commonly termed dilation)
      2. Concentric hypertrophy: pressure overload ventricular hypertrophy (thickened ventricular myocardium)
   C. Abnormal ventricular movement (hypo- or hyperkinetic wall motion)
   D. Fluid accumulation (pericardial, pleural)
 VII. Possible laboratory abnormalities (clinical pathology)
   A. Low venous oxygen tension
   B. Low arterial oxygen tension
   C. Increased blood lactate concentration
   D. Pre-renal azotemia (severe hypoperfusion or inadequate water intake secondary to malaise)
   E. Mild elevation of liver enzymes
   F. Hypoproteinemia (right-sided CHF)
   G. Elevated serum thyroxine concentration (cats)
   H. Low plasma and/or whole blood taurine concentration (cats, some canine breeds)
   I. Low plasma carnitine concentration (some dogs)
   J. Electrolyte abnormalities
   K. Positive heartworm test
   L. Positive blood culture (endocarditis)

DEFINITIVE DIAGNOSTIC CRITERIA OF HEART FAILURE

   I. Measurement of elevated pulmonary capillary wedge pressure (PCWP) with a Swan-Ganz or other end-hole cardiac catheter in a patient with left-heart disease (congestive left-heart failure) or measurement of increased central venous or right atrial pressure in a patient with right-heart disease (congestive right-heart failure).
  II. Identification of pulmonary edema in a patient with moderate-to-severe left atrial enlargement (congestive left-heart failure).
 III. Identification of pulmonary edema in a patient with confirmed acute mitral regurgitation or aortic regurgitation (acute congestive left-heart failure).
  IV. Identification of ascites (and rarely peripheral edema) in a patient with enlarged hepatic veins on ultrasound or obviously distended jugular veins (congestive right-heart failure).
   V. Identification of ascites (and rarely clinically significant peripheral edema)

in a patient with moderate-to-severe right heart enlargement (congestive right-heart failure).

VI. Identification of ascites (and less commonly peripheral edema) in a patient with pericardial disease (congestive right-heart failure).

VII. Identification of pleural effusion in a patient with right and/or left heart disease (congestive right and/or left heart failure).

VIII. Measurement of a low cardiac output or cardiac index in a patient with heart disease (low-output heart failure).

IX. Measurement of increased blood lactate or low venous oxygen tension at rest or with mild exercise in a patient with congestive heart failure or severe cardiac disease (low-output heart failure).

Notes: It should be remembered that noncardiogenic (low venous or capillary pressure) ascites, pleural effusion, pulmonary edema, or peripheral edema can be found in patients that do not have heart failure. In these cases, PCWP and CVP will be normal and other diagnoses should be pursued.

Cardiogenic pleural effusion in cats may be pseudochylous or truly chylous and respond to therapy for congestive heart failure.

ACQUIRED HEART DISEASES

The most common acquired heart diseases in dogs and cats are as follows

I. Chronic, acquired degeneration of the AV valves (common in dogs; rare in cats)

II. Cardiomyopathy (primary myocardial disease of unknown etiology)
   A. Dilated cardiomyopathy (common in dogs; rare in cats)
   B. Hypertrophic cardiomyopathy (common in cats; rare in dogs)
   C. Unclassifiable cardiomyopathies (cats)
   D. Restrictive cardiomyopathy (cats)

III. Dirofilariasis (and other causes of cor pulmonale) (common in dogs; uncommon in cats)

IV. Pericardial disease/effusion (common in dogs, rarely clinically significant in cats)

V. Rhythm and conduction abnormalities (dogs and cats)

VI. Hyperthyroid heart disease (common in cats)

VII. Hypertensive heart disease (dogs and cats)

VIII. Bacterial endocarditis (dogs and cats)

IX. Cardiac tumors (common in dogs; rare in cats)

CARDIOVASCULAR DISEASES THAT COMMONLY LEAD TO HEART FAILURE

The remainder of this document provides summary information on some of the aforementioned diseases that commonly lead to heart failure, and delineates the recommendations of the International Small Animal Cardiology Health Council for therapy for each stage of heart failure.

CHRONIC ACQUIRED DEGENERATIVE VALVULAR
DISEASE (SOMETIMES CALLED ENDOCARDIOSIS)

I. Definition
   A. Chronic acquired degenerative valvular disease is an idiopathic, myxoma-
      tous degenerative disease of the atrioventricular valves that leads to valvu-
      lar insufficiency.
   B. A common cause of cardiac disease in the dog characterized by nodular
      thickening of the edges of the atrioventricular valves. (Bailliere's Compre-
      hensive Dictionary, Blood and Studdent, (eds), 1988.)
II. Pathology
   The mitral valve and tricuspid valve are most commonly affected (uncommonly the aortic valve is affected). A spectrum of atrioventricular valve lesions may be observed; however, the most common change is a shortening
   and thickening of the valves leading to incompetency. Chordae tendineae
   often shorten, become thick and nodular, and may rupture. Histologic
   changes in the valve and chordae tendineae include proliferation of the spongi-
   osa layer due to infiltration and increased deposition of an extracellular matrix
   material called glycosaminoglycans. This myxomatous change is degenerative
   in nature. Pathologic consequences of chronic atrioventricular valve insufficiency include dilation of the atria, dilation and hypertrophy (volume overload
   hypertrophy) of the ventricles, endocardial fibrosis of the atrium (jet lesions),
   and occasionally a full thickness left atrial tear.
III. Pathophysiology
   The atrioventricular valves are involved and the lesions result in an orifice
   (hole) where the valve leaflets normally meet. The orifice permits regurgitation of blood from the ventricle into the atrium during ventricular contraction.
   For any given size defect, the magnitude of blood regurgitating back across
   the mitral valve is worse than it would be across a similar sized defect in the
   tricuspid valve because the left ventricle develops much greater force than
   the right ventricle. Consequently left-heart failure due to mitral regurgitation
   is much more common than right-heart failure due to tricuspid regurgitation.
   The valvular leak initially leads to a decrease in the amount of blood pushed
   forward into the aorta (note: the reduced cardiac output is clinically significant
   only because of the compensatory mechanisms that it initiates, not because
   it is of sufficient magnitude to cause clinical signs in most patients at this
   stage). To compensate, the kidneys sense this decrease in systemic blood flow
   and retain sodium and water to increase blood volume. This action increases
   venous return to the heart, which initially "stretches" the myocardium in the
   affected ventricle. The affected ventricle responds to this stretch by growing
   larger to increase the end-diastolic volume (volume overload). As a result of
   this eccentric (volume overload) hypertrophy, the ventricle is able to pump
   a greater quantity of blood to compensate for the blood lost through the leak
   in the valve without a significant increase in the end-diastolic pressure within
   the ventricle, atria, pulmonary veins, or capillaries. Typically, this condition
   worsens over time, with the ventricle growing larger as the mitral orifice
   enlarges and the regurgitation worsens. The volume overload hypertrophy of
   the left ventricle continues to compensate for the leak, and the left atrium

dilates to accommodate the increased amount of systolic blood flow into it. When the leak becomes severe, the compensatory mechanisms to maintain adequate forward blood flow without increasing left atrial (and therefore pulmonary capillary) pressure beyond that which can be compensated for by enhanced pulmonary lymphatic drainage become overwhelmed and left atrial pressure increases to the point that pulmonary edema is produced. Clinical consequences of advanced mitral valve insufficiency include elevated pulmonary venous pressure, pulmonary edema, left atrial enlargement with bronchial compression, and, late in the course of the disease, ventricular myocardial dysfunction. Consequences of right atrioventricular valve (tricuspid) regurgitation are usually related to elevated systemic venous pressures with hepatomegaly, ascites, and rarely subcutaneous edema. Because normal right ventricular systolic pressure is low (<30 mmHg), regurgitant flow across all but the most severe lesions is not very large in magnitude, and congestive heart failure secondary to isolated right atrioventricular valve (tricuspid) regurgitation is uncommon. In most cases, where signs of right-heart failure are identified, an obstruction to right ventricular outflow (pulmonic stenosis or pulmonary hypertension) is also present. Biventricular heart failure may be manifested as pleural effusion. The most common clinical signs associated with severe mitral regurgitation include exercise intolerance, coughing, and respiratory distress (dyspnea). Syncope can occur in advanced valvular heart disease and may be related to paroxysmal arrhythmias, or vigorous coughing with reduced venous return. Syncope may occur in patients that do or do not have clinical signs of heart failure.

IV. Signalment
  A. This disease spans a very broad range of breeds and ages; however, degenerative AV valve disease is most commonly seen in middle-aged or older small-breed dogs.
  B. For reasons stated above, clinical signs are more common in acquired left AV valve disease; therefore, the following discussion describes left AV valve myxomatous degeneration. Extrapolation to right AV valve myxomatous degeneration is straightforward.
  C. Presumptive diagnostic criteria of left atrioventricular valvular insufficiency due to myxomatous degeneration of the mitral valve are as follows
    1. A systolic murmur over the left cardiac apex in a mature individual
    2. Radiographic, echocardiographic, and/or ECG evidence of left-heart enlargement
    3. Radiographic evidence of pulmonary venous distention or pulmonary infiltrates

V. Definitive diagnostic criteria
  Definitive diagnosis of myxomatous mitral valve degeneration and regurgitation is made with the following
  A. Evidence of left ventricular and left atrial enlargement, thickened mitral valve leaflets, and normal-to-increased shortening fraction on an echocardiogram.
  B. Presence of a regurgitant jet across the mitral valve on spectral or color flow Doppler in conjunction with criteria in V.A.
  C. Regurgitation of radiopaque dye into the left atrium after dye injection

into the left ventricle at the time of cardiac catheterization in conjunction with criteria in V.A.

VI. Differential diagnoses

In patients with clinical signs suggestive of mitral insufficiency secondary to myxomatous degeneration of the left atrioventricular mitral valve differential diagnoses include the following

A. Previously unrecognized congenital malformation of the atrioventricular valve apparatus—similar pathophysiology and clinical signs from a congenital etiology.

B. Bacterial endocarditis of the left AV valve—similar pathophysiology and clinical signs from an infectious etiology.

C. Dilated cardiomyopathy—may have similar clinical, electrocardiographic, and radiographic appearance.

D. Primary respiratory diseases, especially tracheal collapse, chronic bronchitis, and pulmonary fibrosis—may manifest cough and exercise intolerance

E. Neurologic and metabolic disorders—resulting in episodes similar to syncope seen in some dogs with mitral insufficiency.

The Asymptomatic Patient

I. History

No visible signs of heart disease are present.

II. Clinical findings

A. Physical examination

Detection of a cardiac murmur during a routine examination is often the first clue that valvular degeneration has begun. Cardiac findings are typically restricted to auscultation, which reveals a systolic murmur heard best over the left cardiac apex (mitral regurgitation) or possibly the tricuspid valve region (tricuspid regurgitation). Typically, the murmur is softer in the early stages of valve incompetency. It is common for the murmur to become louder and pansystolic (starting immediately after the first heart sound and persisting through the second heart sound) as valvular regurgitation progresses. While loud holosystolic (lasting from the onset of the first heart sound to the second heart sound) and pansystolic murmurs are typical of more advanced disease, one cannot reliably predict severity of mitral regurgitation by auscultation alone.

B. Radiography

The thoracic radiograph during this stage may be normal or may show mild-to-moderate left atrial and left ventricular enlargement. Thoracic radiography is particularly valuable in following the progression of valvular incompetency and the accompanying cardiomegaly that develops with more advanced disease.

C. Electrocardiography

The electrocardiogram is usually normal in this stage although P wave abnormalities may occur and evidence of left ventricular enlargement may become apparent if the disease has progressed to the moderate stage.

D. Echocardiography

The echocardiogram reveals no or moderate left atrial and left ventricular enlargement depending on the severity of the disease. The mitral valve leaflets may appear thickened.

E. Therapy

1. See Appendix 2 for specific medicaments and dosage recommendations
2. International Small Animal Cardiac Health Council (ISACHC) recommendations for therapy in the asymptomatic patient:
   a) Angiotensin converting enzyme (ACE) inhibition therapy: In the absence of cardiac enlargement (Class 1A), there is no evidence that ACE inhibitors are beneficial.
   b) In the presence of moderate-to-severe cardiomegaly (Class 1B), ACE inhibition therapy may be beneficial, but evidence is lacking in dogs. The Council will continue to review this issue as new data become available from ongoing clinical studies.

Mild-to-Moderate Signs of Heart Failure

The mild-to-moderate class of heart failure can be differentiated from the asymptomatic class in that signs of heart failure are evident to the client and may be visible at presentation.

I. History

Client complaints generally include reports of episodic cough, exercise intolerance, lethargy, difficult breathing, tachypnea, and nocturnal restlessness.

II. Clinical findings

A. Physical examination

The dog may appear normal, particularly in the mildest phases of congestive heart failure. This is particularly true if the clinical sign of coughing is caused by left mainstem bronchial compression (not a sign of heart failure) and not by overt pulmonary edema. A systolic cardiac murmur is always present, usually loudest over the left apex. In many cases palpable precordial thrills associated with mitral and/or tricuspid regurgitation are evident. The cardiac rhythm may be regular or irregular. Isolated atrial premature complexes are common in this disease. More advanced arrhythmias may be anticipated in some dogs. The arterial pulse may be normal or brisk. Irregularities of the pulse are expected with cardiac arrhythmias. Left-sided congestive heart failure is evident as tachypnea, possible inspiratory and early expiratory crackles (Caution: absence of these sounds does not rule out pulmonary edema and presence of pulmonary crackles is more commonly identified in older dogs with primary lung disease), and exercise intolerance. A wheeze may be detected in dogs with compression of the left mainstem bronchus by the left atrium. When tricuspid regurgitation is prominent, hepatomegaly and possible ascitic fluid accumulation may be noted.

B. Radiography

Cardiomegaly—usually left sided—is evident. Dorsal deviation of the trachea in dogs that are not flat chested, and elevation and compression of the left mainstem bronchus are common findings. Presence of left atrial and left auricular appendage enlargement is expected on both DV and lateral thoracic radiographs. Pulmonary edema is characterized most frequently by increased perihilar and caudodorsal lung densities.

C. Electrocardiography

The ECG rate and rhythm may be normal. Atrial premature complexes may be observed with progressive atrial distention. Ventricular extrasystoles may be observed but are less common than in dogs with dilated cardiomyopathy. Changes in the P-waves are common and include widened P waves ("P mitrale") and increased amplitude P waves ("P pulmonale"). The frontal mean electrical axis is typically normal but increased amplitude R waves are sometimes observed in Leads II and aVF.

D. Echocardiography

Typical echocardiographic changes include moderate to severe left atrial enlargement, left ventricular volume overload (eccentric) hypertrophy (LV chamber dilation with normal LV wall thickness), and a hyperdynamic left ventricular motion (shortening fraction exceeding 40 percent and commonly >50 percent). Myocardial function is usually normal at this stage as evidenced by a normal end-systolic diameter. The increased shortening fraction is due to the increase in end-diastolic diameter with the normal end-systolic diameter. Exuberant mitral valve excursion and thickening of the mitral valve leaflets are typical findings. Progressive mitral regurgitation is associated with increasing cardiac dimensions and left ventricular shortening fraction. Doppler echocardiography (spectral or color flow) may be used to document the presence of mitral regurgitation and may be useful in semiquantitating the severity of the regurgitation.

E. Therapy

1. See Appendix 2 for specific medicaments and dosage recommendations
2. The ISACHC recommendations for canine patients with mitral insufficiency secondary to chronic degenerative atrioventricular valvular disease with mild-to-moderate heart failure are as follows:
   a) Diuretic therapy
   b) ACE inhibitor therapy
   c) Sodium-restricted diets, if tolerated by the patient
   d) Digitalis glycoside therapy: the Council could not reach a consensus regarding digitalis therapy for this class of canine patient

Advanced Heart Failure

What differentiates mild-to-moderate heart failure from advanced heart failure is the more severe and obvious nature of the clinical signs of disease. Clinical findings such as dyspnea at rest, markedly diminished exercise tolerance, alveolar pulmonary edema, cachexia, or obvious ascites indicate a patient with advanced congestive heart failure. Pallor of the mucous membranes secondary to low cardiac output and pronounced vasoconstriction may occur, although normal mucous membrane color and refill time do not rule out heart failure or systemic hypoperfusion.

I. History

Client complaints generally include reports of frequent cough, exercise intolerance, lethargy, difficult breathing, tachypnea, and nocturnal restlessness.

II. Clinical findings

A. Physical examination

Unless associated with a peracute incident such as a choradal rupture, most dogs with advanced heart failure are in poor body condition and have experienced weight loss. Respiratory distress and tachypnea are typical clinical findings. In biventricular failure or right-sided failure, the patient may have abdominal distention owing to ascites. Systolic murmurs, as previously described, are present. The arterial pulse may be weak or normal and may be irregular due to premature complexes or development of atrial fibrillation. Dogs with respiratory distress may have crackles due to pulmonary edema, but oftentimes have only increased bronchointerstitial sounds due to hyperpnea. In advanced cases of right-heart failure, there will be considerable ascites, as well as hepatomegaly. Jugular venous pressure is often elevated and jugular pulsations may be evident. Arrhythmias are very common in this phase, and atrial fibrillation is a frequent cause of deterioration in class from moderate to severe heart failure. It is common to see older small breed dogs with pulmonary crackles and a murmur of mitral regurgitation. It should be noted that most of these dogs have primary respiratory disease rather than heart failure (pulmonary edema) and an incidental finding of the heart murmur.

B. Radiography

In addition to radiographic abnormalities previously mentioned, alveolar infiltrates typical of cardiogenic pulmonary edema will be observed. These infiltrates are usually most evident in the hilar region, but are often diffuse. There may also be asymmetry in infiltrates in some dogs (right side more dense than left side). Cardiomegaly may be extreme and may mimic pericardial effusion in some cases although usually the markedly enlarged left atrium can be identified. Abdominal x-rays will demonstrate hepatomegaly and may show fluid accumulation if right-heart failure is also present.

C. Electrocardiography

In addition to the abnormalities mentioned previously, cardiac arrhythmias are quite common. Atrial fibrillation is probably the most frequently encountered sustained cardiac arrhythmia. Ventricular arrhythmias also may be observed.

D. Echocardiography

The mitral valve leaflets usually are markedly thickened and there may be evidence of mitral valve prolapse. Some dogs may demonstrate evidence of chordae tendineae rupture. Severe left atrial and left ventricular enlargement are present at this stage. Global left ventricular function (shortening fraction) is usually well preserved although myocardial function (contractility) may actually be decreased in some dogs (especially large breed dogs) at this stage. In severe mitral regurgitation, decreased myocardial function is characterized by a normal or below normal shortening fraction, increased separation between the mitral valve opening point (E point) and ventricular septum, and an increased end-systolic diameter. It should be emphasized that the increase in end-systolic diameter denotes the decrease in myocardial function seen in late stage mitral regurgitation, and that the increase in end-diastolic diameter usually keeps shortening fraction in the normal range or above.

   E. Therapy

    I. Advanced heart failure is divided therapeutically into two subclasses as mentioned earlier

        a) Home care is possible at this time

        b) Hospitalization is mandatory for patient stabilization

          This subclass is assigned when the patient exhibits cardiogenic shock or has developed life-threatening pulmonary edema or pleural effusion. Dogs with refractory ascites also may be assigned to this subclass pending improvement of their heart failure state.

   II. Therapy of advanced heart failure—home care possible (See Appendix 2 for specific medicaments and dosage recommendations)

      A. The ISACHC recommendations to treat canine patients with advanced heart failure (home care) are as follows

        1. Diuretic therapy

        2. ACE inhibition

        3. Digitalization

        4. Hydralazine titration*

      B. Possible use of the following

        1. Sodium restriction, if the dog will accept it

        2. Antiarrhythmic therapy, if needed

        3. Nitrates

        4. Theophylline

        5. Codeine or other cough suppressants

  III. Therapy of advanced heart failure—hospitalization mandatory for stabilization (See Appendix 2 for specific medicaments and dosage recommendations)

      A. The ISACHC recommendations to treat canine patients with advanced heart failure (requiring hospitalization) include

        1. Oxygen therapy

        2. Intravenous furosemide or another loop diuretic†

        3. Preload reduction with topical nitroglycerine or nitroprusside (blood pressure must be monitored if nitroprusside is to be used)

        4. Afterload reduction with hydralazine or sodium nitroprusside to reduce mitral regurgitant fraction†

        5. Amrinone infusion

        6. Dobutamine

        7. Morphine

        8. Theophylline

---

* In the presence of left mainstem bronchial compression, refractory or progressive left-sided heart failure, or insufficient response to ACE inhibitor therapy, consider the addition of hydralazine. If added onto ACE inhibitor therapy, care must be taken not to induce profound hypotension. The drug should generally be titrated using blood pressure (systolic or mean) as the monitoring tool. A broad certified cardiac specialist should be consulted.

† Most effective at reducing life-threatening pulmonary edema

     9. Antiarrhythmic therapy (if needed)
    10. Pleurocentesis (if needed)‡
B. If ascitic fluid accumulation or pulmonary edema are refractory to therapy with one diuretic, consider adding a second diuretic. This can include hydrochlorothiazide or a combination of hydrochlorothiazide plus spironolactone (if the patient is not currently receiving an ACE inhibitor). Also consider the addition of hydralazine as outlined above in refractory left heart failure.

Canine Dilated Cardiomyopathy (DS)

I. Definition and etiology

Dilated cardiomyopathy is a condition characterized by decreased myocardial contractility (primary myocardial failure) and volume overload hypertrophy (dilation) of one or both ventricles.

Most cases of cardiomyopathy in the dog are considered idiopathic; however, a variety of definable conditions may lead to myocardial failure and produce clinical signs indistinguishable from idiopathic DC. Recent investigations have indicated that the likely site of disease is subcellular, and in some cases dilated cardiomyopathy is reversible upon supplementation of a deficient micronutrient. American cocker spaniels with DC are taurine and possibly carnitine deficient and usually respond to supplementation. Some large breed dogs (a family of boxer dogs has been reported) are carnitine deficient and responsive to supplementation.

II. Pathology

Global dilation of all four cardiac chambers is common. Marked volume overload ventricular hypertrophy creates the ventricular chamber enlargement and is characterized by a marked increase in heart weight and chamber enlargement, with wall thicknesses that are normal to thinner than normal. Endomyocardial fibrosis may be present, as well as dilatation of the atrioventricular valve annuli. The AV valves are generally normal or show minimal degenerative change. Histologic manifestations of idiopathic DC are nonspecific. The cells are longer than normal, characteristic of eccentric hypertrophy. Myocardial degeneration, cytoplasmic vacuolization, necrosis, and fibrosis can usually be found, but the most remarkable finding usually is the vast amount of relatively normal appearing myocardium present. Except in rare cases of myocarditis (e.g., Chagas disease), inflammatory cells are sparse or absent.

III. Pathophysiology

Dilated cardiomyopathy is idiopathic primary myocardial failure. It occurs when a primary disease of the myocardium results in a decrease in myocardial contractility (myocardial failure). This disease progresses insidiously over a number of years. In the early and middle stages of the disease, the dog appears normal. The disease can usually only be identified by echocardiographic examination at this stage. As a consequence of the depression in myocardial

---

‡ Most effective at reducing life-threatening pleural effusion

contractility, end-systolic diameter and volume initially increase. The chamber eccentrically hypertrophies secondary to renal salt and water retention to increase end-diastolic diameter and volume (volume overload hypertrophy). This allows the heart to compensate for the depression in contractility and to maintain a normal stroke volume (amount of blood pumped with each beat) at a normal end-diastolic intraventricular pressure. As the disease progresses, myocardial contractility is further depressed and the heart grows even larger. At the end stage of the disease, the ability of the heart to hypertrophy further becomes markedly limited. As the kidneys retain more sodium and water, and as blood volume continues to increase without further chamber enlargement, the diastolic pressure in the ventricle increases. This increase in diastolic pressure backs up into the atrium, veins, and capillary bed behind the affected ventricle, causing edema. When the ventricular size is increased, AV valvular regurgitation commonly occurs, which may further aggravate the increase in atrial, venous and capillary pressures (although the amount of regurgitation is usually mild). Cardiac output may also become inadequate at this stage, resulting in clinical signs of hypoperfusion. Tachyarrhythmias, such as atrial fibrillation, may result in worsened hemodynamics and may promote further myocardial deterioration.

IV. Signalment

Affected dogs are predominantly male, middle-aged to geriatric, and large or giant breeds (Doberman pinschers, Great Danes, Irish wolfhounds, St. Bernards). Spaniels are a notable exception, with springer spaniels and cocker spaniels sometimes affected with this disease. A wide range of age groups may be affected, and dogs as young as 6 months of age or older than 10 years of age are recognized.

V. Diagnostic criteria of dilated cardiomyopathy

    A. The echocardiogram is considered the gold standard for diagnosis of dilated cardiomyopathy. Ventricular chamber enlargement with decreased ventricular shortening fraction is the feature most characteristic of this disorder.

    B. A presumptive diagnosis of dilated cardiomyopathy can usually be made under the following conditions

        1. Identification of a typical breed (dilated cardiomyopathy is unusual in an atypical or mixed breed dog)

        2. Radiographic evidence of generalized cardiomegaly

        3. Auscultation of a gallop sound (rhythm)

        4. Demonstration of objective signs of congestive heart failure on physical examination and radiography

        5. Evidence of cardiac arrhythmias (atrial fibrillation and ventricular tachyarrhythmias are most characteristic)

VI. Differential diagnoses

    1. Previously unrecognized congenital heart disease (especially PDA and mitral valve dysplasia)§

---

§ Most common and often difficult to differentiate in later stages when myocardial failure may be a prominent component

2. Mitral regurgitation due to degenerative valve disease in a larger breed dog§
3. Pericardial disease
4. Bacterial endocarditis
5. Primary cardiac arrhythmia
6. Severe endocrine deficiency (hypothyroidism, Addison's disease)
7. Neurologic disease (in the patient with syncope)

The Asymptomatic Patient

 I. History
    No visible signs of disease are present.
II. Clinical findings
    A. Physical examination
       Serendipitous detection of a systolic heart murmur (usually soft), an audible third heart sound (gallop sound), or an arrhythmia should prompt consideration of occult cardiomyopathy. The detection of cardiomegaly during routine thoracic radiography or during evaluation of another condition may be an early clue to the presence of myocardial disease. Occasionally an affected dog is identified via echocardiographic screening.
    B. Radiography
       The thoracic radiograph may be normal, or generalized mild-to-moderate cardiomegaly, most commonly left-sided, may be evident. Pulmonary venous distention may indicate incipient heart failure.
    C. Electrocardiography
       The ECG may be normal or demonstrate left-heart enlargement, a ventricular conduction abnormality, or isolated atrial or ventricular premature complexes.
    D. Echocardiography
       End-systolic diameter is always increased because of the decrease in myocardial contractility. End-diastolic diameter is usually increased to compensate for the myocardial failure. In most cases where echocardiographic evidence of myocardial failure is present in the absence of clinical signs, the cardiac chambers are usually at or slightly above the upper limits of normal for end-diastolic diameter, and left ventricular shortening fraction (SF) is depressed (SF usually is between 15 and 25 percent) due to the increase in end-systolic diameter. However, a lower SF may occasionally be observed in asymptomatic patients.
    E. Therapy
       1. See Appendix 2 for specific medicaments and dosage recommendations
       2. The ISACHC recommendations to treat canine patients with dilated cardiomyopathy in asymptomatic heart failure are not agreed upon at present.
          a) Some members believe therapeutic intervention is appropriate at this stage (Class 1A) in light of convincing data from other species. Others decline to recommend therapy at this point since there are no canine studies from which to base a therapeutic recommendation.

    b) Those Council members in favor of intervening therapeutically in echocardiographically confirmed cases of dilated cardiomyopathy (Class 1B) suggest one or more of the following medicaments:

       (1) ACE inhibitors

       (2) Digitalis

       (3) L-carnitine or taurine supplementation can be supplemented if a deficiency is clearly documented. Studies are in progress to determine the benefits of supplementation of both in American cocker spaniels with the disease. Preliminary results of this study are promising. Further studies will be needed before a consensus can be reached by the council members.

Mild-to-Moderate Signs of Heart Failure

What differentiates the mild-to-moderate class of heart failure from the asymptomatic class is that signs of heart failure have become evident to the client and are often visible at the time of presentation.

I. History

Common historical findings include dyspnea, cough, weight loss, exercise intolerance, lethargy, and depression. The onset of left-sided congestive heart failure is heralded by tachypnea and respiratory distress. Affected dogs may exhibit a mild or intermittent cough. Dogs with right-heart failure commonly have ascites.

II. Clinical findings

A. Physical examination

Dogs with mild-to-moderate heart failure due to dilated cardiomyopathy are often thin and may have experienced significant weight loss. Lack of weight loss does not rule out the disease, however. Careful auscultation usually indicates the presence of a gallop sound (rhythm) or a murmur of mitral or tricuspid regurgitation. Cardiac rhythm abnormalities may be evident on auscultation and palpation of the femoral pulse. The arterial pulse is normal to hypokinetic. Jugular venous pressure is usually normal in mild heart failure but may become elevated with progression of disease. Left-sided congestive heart failure is typical and is characterized on physical examination by an increased respiratory rate. End-inspiratory crackles may sometimes be identified. Early signs of right-heart failure include elevated jugular venous pressure, hepatomegaly, and a suspicion of ascites.

B. Radiography

Typical findings are of left-sided or generalized cardiomegaly with left atrial enlargement, pulmonary venous distention, and increased pulmonary densities typical of pulmonary edema. A small pleural effusion also may be evident. Hepatomegaly is a common finding on abdominal radiography.

C. Electrocardiography

Cardiac rhythm disturbances are common and include atrial premature complexes, ventricular premature complexes, paroxysmal ventricular tachycardia, and more sustained tachyarrhythmias. Atrial fibrillation may be evident in some cases; however, in dogs with myocardial failure, atrial fibrillation usually leads to signs of advanced congestive heart failure. P waves may be abnormal (usually widened) and alterations in the QRS morphology are expected. Changes may include deep Q waves, increased amplitude R waves, widened QRS complexes, and slurring of the R wave descent. Nonspecific ST segment and T wave changes are also commonplace.

D. Echocardiography

Characteristic features are a marked increased in end-systolic diameter with secondary left ventricular eccentric (volume overload) hypertrophy (moderately increased end-diastolic diameter) resulting in left ventricular hypokinesis (SF usually <15 percent), increased separation between the ventricular septum and opening (E point) of the septal mitral leaflet, and varying degrees of regional left ventricular wall dysfunction. Variable and chaotic contraction of the ventricular walls is typical in patients with atrial fibrillation. Color flow Doppler echocardiography usually reveals a small mitral regurgitant jet. Ultrasound of the liver in cases with right-heart failure demonstrates enlarged hepatic veins.

E. Therapy

1. See Appendix 2 for specific medicaments and dosage recommendations
2. Treatment recommendations by ISACHC for this mild-to-moderate class of heart failure are as follows
   a) Digitalis glycosides
   b) Diuretic therapy
   c) ACE inhibitor
   d) Antiarrhythmic therapy when indicated (digoxin, beta blocker, diltiazem for atrial fibrillation; ventricular antiarrhythmic drugs for ventricular arrhythmias)
   e) Dietary sodium restriction, if tolerated
   f) L-carnitine or taurine may be supplemented when appropriate based on suitable laboratory tests. Both should be administered to American cocker spaniels with DC
   g) Beta blockers‖

Advanced Heart Failure

I. History

This is the most common presentation for the canine patient with this disease. Onset of the disease oftentimes appears acute to the owner even though the disease has been progressing for years. What differentiates advanced heart failure from mild-to-moderate heart failure is the more severe and obvious nature of the clinical signs of disease. Clinical findings such as dyspnea at rest,

---

‖ The Council could not reach a consensus regarding the efficacy and advisability of low-dose beta blocker therapy. Beta blockers are efficacious at improving myocardial function in some people with dilated cardiomyopathy. No studies have shown efficacy of this approach in the dog and pilot studies have not been encouraging.

markedly diminished exercise tolerance, or severe ascites or pleural effusion indicates a patient with advanced congestive heart failure. Pallor of the mucous membranes, weak femoral pulses, and cold extremities may be evident and indicate poor peripheral perfusion.

II. Clinical findings

A. Physical examination

Dogs with dilated cardiomyopathy in advanced heart failure are oftentimes cachectic, weak, lethargic, anorectic, and dyspneic. Dogs in cardiogenic shock from severe hypoperfusion may be moribund. Sinus tachycardia, atrial fibrillation, or sinus rhythm with premature ventricular complexes are usually detected. A gallop sound (rhythm) is a consistent finding but may be difficult to detect in arrhythmic patients and by untrained personnel. Systolic murmurs of mitral or tricuspid regurgitation may be heard. The arterial pulse may be hypokinetic and may be irregular, owing to a cardiac arrhythmia. Elevated jugular venous pressure is possible. Most cases of advanced heart failure manifest severe left-sided or biventricular heart failure; and the physical findings of pulmonary edema (respiratory distress, tachypnea), pleural effusion (respiratory distress, tachypnea, muffled heart sounds), or both, will be evident.

B. Radiography

Cardiomegaly is usually moderate to severe and the heart is usually globally enlarged. Cardiomegaly may be difficult to appreciate in some deepchested cases, especially in Doberman pinschers. Pulmonary venous distention, alveolar lung infiltrates of pulmonary edema, and/or pleural effusion will be evident.

C. Electrocardiography

Previously described electrocardiographic abnormalities are expected. Atrial fibrillation or sinus rhythm with paroxysmal ventricular tachycardia is very common at this stage.

D. Echocardiography

Previously described echocardiographic abnormalities are present. Moreover, pleural and small pericardial effusions secondary to heart failure may be observed.

E. Therapy

Dilated cardiomyopathy is associated with a higher mortality rate than other diseases that lead to heart failure. ACE inhibitors have been shown to prolong survival in both dogs and other species with dilated cardiomyopathy. Beta blockers have been shown to prolong survival in other species with dilated cardiomyopathy; however, studies in dogs are lacking and preliminary studies are discouraging. Dogs with dilated cardiomyopathy die from heart failure and die suddenly (presumably from ventricular arrhythmias deteriorating into ventricular fibrillation). Therapy outlined here is for heart failure. Effective therapy to prevent sudden death has not been elucidated in dogs. Typical ventricular antiarrhythmics can be tried but are oftentimes disappointing.

Advanced heart failure is subdivided therapeutically into two subclasses: home care is possible at this time and hospitalization is mandatory for patient stabilization.

This subclass is assigned when the patient has developed life-threatening pulmonary edema or pleural effusion, or exhibits cardiogenic shock. Dogs with refractory ascites also may be assigned to this sublcass pending improvement of their heart failure state.

1. Therapy—home care is possible
    a) See Appendix 2 for specific medicaments and dosage recommendations
    b) The ISACHC recommendations to treat canine patients with advanced heart failure due to dilated cardiomyopathy (home care)
        (1) Digitalis
        (2) Diuretic therapy
        (3) ACE inhibitor
        (4) Dietary sodium restriction, if diet is accepted
        (5) Antiarrhythmic drug therapy, when appropriate, to control heart rate in atrial fibrillation (e.g. digoxin, diltiazem, beta-blocker) or when required to suppress ventricular ectopia (e.g. procainamide, tocainide, etc.)
        (6) No consensus was reached regarding the use of low-dose beta blockade therapy in this stage of cardiomyopathy. There was a consensus, however, that beta blockade was appropriate if used to control ventricular rate response in dogs with atrial fibrillation.
    c) Alternative therapies
        (1) Hydralazine
        (2) Nitrates
        (3) Bronchodilators (theophylline and related compounds)
            Note: Alternative therapy is generally added in step-wise fashion in those cases where additional drug therapy is warranted due to progressive signs of cardiac failure. Hydralazine is particularly likely to be helpful when there is concurrent moderate mitral regurgitation. When combination vasodilator therapy is contemplated, the clinician should be mindful that this therapy may be associated with clinically significant hypotension and impaired renal perfusion. Blood pressure monitoring should be available. Consultation with a board certified cardiologist is encouraged.
2. Therapy—hospitalization is mandatory
    a) See Appendix 2 for specific medicaments and dosage recommendations
    b) ISACHC recommendations
        (1) Intravenous diuretic therapy (furosemide¶ or another loop diuretic)
        (2) Dobutamine¶ or amrinone infusion
        (3) Oxygen therapy
        (4) Preload reduction using nitroglycerine ointment or sodium nitroprusside¶ (arterial blood pressure must be monitored during sodium nitroprusside therapy)

¶ Most effective drugs for controlling severe pulmonary edema

     (5) Morphine

     (6) Theophylline may be considered (beware of aggravation of cardiac arrhythmias)

     Cautionary note: Arterial blood pressure should be critically evaluated in these cases.

  c) Cardiac arrhythmias represent a special concern in dilated cardiomyopathy, and, when present, antiarrhythmic drug therapy should be prescribed.

     (1) Atrial arrhythmias (particularly atrial fibrillation)

       i) Digoxin

       ii) Beta blockade

       iii) Diltiazem

         Cautionary notes: Both diltiazem and beta blockers depress myocardial contractility at higher doses. In using these drugs to control ventricular rate response, a low initial starting dose should be chosen (01. to 0.2 mg/kg PO TID for propranolol and 0.5 mg/kg PO TID for diltiazem). Incremental doses should be used to gradually obtain the desired heart rate effect.

     (2) Ventricular arrhythmias

       i) Isolated or periodic ventricular extrasystoles

         No consensus was reached by the Council regarding the treatment of these isolated rhythm disturbances; however, the use of Holter monitoring or additional consultation was believed to be worthwhile.

       ii) Sustained ventricular arrhythmias

         (*A*) Lidocaine

         (*B*) Procainamide

         (*C*) Tocainide

         (*D*) Mexiletine

         (*E*) Quinidine

CANINE DIROFILARIASIS

  I. Definition

    Heartworm disease is the clinical manifestation of *Dirofilaria immitis* parasitism (dirofilariasis). Adult filariae injure the pulmonary vascular tree and the lung, leading to pulmonary artery injury and, when severe, pulmonary hypertension and a pressure overload on the right ventricle. The heart and lung are usually the principal organs injured in advanced dirofilariasis.

  II. Pathology

    The parasite *Dirofilaria immitis* injures the pulmonary artery endothelium, resulting in swelling, altered intracellular junctions, and platelet and leucocyte activation. These activated cells release factors that stimulate collagen formation, intimal thickening and proliferation, and medial hypertrophy of the pulmonary arteries. Intimal smooth muscle cells proliferate and migrate toward the surface producing villus proliferation from the pulmonary arterial surface.

Consequent to these changes, the pulmonary arteries enlarge and narrow. Pulmonary thromboemboli (presumably secondary to dead adult worms) and exuberant microvillus formation may produce blunting of (blockage of blood flow through) the pulmonary arteries. This is most commonly associated with the development of pulmonary hypertension. Pulmonary parenchymal reactions also may occur in heartworm disease. Sequestration and reaction to sequestered microfilaria in the lung parenchyma may cause pneumonitis. The exact mechanisms of pulmonary injury are not fully elucidated but include eosinophilic pneumonitis, as well as pulmonary thrombosis and infarction secondary to worm death and pulmonary fibrosis. The severity of heartworm disease is often, but not always, related to the parasite burden. Dogs that are severely allergic to the parasites commonly have severe pulmonary arterial and pulmonary parenchymal disease and are commonly amicrofilaremic. In cases of large numbers of adult parasites, retrograde migration of worms into the right atrium and tricuspid valve apparatus may occur (caval syndrome).

III. Pathophysiology

The presence of adult heartworms in the pulmonary arteries leads to the aforementioned anatomic changes in those pulmonary arteries infested by the adult worms. Pulmonary artery changes in the areas where the heartworms lie can be identified radiographically. The result of these vascular changes include narrowing of the vascular lumina and limitation of pulmonary blood flow. If the pulmonary artery disease is severe and especially if thromboemboli are present, pulmonary vascular resistance increases to the point that significant pulmonary hypertension develops. If severe pulmonary hypertension develops, right heart enlargement (eccentric hypertrophy) and right heart failure may ensue. Why the heart develops eccentric—rather than the expected concentric—hypertrophy is unknown. Pulmonary parenchymal reaction, which may lead to alveolar hypoxia, adds a reversible aspect of vasoconstriction which further increases pulmonary vascular resistance. In the most advanced cases of dirofilariasis, the affected dog has marked exercise intolerance and may develop right-sided congestive heart failure.

IV. Signalment

There are no age or breed predilections per se; however, large breed, male dogs are predisposed epidemiologically to this condition. This predisposition is probably related to the more frequent use of such dogs in outdoor environments. Owing to the life cycle of this parasite, the earliest signs of heartworm disease are not likely to be seen prior to 7 months of age.

V. Diagnostic criteria

A. Identification of circulating microfilaria of *Dirofilaria immitis* (in the absence of probable transplacental transfer of microfilaria) (microfilaria must be differentiated from those of *Dipetalonema reconditum*)

B. A positive serologic test for adult heartworm antigen, especially with typical signs and/or radiographic changes of heartworm disease

C. Clinical signs of exercise intolerance, coughing, or right-sided congestive heart failure in the face of compatible radiographic changes (a heartworm antigen test is also recommended to verify the diagnosis)

VI. Differential diagnoses

A. Primary respiratory disorders including infectious, parasitic, inflammatory, and neoplastic disease

B. Pulmonary neoplasia—primary or metastatic
C. Other forms of cardiac disease (dilated cardiomyopathy, tricuspid valve malformation or endocardiosis, congenital heart disease, pericardial disease)

The Asymptomatic Patient

I. History
Diagnosis of asymptomatic dirofilariasis is most often made during routine screening for heartworm disease (microfilaria detection and serum heartworm antigen detection). Asymptomatic dogs show absolutely no clinical signs of heartworm disease.
II. Clinical findings
A. Physical examination
No abnormalities are usually identified on physical examination.
B. Radiography
Thoracic radiographs may be normal or may show varying degrees of pulmonary artery enlargement, pulmonary artery blunting, pulmonary artery tortuosity, main pulmonary artery enlargement, and right heart enlargement.
C. Electrocardiography
The electrocardiogram is usually normal at this stage.
D. Echocardiography
The echocardiogram is usually normal at this stage although mild right-heart enlargement and main pulmonary artery enlargement may be identified.
E. Therapy
Follow the recommendations of the American Heartworm Society

Mild-to-Advanced Heart Failure

I. History
Historical complaints usually include exercise intolerance, possible syncope, and loss of condition. If there are concurrent pulmonary parenchymal complications, then difficult breathing, tachypnea, and coughing are frequent signs. The opportunity for frequent exposure to mosquitoes and a lax preventative program are obvious risk factors for development of advanced dirofilariasis.
II. Clinical findings
A. Physical examination
1. Clinical signs of advanced heartworm disease can generally be grouped into respiratory signs, cardiovascular signs, signs referable to caval syndrome, and signs secondary to other disorders occurring secondary to heartworm infestation (renal disease, disseminated intravascular coagulopathy, anemia, dysproteinemia)
2. Respiratory signs generally include tachypnea, dyspnea, coughing, and occasionally hemoptysis (probably related to rupture and hemorrhage

of bronchial or pulmonary arteries into the lung parenchyma). These signs are due to heartworm infestation, not to heart failure. Cardiovascular signs which are related to pulmonary vascular changes and pulmonary hypertension include weakness (oftentimes episodic), exercise intolerance, syncope, and clinical signs of right-sided congestive heart failure.

Dogs with advanced heartworm disease have generally lost weight and have a poor hair coat. Auscultation of the heart may demonstrate a normal heart rhythm or occasionally premature complexes or even atrial fibrillation. The second heart sound may be normal, louder than normal, or rarely even split, a consequence of pulmonary hypertension. A systolic murmur of tricuspid regurgitation may be evident over the right hemithorax. The arterial pulse is usually normal but the central venous pressure will be increased when heart failure has occurred. Jugular vein distension and pulsations are common in advanced dirofilariasis. Auscultation of the lungs may demonstrate increased bronchial sounds or crackles if there is pulmonary parenchymal reaction to the parasite or if there has been substantial pulmonary thromboembolism. Clinical signs of right-sided congestive heart failure include hepatomegaly and ascites.

B. Radiography

Radiographic changes include right ventricular and possibly right atrial enlargement. Increased size of the main pulmonary artery commonly occurs. In advanced cases, a reversed "D" configuration to the cardiac silhouette is evident. Lobar pulmonary arteries become dilated, tortuous, and blunted (pruning of the arteries). These changes are typically most severe in the dorsal regions of the caudal lung lobes. Increased lung densities are often evident and may be related to noncardiogenic edema, eosinophilic infiltrates, pulmonary embolism and infarction, or pulmonary fibrosis.

C. Electrocardiography

The electrocardiogram is often normal in heartworm disease; however, with pulmonary hypertension sufficient to cause right-heart failure, changes in the P waves and QRS complexes may occur. Interestingly, P pulmonale (increased P wave voltage) is relatively uncommon in heartworm disease; however, widening of the P wave may be an indication of right atrial enlargement or conduction delay. An axis deviation to the right, characterized by prominent S waves in leads I, II, aVF, and the lower left chest leads, is usually observed in those cases with severe right ventricular enlargement and/or right-heart failure. Rhythm disturbances ranging from sinus tachycardia to more profound irregularities, including right ventricular extrasystoles and atrial fibrillation, may be present.

D. Echocardiography

1. Echocardiography can be used to document enlargement of the right ventricle. Clinical usefulness of echocardiography is more evident in cases of caval syndrome where masses of heartworms can be readily identified in the tricuspid valve orifice or in some cases of occult dirofilariasis where adult heartworms may be visible in the pulmonary arteries

by high-quality, two-dimensional echocardiograms. Echocardiography may attain greater prominence with the use of flexible alligator forceps to manually remove heartworms from the pulmonary arteries.

2. Echocardiographic manifestations of advanced heartworm disease leading to right heart-failure include right atrial, right ventricular, and pulmonary artery dilation. Flattening and abnormal motion of the ventricular septum is typical of right ventricular pressure or volume overload. Linear echogenic densities compatible with those of adult heartworms may be evident in the main pulmonary artery or occasionally in the heart chambers proper. Left ventricular contractility is preserved but the left ventricular luminal dimensions are usually decreased in size which may decrease shortening fraction.

E. Therapy
   1. See Appendix 2 for specific medicaments and dosage recommendations
   2. Therapy for dogs presented in moderate-to-severe heart failure
      a) Diuretic therapy: Maintenance therapy with a loop diuretic such as furosemide is recommended as initial treatment for congestive heart failure. The council recommends the administration of a second diuretic (hydrochlorothiazide or hydrochlorothiazide plus spironolactone, or triamterene) in the event of refractory ascites. The possibility of malabsorption of orally administered diuretics must also be considered, and parenteral administration of loop diuretics maybe highly effective in some patients.
      b) Cage rest is essential in dogs with heart failure caused by dirofilariasis. Benefits include improved mobilization of edema and possibly increased survival following adulticide administration.
      c) Digitalis glycosides may be beneficial in treatment of heart failure caused by dirofilariasis. While the use of digitalis glycosides has been controversial in this setting, the Council believes the drug may be effective and may be safe provided careful monitoring of serum digoxin levels occurs and conservative doses are provided initially.
      d) Aspirin therapy: Although commonly recommended to reduce pulmonary vascular reaction, no consensus was reached by the Council regarding the benefits of aspirin use. When aspirin is prescribed, strict attention must be directed to the possible development of gastric ulceration.
      e) Flexible forceps catheters that can be advanced into the pulmonary artery have been employed successfully for manual removal of heartworms in other parts of the world. This procedure may become standard treatment in the United States in the future.
      f) Antiarrhythmic therapy: Occasionally antiarrhythmic drug therapy is required in the management of arrhythmias associated with heartworm disease.
      g) ACE inhibitor therapy: Although the benefits of ACE inhibitor therapy in left-sided and biventricular heart failure have been documented, the benefits in isolated right-heart failure caused by pulmonary hypertension have not been studied. For this reason, the Council recommends careful monitoring of any patients receiving this form of therapy.

h) Thiacetarsemide administration should be attempted if and when heart failure is stabilized. Successful adulticide therapy may result in significant regression of the pulmonary hypertension. Consequently, successful adulticide therapy may result in regression of signs of heart failure.

FELINE HYPERTROPHIC CARDIOMYOPATHY

I. Definition
Feline hypertrophic cardiomyopathy is an idiopathic myocardial disorder characterized by concentric hypertrophy (thickened walls with a normal to small size chamber) of the left ventricle. The diagnosis of feline hypertrophic cardiomyopathy is one of exclusion. Other potential known causes of left ventricular concentric hypertrophy in the cat include congenital subaortic stenosis, congenital aortic stenosis, hyperthyroid heart disease, systemic hypertension, and acromegaly.

II. Pathology
Left ventricular concentric hypertrophy is the essential feature of this condition. The ventricular free wall and ventricular septum are most commonly thickened symmetrically but there may be asymmetric thickening of either the ventricular septum or the left ventricular free wall. Papillary muscle thickening is typical. In some cases, the left ventricular outlet appears narrowed, as a consequence of septal hypertrophy adjacent to the septal mitral leaflet. Histologically, myocardial hypertrophy is the primary abnormality. In 30 percent of cats, disorganization of myocytes may be observed. Interstitial and interfibral fibrosis may be observed and may particularly involve the conduction system of the ventricles. Sclerosis and narrowing of intramural coronary arteries is a frequent microscopic feature. The left atrium is commonly distended and also hypertrophied, and thrombi may be observed in this chamber or remote to the heart. A frequent complication of feline hypertrophic cardiomyopathy is a distant thromboembolus which typically lodges at the iliac trifurcation.

III. Pathophysiology
Hypertrophic cardiomyopathy is a disease characterized by diastolic dysfunction of the left ventricle. As a consequence of many factors—gross hypertrophy of the wall, myocardial fibrosis, possibly insufficient coronary perfusion—the left ventricle becomes stiff and less distensible. Elevated left atrial pressure is required to fill this chamber and leads to dilation and hypertrophy of the left atrium. Chronic elevations in left ventricular diastolic pressure are translated into the pulmonary vascular tree, leading to pulmonary venous congestion and edema. The two major syndromes recognized in cats with feline hypertrophic cardiomyopathy are congestive heart failure and aortic thromboembolism. Stresses that lead to tachycardia may abruptly increase left ventricular stiffness by increasing myocardial oxygen demand. Functional abnormalities of relaxation may ensue, which further impair ventricular filling. This may explain some cases of acute pulmonary edema that develop in cats that were previously well compensated for their disease.

Additional functional abnormalities may develop during systole. Mitral regurgitation is common in cats with hypertrophic cardiomyopathy and may be explained by either geometric changes in the left ventricle and papillary muscles, or systolic anterior motion of the mitral valve during systole. Movement of the anterior (septal) mitral valve towards the ventricular septum in systole may be associated with narrowing of the left ventricular outlet, generation of a pressure gradient, and a functional outflow obstruction. The overall significance of outflow obstruction in this disease is at this time unresolved.

IV. Signalment

The age range of this disease complex is very broad, ranging from 5 months of age to 14 years. Males are affected far more commonly than females. Domestic short-hair cats, followed by domestic long-hair cats, appear to be most frequently affected. This disease prevalence is due to breed prevalence. A genetic form of the disease is present in Maine coon cats and may be present in other breeds as well.

V. Diagnostic criteria

A. Hypertrophic cardiomyopathy should always ruled out whenever cardiomegaly (especially left atrial enlargement), a gallop rhythm or murmur of mitral insufficiency, and typical signs compatible with the disease, including thromboembolism and left-sided congestive heart failure, are identified. Definitive diagnosis of hypertrophic cardiomyopathy must rely on either echocardiographic or angiographic evidence of left ventricular hypertrophy. Moreover, other known causes of left ventricular hypertrophy must be excluded before this diagnosis can be made.

B. Echocardiographic evidence of left ventricular hypertrophy, generally associated with left atrial enlargement, is sufficient evidence of hypertrophic cardiomyopathy in an absence of other causes of ventricular hypertrophy.

C. Selective or nonselective angiography may be used to demonstrate left ventricular hypertrophy; however, these techniques are invasive and are not recommended when echocardiography is available.

VI. Differential diagnoses

A. Other forms of cardiomyopathy (restrictive, dilated)
B. Myocarditis
C. Hyperthyroidism
D. Hypertensive heart disease
E. Congenital or acquired valvular disease
F. Congenital heart disease
G. Peritoneal-pericardial diaphragmatic hernia

The Asymptomatic Patient

I. History

These cats do not exhibit any historical or clinical signs of disease. The diagnosis is most commonly made after the serendipitous detection of a systolic cardiac murmur or gallop rhythm during the course of a clinical examination. Some cats are recognized when cardiomegaly is detected when thoracic radiography is undertaken for another reason. Others may be identified because of echocardiographic screening for the disease.

II. Clinical findings

  A. Physical examination

    The most frequent clinical findings in asymptomatic cats are the presence of a left apical/sternal border systolic murmur of mitral regurgitation or a gallop sound (rhythm).

  B. Radiography

    The thoracic radiograph may appear normal or may show evidence of left atrial and left ventricular enlargement. No pulmonary edema is present.

  C. Electrocardiography

    The electrocardiogram may be normal or show evidence of left ventricular enlargement or left axis deviation.

  D. Echocardiography

    The diagnosis of hypertrophic cardiomyopathy relies on echocardiography. At this stage there may be very mild left ventricular wall thickening that may be diffuse or focal. However, there may also be severe left ventricular wall thickening with or without mild left atrial enlargement or there may be anything in between these two extremes.

  E. Therapy

    1. See Appendix 2 for specific medicaments and dosage recommendations

    2. The ISACHC recommendations to treat feline patients with hypertrophic cardiomyopathy that are asymptomatic include the following:

      a) Diltiazem or a beta blocker (propranolol or atenolol): The Council could not reach a consensus regarding the superiority of either agent in this circumstance, but the members believe that one of these two medicaments should be prescribed.

      b) Aspirin therapy, administered orally every third day: The Council could not reach a consensus of opinion regarding the efficacy of this therapy.

Mild-to-Moderate Signs of Heart Failure

  I. History

Clinical signs of mild-to-moderate heart failure generally include decreased activity (difficult to document in a cat), tachypnea, exertional dyspnea, and nonspecific signs of anorexia, listlessness, and sometimes coughing. Coughing is usually mistaken for vomiting by the owner. Some cats with hypertrophic cardiomyopathy may be affected by aortic thromboembolism; yet, minimal, if any, signs of congestive heart failure may occur.

II. Clinical findings

  A. Physical examination

    Cats, unlike dogs, often maintain body condition, and may, in fact, be overweight. Many cats have abnormal cardiac auscultation that is characterized by either sinus tachycardia, the presence of occasional premature beats, a systolic murmur near the left apex and along the sternal border, or a gallop sound (rhythm). Arterial pulses are usually normal, unless there is an aortic thromboembolus. The jugular venous pressure is usually normal. Cats with left-sided heart failure rarely cough (although they may with tracheal palpation in the exam room), but most demonstrate tachypnea. Auscultation of the lungs may reveal fine inspiratory crackles related to pulmonary edema, or simply harsh bronchointerstitial sounds. If an aortic thromboembolus is present, typical vascular, musculoskeletal, and neurologic deficits will be evident. Typical features include cold limbs, absent or very weak pulses, paresis, contracture of effected muscle groups, pain, and progressive lower motor neuron neuropathy.

B. Radiography

Cardiomegaly is evident, and is most prominent on the dorsoventral view where the left auricle will be increased in size. Generally, there is mild elongation of the cardiac silhouette compatible with left ventricular hypertrophy. In some—but not all—cats, the heart assumes a valentine appearance on the dorsoventral projection. Pulmonary edema is evident as an increased interstitial or alveolar pattern and is frequently patchy and focal in appearance. Unlike the dog, perihilar lung edema is not a consistent feature of congestive heart failure in cats.

C. Electrocardiography

A wide variety of electrocardiographic abnormalities have been detected in this disease. In some cats the ECG is normal. Other cats manifest increased amplitude or duration P waves compatible with atrial enlargement. Increased amplitude R waves or a left cranial axis deviation may be observed and are suggestive of left ventricular hypertrophy or left anterior fascicular block. Increased duration of the QRS complex also may be recognized.

D. Echocardiography

This modality is the most accurate technique for diagnosing hypertrophic cardiomyopathy and is also helpful in assessing the severity of disease. Typical echocardiographic findings include ventricular septal, left ventricular wall, and papillary muscle hypertrophy. Left ventricular luminal size is usually—but not always—decreased. The left atrium is enlarged in symptomatic cats. The shortening fraction is usually normal to elevated, indicating maintenance of systolic contractile function. Abnormal systolic motion of the septal (anterior) mitral leaflet may be observed, particularly in cats with a narrowed left ventricular outflow tract. Thrombi may occasionally be identified in the left atrium or left atrial appendage.

E. Therapy

1. See Appendix 2 for specific medicaments and dosage recommendations
2. The ISACHC recommends to treat feline patients with hypertrophic cardiomyopathy and mild-to-moderate heart failure as follows
   a) Furosemide
   b) Minimize stress
   c) Diltiazem or a beta blocker: the Council could not reach a consensus regarding the superiority of one of these treatments over the other. *Note:* The use of nonspecific beta blockers should be avoided in the presence of pulmonary edema. Beta blockers may be prescribed, however, following resolution of pulmonary edema

d) Nitrates: Nitrates may be beneficial as supplemental treatment for pulmonary edema or if the cat is resistant to oral administration of medicaments

e) Antiarrhythmic therapy if an abnormal cardiac rhythm is identified and is sustained

f) Dietary sodium restriction, if tolerated by the cat

Advanced Heart Failure

To be classified with advanced heart failure, the cat must demonstrate obvious signs of congestive heart failure, usually characterized as respiratory distress. Respiratory distress can usually be traced to the presence of alveolar pulmonary edema and occasionally pleural effusion, or both.

 I. History
II. Clinical findings
   A. Physical examination
      The physical findings of advanced heart failure in cats are an extension of those previously noted. Severe pulmonary edema will be manifested as dyspnea, tachypnea, cyanosis, and possibly identification of widespread pulmonary crackles. Some cats may have evidence of a pleural fluid line, muffling of heart sounds, and dullness to percussion if pleural effusion is present. Signs of thromboembolism are evident in some cats. A systolic murmur or gallop rhythm is almost always evident, and sinus tachycardia or even atrial fibrillation may be identified.
   B. Electrocardiography
      Electrocardiographic findings are typical of those previously mentioned. In addition, there is a greater tendency toward atrial and ventricular dysrhythmias. Cats with massive left atrial dilation may develop atrial fibrillation, which is poorly tolerated in cats with this disease.
   C. Radiography
      Radiography demonstrates cardiomegaly, which may be more generalized. There is usually marked left atrial and auricular appendage enlargement. Diffuse alveolar infiltrates of pulmonary edema or pleural effusion are evident.
   D. Echocardiography
      The echocardiographic features are those previously mentioned. Left atrial enlargement is usually more severe.
   E. Therapy
      1. See Appendix 2 for specific medicaments and dosage recommendations
      2. As a general rule, the hospital and home care of cats with hypertrophic cardiomyopathy and severe congestive heart failure is qualitatively similar
      3. The ISACHC recommendations to treat feline patients with advanced heart failure due to hypertrophic cardiomyopathy include the following
         a) Oxygen therapy

b) Diltiazem with or without a beta blocker: the Council generally agreed that diltiazem was preferable to a beta blocker in this setting.
c) Furosemide
d) Nitrate and/or ACE inhibitor
e) Thoracocentesis if pleural effusion is present
f) Referral if the patient is persistently difficult to manage

Appendix 2
Common Cardiovascular Drugs*
Francis W. K. Smith, Jr.

Advancing technology has provided clinicians with ever more powerful and effective drugs for treating diseases. As more drugs become available, it becomes progressively more difficult for practitioners to make rational choices between similar drugs. It is also difficult to be aware of the numerous side effects, contraindications, and drug interactions of the many cardiopulmonary drugs available. The following tables and charts have been designed and provided in the hope of facilitating rational drug selections for the treatment of cardiopulmonary disease.

An attempt has been made to make these tables as complete as possible, while focusing on the more common or serious side effects and drug interactions. For a more exhaustive review of individual drugs, the reader should refer to the package insert and drug chapters in this book. The reader should also follow the current veterinary literature, as new dosing recommendations may become available as a result of clinical use and scientific research. This advice is especially appropriate for new or infrequently used drugs.

DISCLOSURE

Medicine is a science that is constantly changing. Changes in treatment and drug therapy are required with new research and clinical experiences. The author, editor, and publisher of this book have made every effort to ensure that the drug dosage schedules are accurate. The drug dosages are based on the standards accepted at the time of publication. The product information sheet included in the package of each drug should be checked before the drug is administered to be certain that changes have not been made in the recommended dose of or in the contraindications for administration. Primary responsibility for decisions regarding treatment of patients remains with the attending clinician. All patients should be carefully monitored for desired efficacious and undesired toxic effects while instituting, titrating, and maintaining therapy.

Drugs are listed in alphabetical order by generic name. The order of presentation in no way reflects the preference for use. General recommendations for therapy may be found in the main body of this document.

---

* The tables in this appendix are adapted from Tilley LP, Smith FWK, Miller MS: Cardiology Pocket Reference. 2nd Ed. American Animal Hospital Association, 1990, with permission.

FUNCTIONAL CLASSIFICATION OF CARDIOPULMONARY DRUGS

Antiarrhythmic Class 1
    Class 1A
        Disopyramide*
        Procainamide
        Quinidine gluconate
        Quinidine polygalacturonate
        Quinidine sulfate
    Class 1B
        Lidocaine
        Mexiletine
        Phenytoin
        Tocainide
    Class 1C
        Flecanide*

Antiarrhythmic Class 2
    Nonselective β blocker
        Nadolol*
        Pindolol*
        Propranolol
        Timolol*
    Selective β1 blocker
        Atenolol
        Metoprolol

Antiarrhythmic Class 3
        Amiodarone*
        Bretylium tosylate*

Antiarrhythmic Class 4
    Calcium Entry Blocker
        Diltiazem
        Verapamil

Anticholinergic
        Atropine sulfate
        Glycopyrrolate
        Isopropamide iodide
        Propantheline bromide

Antithrombotic
    Anticoagulant
        Heparin
        Warfarin
    Platelet inhibitor
        Acetylsalicylic acid

Bronchodilator
    Catecholamine
        Albuterol
        Terbutaline
    Combination
        Marax
    Xanthine
        Aminophylline
        Oxtriphylline
        Theophylline

Cardiac inotropic agent
    Bipyrimidine derivative
        Amrinone
        Milrinone*

    Catecholamine
        Dobutamine HCl
        Dopamine HCl
        Epinephrine
        Isoproterenol
    Digitalis glycoside
        Digitoxin
        Digoxin

Cough suppressant
    Narcotic
        Butorphanol tartrate
        Hydrocodone bitartrate
    Nonnarcotic
        Dextromethorphan

Diuretic
    Loop
        Bumetanide*
        Furosemide
    Potassium sparing
        Spironolactone
        Triamterene
    Thiazide
        Chlorothiazide
        Hydrochlorothiazide

Heartworm medications
    Adulticide
        Thiacetarsamide
    Preventive
        Diethylcarbamazine
        Ivermectin
        Milbemycin oxime

Nutritional supplement
    Amino acid
        Carnitine
        Taurine

Respiratory stimulant
        Doxapram HCl

Vasodilator—Arteriolar
        Hydralazine HCl

Vasodilator—Balanced
    ACE inhibitor
        Benazepril
        Captopril
        Enalapril
    Alpha-1 adrenergic blocker
        Prazosin HCl
    Nitrate
        Nitroprusside sodium

Vasodilator—Venous
    Narcotic
        Morphine sulfate
    Nitrate
        Isosorbide dinitrate
        Nitroglycerin

* Rarely used in veterinary medicine or not commercially available (milrinone) and not included in the drug formulary.

TRADE NAME LISTING

Trade Name	Drug Name	Trade Name	Drug Name	Trade Name	Drug Name
Adrenalin	Epinephrine	Dilantin	Phenytoin	Lotensin	Benazepril
Aldactone	Spironolactone	Diuril	Chlorothiazide	Marax	Marax
Aminophyllin	Aminophylline	Dobutrex	Dobutamine	Mexitil	Mexiletine
Apresoline	Hydralazine		HCl	Minipress	Prazosin HCl
	HCl	Dopram	Doxapram HCl	Nipride,	Nitroprusside
Aspirin	Acetylsalicylic	Dyrenium	Triamterene	Nitropress	sodium
	acid	Enacard	Enalapril	Nitro-Bid,	Nitroglycerin
Brethine	Terbutaline	Filaribits	Diethylcarba-	Nitrol	
Calan	Verapamil		mazine	Pro-Banthine	Propantheline
Caparsolate	Thiacetarsa-	Heartgard-30	Ivermectin		bromide
	mide	Hycodan	Hydrocodone	Procan SR,	Procainamide
Capoten	Captopril		bitartrate	Pronestyl	
Caracide	Diethylcarba-	Hydrodiuril	Hydrochloro-	Proventil	Albuterol
	mazine		thiazide	Quinaglute	Quinidine
Cardioquin	Quinidine	Inderal	Propranolol	Dura-tabs	gluconate
	polygalactur-	Inocor	Amrinone	Quinidex	Quinidine
	onate	Interceptor	Milbemycin		sulfate
Cardizem	Diltiazem		oxime	Robinul	Glycopyrrolate
Cardoxin	Digoxin	Intropin	Dopamine HCl	Stadol	Butorphanol
Carnitor	Carnitine	Isoptin	Verapamil		tartrate
Choledyl	Oxtriphylline	Isordil	Isosorbide	Taurine V	Taurine
Coumadin	Warfarin		dinitrate	Tenormin	Atenolol
Crystodigin	Digitoxin	Isuprel	Isoproterenol	Theo-Dur	Theophylline
Darbid	Isopropamide	Lanoxin	Digoxin	Tonocard	Tocainide
	iodide	Lasix	Furosemide	Torbutrol	Butorphanol
Difil	Diethylcarba-	Liquaemin	Heparin		tartrate
	mazine	Lopressor	Metoprolol	Ventolin	Albuterol
				Xylocaine	Lidocaine

CARDIOPULMONARY DRUGS

Drug Trade Name	Formulation	Indications	Dog Dose (D) Cat Dose (C)	Comments
Acetylsalicylic acid* Aspirin	Tab: 81, 325 mg	Prevention of thromboembolism	D: 5–10 mg/kg PO SID C: 25 mg/kg PO q 3 days	Start 1 week prior to and continue 3–4 weeks post adulticide therapy in dogs with severe pulmonary vascular disease Not 100% effective in preventing emboli
Albuterol* (Proventil, Ventolin)	Tab: 2, 4 mg Syrup: 0.4 mg/ml	Bronchodilation in patients with reversible obstructive lung disease and asthma	D: 0.02–0.05 mg/kg PO TID C: None	Can be used in combination with xanthine bronchodilators β_2 agonist Decrease dose with renal disease
Aminophylline* (Aminophyllin)	Tab: 100, 200 mg Ampules: 25 mg/ml Oral solution: 21 mg/ml	Asthma, COPD	D: 11 mg/kg TID–QID, PO, IV, IM (slowly IV) C: 5 mg/kg BID–TID; PO, IV, IM (slowly IV) See comments	Reduce dose with CHF, liver disease, cimetidine, erythromycin, propranolol Therapeutic range as theophylline: 10–20 μg/ml Toxicity common with IV administration Dose on lean body weight
Amrinone (Inocor)	Ampul: 5 mg/ml	Short-term management of severe myocardial failure	D: 1–3 mg/kg bolus, then 30–100 μg/kg/min CRI (titrate up to effect) C: Same	Can use with digoxin and catecholamines Also has arteriolar dilating properties Do not administer in solutions with dextrose Pretreat with digitalis in patients with atrial fibrillation
Atenolol (Tenormin)	Tab: 25, 50, 100 mg	Atrial and ventricular arrhythmias, hypertrophic cardiomyopathy, hypertension	D: 0.25–1.0 mg/kg PO BID C: 6.25–12.5 mg PO SID	Less bronchoconstriction, vasoconstriction, and interference with insulin therapy than with nonselective beta blockers Taper dose when discontinue therapy Decrease dose with renal disease

Drug	How supplied	Indications	Dosage	Comments
Atropine sulfate*	Inj: 0.05, 0.1, 0.3, 0.4, 0.5, 0.8, 1.0 mg/ml	Sinus bradycardia, AV block, sick sinus syndrome, cardiac arrest	D: 0.01–0.04 mg/kg IV, IM, IO; 0.02–0.04 mg/kg SC TID–QID (IT: double dose); C: Same	May transiently worsen bradyarrhythmia; More potent chronotropic effects than glycopyrrolate
Benazepril (Lotensin)	Tab: 5, 10, 20, 40 mg	Balanced vasodilation in CHF, hypertension	D: 0.25–0.5 mg/kg PO SID; C: None	Monitor electrolytes and renal function; Excreted equally in bile and urine
Butorphanol tartrate (Torbutrol, Stadol)	Inj: ½, 1, 2 mg/ml; Tab: 1, 5, 10 mg (Torbutrol)	Nonproductive cough (COPD, tracheal collapse)	D: 0.055–0.11 mg/kg SC BID–QID; 0.55 mg/kg BID–QID PO; C: None	More potent cough suppressant than dextromethorphan
Captopril (Capoten)	Tab: 12.5, 25, 50, 100 mg	Balanced vasodilation in CHF, hypertension	D: 0.5–2.0 mg/kg PO TID (titrate up to effect); C: Same	Doses exceeding 2 mg/kg have caused renal failure; Monitor electrolytes and kidney function; Increased survival in heart failure patients; Decrease dose with renal disease
Carnitine* (Carnitor)	Tab: 330 mg; Can be purchased in bulk as powder	Canine dilated cardiomyopathy accompanied by carnitine deficiency	D: 2 Gr PO TID; C: None	L isomer is active form; Not effective in all cases
Chlorothiazide* (Diuril)	Tab: 250, 500 mg; Oral suspension: 50 mg/ml	Diseases associated with fluid retention (CHF, hepatic disease, nephrotic syndrome, hypertension)	D: 20–40 mg/kg PO BID; C: Same	Less potent than loop diuretics; Not effective with low GFR (renal failure); Can use with loop diuretics for increased diuresis; May precipitate hepatic encephalopathy in patients with severe liver disease
Dextromethorphan*	In many OTC cough formulas	Nonproductive cough (COPD, tracheal collapse)	D: 2 mg/kg PO TID–QID; C: Same	Only cough suppressant safe for use in cats

* Available in a generic preparation

(Continues)

CARDIOPULMONARY DRUGS (Continued)

Drug Trade Name	Formulation	Indications	Dog Dose (D) Cat Dose (C)	Comments
Diethylcarbamazine* (Caracide, Filaribits, Difil)	Tab: 30, 50, 90, 200, 300, 400 mg Chew-tab: 120, 180 mg Syrup: 60 mg/ml	Heartworm prevention	D: 6–7 mg/kg PO SID C: Same	Give daily starting 1 month prior to and continuing 1 month beyond mosquito season Do not start in microfilaremic animals (may cause shock) Can continue, if microfilaremia developed while on DEC
Digitoxin* (Crystodigin)	Tab: 0.05, 0.1 mg	Supraventricular arrhythmias, myocardial failure	D: 0.02–0.03 mg/kg PO TID C: None	GI side effects less common than with digoxin Dose based on total body weight Toxicity potentiated by hypokalemia, hyponatremia, hypercalcemia, thyroid disorders, hypoxia Preferred to digoxin in renal failure Use lower end of dose range in large dogs
Digoxin* (Cardoxin, Lanoxin)	Tab: 0.125, 0.25, 0.5 mg Inj: 0.25 mg/ml Elixir: 0.05 mg/ml, 0.15 mg/ml Cap: 0.05, 0.1, 0.2 mg	Supraventricular arrhythmias, myocardial failure	D: *Maintenance dose:* 0.22 mg/m² PO BID 0.0055–0.01 mg/kg PO BID See dosing chart (p. 517) *IV loading dose:* 0.02 mg/kg IV, $\frac{1}{4}$ q 1 hr to effect. Begin oral therapy 12 hours later *Oral loading dose:* Twice the maintenance dose for the first 24–48 hours C: 0.01 mg/kg PO QOD (Tab preferred) 0.007 mg/kg PO QOD (w/Lasix and aspirin)	Toxicity potentiated by hypokalemia, hyponatremia, hypercalcemia, thyroid disorders, hypoxia Dose on lean body weight, reduce dose 10%–15% with elixirs Therapeutic range 1–2.4 ng/ml; 8 hours after a dose Rapid digitalization not recommended except in emergency Reduce dose 50% with quinidine

Drug	Preparation	Indications	Dose	Comments
Diltiazem (Cardizem)	Tab: 30, 60, 90, 120 mg Inj: 5 mg/ml	Supraventricular arrhythmias, hypertrophic cardiomyopathy, hypertension	D: 0.5–1.5 mg/kg PO TID (titrate up to effect) C: 1.0–2.5 mg/kg PO TID	Less myocardial depression than verapamil
Dobutamine HCl (Dobutrex)	Inj: 12.5 mg/ml	Short-term management of severe myocardial failure	D: 2.5–20 µg/kg/min (titrate up to effect). Administer in D5W C: 1–10 µg/kg/min (titrate up to effect). Administer in D5W	Monitor ECG, BP, and pulse quality Preferable to dopamine in CHF, but more expensive Inotropic effect is dose dependent Less arrhythmigenic than most other catecholamines Intermittent use may cause sustained improvement Use with caution in cats
Dopamine HCl* (Intropin, Dopastat)	Inj: 40, 80, or 160 mg/ml	Shock, short-term management of severe myocardial failure	D: 2–20 µg/kg/min (titrate up to effect). Administer in D5W, saline, or LRS C: 2–10 µg/kg/min (titrate up to effect)	Monitor ECG, BP, and pulse quality May cause tissue necrosis if extravasation occurs Can administer intraosseously
Doxapram HCl (Dopram)	Inj: 20 mg/ml	Respiratory arrest or depression	D: 5–10 mg/kg IV C: Same	
Enalapril (Enacard)	Tab: 1, 2.5, 5, 10, 20 mg Inj: 1.25 mg enalaprilat per ml	Balanced vasodilation in CHF, hypertension	D: 0.5 mg/kg PO SID–BID (titrate up to effect) C: 0.25–0.5 mg/kg PO SID–QOD (titrate up to effect)	Fewer GI side effects and longer half life than captopril Monitor renal function and electrolytes Increased survival in heart failure patients Decrease dose with renal disease
Epinephrine* (Adrenalin)	Inj: 1:1000 conc (1 mg/ml) 1:10000 conc (0.1 mg/ml)	Cardiac arrest	D: 0.2 mg/kg IV, IO q 3–5 min Double dose for IT administration C: Same	Monitor with ECG Previously recommended dose of 0.02 mg/kg may be a safer starting dose if a defibrillator is not available

*Available in a generic preparation

(Continues)

509

CARDIOPULMONARY DRUGS (Continued)

Drug Trade Name	Formulation	Indications	Dog Dose (D) Cat Dose (C)	Comments
Furosemide* (Lasix)	Tab: 12.5, 20, 40, 50, 80 mg Inj: 10 and 50 mg/ml Oral solution: 10 mg/ml	Diseases associated with fluid retention (CHF, hepatic disease, nephrotic syndrome), hypertension	D: 2–4 mg/kg PO, IM, IV QOD–TID 2–8 mg/kg IV q 1–2 hr for severe pulmonary edema C: 1–4 mg/kg PO, IM, IV QOD–BID	Hypokalemia uncommon in dogs unless anorexic or high dose Decreased oral absorption in decompensated CHF Monitor hydration and electrolytes May precipitate hepatic encephalopathy in patients with severe liver disease Bioavailability reduced with food Titrate to lowest dose that controls edema
Glycopyrrolate* (Robinul)	Inj: 0.2 mg/ml	Sinus bradycardia, AV block, sick sinus syndrome	D: 0.005–0.01 mg/kg IV, IM, 0.01–0.02 mg/kg SC C: Same	Longer duration of action with less of a chronotropic effect than atropine
Heparin* (Liquaemin)	Inj: 1000, 5000, 10000 U/ml	Short-term prevention of thromboembolism	C: 220 units/kg IV followed in 3 hrs by 50–100 U/kg SC TID	Antidote: Protamine sulfate
Hydralazine HCl* (Apresoline)	Tab: 10, 25, 50, 100 mg Inj: 20 mg/ml	Arterial dilation in CHF, hypertension	D: 1–3 mg/kg PO BID (titrate up to effect) C: 0.5–0.8 mg/kg PO BID	Causes sodium retention, requiring increased diuretic doses Reflex tachycardia can be controlled with digitalis Decreasing dose 50%–75% for 1–2 weeks and then titrating upward may control vomiting Can use injectable formulation orally for more accurate dosing in small patients

Drug (Brand)	Formulations	Indications	Dosage	Comments
Hydrochlorothiazide* (Hydrodiuril)	Tab: 25, 50, 100 mg Solution: 10, 100 mg/ml	Diseases associated with fluid retention (CHF, hepatic disease, nephrotic syndrome), hypertension	D: 2–4 mg/kg PO BID C: 1–2 mg/kg PO BID	Less potent than loop diuretics Not effective with low GFR (renal failure) Can combine with loop diuretics for added diuresis May precipitate hepatic encephalopathy in patients with severe liver disease
Hydrocodone bitartrate* (Hycodan)	Tab: 5 mg Syrup: 1 mg/ml	Nonproductive cough (COPD, tracheal collapse)	D: 0.22 mg/kg PO SID–QID C: Do not use	More potent than dextromethorphan
Isopropamide iodide (Darbid)	Tab: 5 mg	Sinus bradycardia, AV block, sick sinus syndrome	D: 0.2–0.4 mg/kg PO BID–TID C: None	
Isoproterenol (Isuprel)	Inj: 1:5000 (0.2 mg/ml)	Short-term management of sinus bradycardia, AV block, sick sinus syndrome	D: 0.04–0.09 µg/kg/min IV (titrate up to effect) 0.1–0.2 mg q 4–6 hr IM, SC C: Same	
Isosorbide dinitrate* (Isordil)	Tab: 5, 10, 20, 30, 40 mg	Venodilation in CHF	D: 0.5–2.0 mg/kg PO BID–TID C: None	Can combine with hydralazine for balanced vasodilation Schedule 12-hour drug-free period to try and avoid tolerance
Ivermectin (Heartgard-30)	Tab: 68, 136, 272 µg	Heartworm prevention	D: Prevention: 0.006–0.012 mg/kg monthly (Heartgard-30) PO C: Prevention: 0.024 mg/kg monthly	Not approved for use in cats Not approved as microfilaricide Adverse reactions have been reported in some members of the collie breed at dosages of 100 µg/kg and higher
Lidocaine* (Xylocaine)	Inj: 5, 10, 15, 20 mg/ml (without epinephrine)	Ventricular arrhythmias	D: 2–8 mg/kg slowly IV or IO (double the dose IT) in 2 mg/kg boluses followed by IV drip at 25–75 (occasionally up to 100) µg/kg/min CRI C: 0.25–0.75 mg/kg IV over 5 min	Use with caution in cats Drug of choice for initial control of ventricular tachycardia Effects increased by high potassium and decreased by low potassium Seizures controlled with diazepam Do not use formulations with epinephrine for arrhythmia control

(Continues)

* Available in a generic preparation

511

CARDIOPULMONARY DRUGS (Continued)

Drug Trade Name	Formulation	Indications	Dog Dose (D) Cat Dose (C)	Comments
Marax	Combination bronchodilator in tablet and syrup formulations	COPD, asthma	D: 1 cc/5 kg PO BID–TID C: None	Contains ephedrine, theophylline, atarax Use with caution in cardiac patients Combination of bronchodilators may have additive effect
Metoprolol (Lopressor)	Tab: 50, 100 mg Inj: 1 mg/ml	Atrial and ventricular arrhythmias, hypertrophic cardiomyopathy, hypertension	D: 0.5–1.0 mg/kg PO TID C: Same	Less bronchoconstriction, vasoconstriction, and interference with insulin therapy than with nonselective beta blockers Taper dose when discontinue therapy
Mexiletine (Mexitil)	Cap: 150, 200, 250 mg	Ventricular arrhythmias	D: 5–8 mg/kg PO BID–TID C: None	Reduce dose with liver disease Take with food to reduce GI side effects
Milbemycin oxime (Interceptor)	Tab: 2.3, 5.75, 11.5, 23 mg	Heartworm prevention Control of adult hookworm infections	D: 0.5–1.0 mg/kg PO monthly C: 0.5 mg/kg monthly	Not approved as microfilaricide Check for microfilaria prior to instituting therapy Not approved for use in cats
Morphine sulfate*	Inj: 0.5, 1, 2, 4, 5, 8, 10, 15 mg/ml	Severe pulmonary edema for venodilator/sedative effects	D: 0.05–0.1 mg/kg IV q 2–3 min to effect 0.2–0.5 mg/kg IM, SC PRN C: Avoid	May raise intracranial pressure
Nitroglycerin* (Nitro-Bid, Nitrol)	2% ointment (1 inch = 15 mg)	Venodilation of CHF	D: 0.25 inch/5 kg cutaneously TID–QID C: $\frac{1}{8}-\frac{1}{4}$ inch cutaneously TID–QID	Can combine with hydralazine for balanced vasodilation Apply to ears if warm to touch, otherwise use shaved area in inguinal or axillary region (use gloves when applying) Schedule 12-hour drug-free period to try and avoid tolerance

Drug	Supplied	Indications	Dosage	Comments
Nitroprusside sodium* (Nipride, Nitropress)	Inj: 50 mg/vial	Short-term balanced vasodilation in severe CHF	D: 1–10 µg/kg/min in D5W C: Unknown	Adjust drip rate to maintain mean arterial pressure of ~70 mmHg Discontinue if metabolic acidosis develops Large dose may cause cyanide toxicity
Oxtriphylline* (Choledyl)	Tab: 100, 200 mg Tab SA: 400, 600 mg Syrup: 10 mg/ml	Asthma, COPD	D: 14 mg/kg PO TID–QID Choledyl SA 30 mg/kg PO BID C: 6 mg/kg PO BID–TID	Reduce dose with CHF, liver disease, cimetidine, erythromycin, propranolol Therapeutic range as theophylline: 10–20 µg/ml Dose on lean body weight
Phenytoin* (Dilantin)	Inj: 50 mg/ml Cap: 30, 100 mg	Arrhythmias due to digoxin toxicity	D: 2 mg/kg IV slowly (3–5 min) up to 10 mg/kg total dose 35 mg/kg PO TID–QID C: None	
Prazosin HCl (Minipress)	Cap: 1, 2, 5 mg	Balanced vasodilation in CHF, hypertension	D: 1 mg/15 kg PO TID Titrate to effect C: None	Tolerance develops
Procainamide* (Procan SR, Pronestyl)	Cap: 250, 375, 500 mg Tab: 250, 375, 500 mg Tab SR: 250, 500, 750, 1000 mg Inj: 100, 500 mg/ml	Ventricular and supraventricular arrhythmias, WPW	D: 8–20 mg/kg IM, PO QID (SR–TID) 2 mg/kg IV over 3–5 min up to total dose of 20 mg/kg 20–50 µg/kg/min CRI C: 3–8 mg/kg PO, IM TID–QID	Beware hypotension with IV administration Effects increased by high potassium and decreased by low potassium Monitor ECG: 25% prolongation of QRS is sign of toxicity Fewer GI and CV side effects than quinidine Use with caution in cats Reduce dose with severe renal and liver disease
Propantheline bromide* (Pro-Banthine)	Tab: 7.5, 15 mg	Sinus bradycardia, AV block, sick sinus syndrome	D: 1–2 mg/kg PO BID–TID C: 7.5 mg PO SID–TID	Sugar-coated tablets difficult to halve

* Available in a generic preparation

(Continues)

513

CARDIOPULMONARY DRUGS (Continued)

Drug Trade Name	Formulation	Indications	Dog Dose (D) Cat Dose (C)	Comments
Propranolol* (Inderal)	Tab: 10, 20, 40, 60, 80, 90 mg Inj: 1 mg/ml Solution: 4, 8, 80 mg/ml	Atrial and ventricular arrhythmias, hypertrophic cardiomyopathy, hypertension, thyrotoxicosis	D: 0.2–1.0 mg/kg PO TID 0.02–0.06 mg/kg IV over 5–10 minutes C: <4.5 kg: 2.5–5 mg PO BID–TID >4.5 kg: 5 mg PO BID–TID 0.02–0.06 mg/kg IV over 5–10 minutes	Nonselective β blocker Start with low dose and titrate to effect Taper dose when discontinue therapy Reduce dose with liver disease
Quinidine gluconate* (Quinaglute Dura-tabs) Quinidine polygalacturonate (Cardioquin) Quinidine sulfate* (Quinidex)	Tab: 324 mg Inj: 80 mg/ml Tab: 275 mg Tab: 100, 200, 300 mg Tab SR: 300 mg Cap: 200, 300 mg Inj: 200 mg/ml	Ventricular and supraventricular arrhythmias, WPW, conversion of atrial fibrillation	D: 6–20 mg/kg PO, IM QID 6–20 mg/kg PO TID with sustained release products 5–10 mg/kg IV (very slowly) C: None Note: Dose calculated for quinidine base equivalent, which varies with each quinidine salt See comment section	Decrease digoxin dose 50% when using quinidine Effects increased by high potassium and decreased by low potassium Monitor ECG: 25% prolongation of QRS is sign of toxicity Has vagolytic, negative inotropic, and vasodilating properties Hypotension is common with IV administration Reduce dose in CHF, hepatic disease, and hypoalbuminemia Quinidine base (%) in each quinidine salt: Quinidine sulfate (83%): 200 mg tab = 166 mg quinidine Quinidine gluconate (62%): 324 mg tab = 200 mg quinidine Quinidine polygalacturonate (60%): 275 mg tab = 166 mg quinidine
Spironolactone* (Aldactone)	Tab: 25, 50, 100 mg	Diseases associated with fluid retention (CHF, hepatic disease, nephrotic syndrome), hypertension, hypokalemia	D: 1–2 mg/kg PO BID C: Same	2–3 days to achieve peak effect Weak diuretic Usually combined with a loop diuretic

Drug	Supplied	Indication	Dose	Comments
Taurine* (Taurine V)	Tab: 250 mg Cap: 500 mg as generic	Dilated cardiomyopathy (cats)	D: 250–500 mg PO BID C: 250 mg PO BID	Clinical improvements noted in 4–10 days Echo improvement usually by 6 weeks Continue supplement for 12–16 weeks while correcting diet
Terbutaline (Brethine; Bricanyl)	Tab: 2.5, 5 mg Inj: 1 mg/ml	Asthma, COPD	D: 0.2 mg/kg PO BID–TID C: 0.1 mg/kg PO BID 0.05 mg/kg SC, IM, IV	Can be used in combination with xanthine bronchodilators β₂ Agonist Decrease dose with renal disease
Theophylline* (Theo-Dur)	Theo-Dur Tab: 100, 200, 300, 450 mg Cap: 50, 75, 125, 200 mg	Asthma, COPD	D: 9 mg/kg PO BID–TID Theo-Dur: 20 mg/kg PO BID C: 4 mg/kg PO BID–TID Theo-Dur: 25 mg/kg PO SID at night	Reduce dose with CHF, liver disease, cimetidine, erythromycin, propranolol Therapeutic range: 10–20 μg/ml Dose on lean body weight
Thiacetarsamide (Caparsolate)	Inj: 10 mg/ml	Heartworm adulticide	D: 2.2 mg/kg IV BID for 2 days Give paired daily injections at 6–8 hr intervals and limit overnight interval to 16 hrs or less C: Same	Feed 30–60 min prior to each treatment Check UA for bilirubin prior to each treatment Not always 100% effective, may need to retreat some cases Treat perivascular injections with topical DMSO TID–QID Stop treatment if icteric, persistent vomiting, or anorexic; retreat in 2–4 weeks
Tocainide (Tonocard)	Tab: 400, 600 mg	Ventricular arrhythmias	D: 10–20 mg/kg PO TID C: None	Oral analog of lidocaine Giving with food may decrease GI upset
Triamterene* (Dyrenium)	Cap 50, 100 mg	Diseases associated with fluid retention (CHF, hepatic disease, nephrotic syndrome), hypertension, hypokalemia	D: 1–2 mg/kg PO BID C: None	Weak diuretic Usually combined with a loop diuretic

*Available in a generic preparation

(Continues)

CARDIOPULMONARY DRUGS (*Continued*)

Drug Trade Name	Formulation	Indications	Dog Dose (D) Cat Dose (C)	Comments
Verapamil* (Calan, Isoptin)	Tab: 80, 120, 240 mg Inj: 2.5 mg/ml	Supraventricular arrhythmias, hypertrophic cardiomyopathy	D: 0.05–0.2 mg/kg slow IV (1–2 min) in boluses of 0.05 mg/kg given at 10–30 minute intervals (to effect) C: None	Diltiazem is a safer alternative in heart failure Potent vasodilator and negative inotrope
Warfarin (Coumadin)	Tab: 2, 2.5, 5, 7.5, 10 mg	Prevention of thromboembolism	D: 0.1–0.2 mg/kg PO SID C: Same	Initiate therapy with 4 days of heparin to prevent initial hypercoaguable state Control animal's lifestyle and environment to minimize risk of trauma Adjust dose to maintain PT at 1.5–2 times baseline value

* Available in a generic preparation

516

CARDOXIN LS DOSAGE TABLE—GUIDELINE[a] TO MAINTENANCE DOSAGE

Weight in Pounds	Milliliters (ml) of Cardoxin LS Every 12 Hours[b]	Milligrams (mg) of Cardoxin LS Every 12 Hours[b]
1	0.08	0.004
2	0.16	0.008
3	0.22	0.011
4	0.30	0.015
5	0.38	0.019
6	0.46	0.023
7	0.54	0.027
8	0.62	0.031
9	0.68	0.034
10	0.76	0.038

[a] Guideline refers to the approximate amount of the glycoside usually required by a dog for each maintenance therapy. The dosage is based on weight; 0.005 mg/lb × lean body weight (total body weight × 85%) − 10%, twice daily. Cardoxin should be used in place of Cardoxin LS for dogs over 20 lbs. The Cardoxin prescribing insert should be carefully reviewed for dosage information for dogs over 20 lbs. prior to administration.

[b] Requires twice daily administration preferably at 12-hour intervals.

(From Drug Insert, Evsco Pharm., Affiliate of IGI, Inc., Buena, New Jersey, with permission.)

CARDOXIN DOSAGE TABLE—GUIDELINE[a] TO MAINTENANCE DOSAGE

Total Body Weight (lbs)	Body Surface Area (m²)	Milliliters (ml) of Cardoxin Every 12 Hours[b]	Milligrams (mg) of Cardoxin Every 12 Hours[b]
5	—	0.13	0.019
10	—	0.25	0.038
15	—	0.38	0.057
20	—	0.51	0.076
25	0.502	0.66	0.099
30	0.566	0.75	0.112
35	0.627	0.83	0.124
40	0.685	0.91	0.136
45	0.740	0.97	0.146
50	0.794	1.05	0.157
Over 60	over 0.895	1.18	0.177
Over 100	over 1.254	1.65	0.248

[a] Guideline refers to the approximate amount of the glycoside usually required by a dog for daily maintenance therapy. From 0–20 pounds the dosage is based on weight; 0.005 mg/lb × lean body weight (total body weight × 85%) − 10%, twice daily. Above 20 lbs. the dosage is based on body surface area; 0.22 mg/m² − 10%, twice daily.

[b] Requires twice daily administration preferably at 12-hour intervals.

(From Drug Insert, Evsco Pharm., Affiliate of IGI, Inc., Buena, New Jersey, with permission.)

ABBREVIATIONS

Routes of	PO	Per os, oral
Administration	IM	Intramuscular
	IV	Intravenous
	SC	Subcutaneous
	IT	Intratracheal
	IO	Intraosseous
Dosage Schedules	QID	Four times daily; every 6 hours
	TID	Three times daily; every 8 hours
	BID	Twice daily; every 12 hours
	SID	Once daily; every 24 hours
	QOD	Once every other day; every 48 hours
	q	Every
	PRN	As needed
Formulations	Tab	Tablet
	Inj	Injectable solution
	Cap	Capsule
Miscellaneous	ACE	Angiotensin converting enzyme
	AV	Atrioventricular
	BP	Blood pressure
	CHF	Congestive heart failure
	CNS	Central nervous system
	COPD	Chronic obstructive pulmonary disease
	CRI	Constant rate infusion
	CV	Cardiovascular
	D5W	5% dextrose in water
	ECG	Electrocardiogram
	ECHO	Echocardiogram
	GFR	Glomerular filtration rate
	GI	Gastrointestinal
	HR	Heart rate
	ITP	Immune-mediated thrombocytopenia purpura
	LRS	Lactated Ringer's solution
	OTC	Over the counter
	NSAID	Nonsteroidal antiinflammatory drugs
	WPW	Wolff-Parkinson-White syndrome

CARDIOPULMONARY DRUGS

Drug	Side Effects	Contraindications	Precautions	Drug Interactions
Acetylsalicylic acid	Vomiting, diarrhea, anorexia, GI bleeding	Bleeding disorders, GI ulcers	Hepatic and renal disease	Steroids increase risk of GI ulcers May decrease vasodilation of ACE inhibitors Decreases effects of spironolactone Increases digoxin levels Increased risk of hemorrhage with heparin and warfarin
Albuterol	Muscle tremors, nervousness restlessness, insomnia, nausea, vomiting, anorexia, tachycardia	Tachyarrhythmias	Diabetes mellitus, hyperthyroidism	Mutual antagonism: β-blockers Decreases theophylline levels
Aminophylline	Tachyarrhythmias, tachypnea, restlessness, insomnia, vomiting, anorexia, seizures (rare)	Tachydysrhythmias, GI ulcers	CHF, liver disease, hyperthyroidism, diabetes mellitus	Levels increased by cimetidine, erythromycin, and propranolol
Amrinone	Tachycardia, hypotension, anorexia, vomiting	None	Renal and hepatic disease Hypertrophic cardiomyopathy	None reported
Atenolol	Hypotension, CHF, bradycardia, heart block, weakness, depression, bronchospasm, diarrhea	Heart block (2nd or 3rd degree), uncompensated CHF, shock	COPD, asthma, renal disease, compensated CHF, diabetes mellitus, peripheral claudication	Decreased bronchodilation: theophyllines Mutual inhibition: sympathomimetics Increased hypotension: vasodilators, anticholinergics Increased hypoglycemic effect: insulin Additive depression of contractility and conduction: verapamil, diltiazem
Atropine sulfate	Tachycardia, constipation, dry mucous membranes	Tachydysrhythmias, GI obstruction, closed angle glaucoma	CHF, COPD, renal disease, hyperthyroidism	Increases arrhythmic potential of epinephrine Antagonizes toxic effects of organophosphates

(Continues)

CARDIOPULMONARY DRUGS (*Continued*)

Drug	Side Effects	Contraindications	Precautions	Drug Interactions
Butorphanol tartrate	Lethargy, depression, anorexia, vomiting, constipation, respiratory depression	Productive cough	Respiratory depression, hepatic or renal disease, increased intracranial pressure	Effects increased with other CNS depressants Cimetidine: narcotic toxicity
Captopril	Hypotension, anorexia, vomiting, diarrhea, azotemia, hyperkalemia, proteinuria	Hypotension	Hyperkalemia, renal disease, collagen vascular diseases, COPD	Hypotension: diuretics, vasodilators, phenothiazines, quinidine, phenytoin, β blockers Hyperkalemia: potassium-sparing diuretics, potassium supplements NSAID may decrease antihypertensive effect
Carnitine	Diarrhea	None	None	None
Chlorothiazide	Hypovolemia, hypokalemia, metabolic alkalosis, vomiting, anorexia, lethargy	Renal failure, anuria	Renal or hepatic disease, hypokalemia, COPD, diabetes mellitus	Increased toxicity of digoxin if hypokelemia develops Hypokalemia: steroids
Dextromethorphan	Nausea	Productive cough		
Diethylcarbamazine	Vomiting, depression, shock in microfilaremic dogs	Microfilaremia		
Digitoxin	Arrhythmias, heart block, anorexia, vomiting, lethargy	Severe ventricular arrhythmias	Hepatic or thyroid disease, AV block, sick sinus syndrome, hypertrophic cardiomyopathy	Hypokalemia and hypomagnesemia (diuretics, steroids) potentiates toxicity Increased levels with spironolactone Levels decreased by anticonvulsants, phenylbutazone
Digoxin	Any arrhythmia, AV block, anorexia, vomiting, depression	Severe ventricular arrhythmias	Renal or thyroid disease, AV block, sick sinus syndrome, hypertrophic cardiomyopathy	Hypokalemia and hypomagnesemia (diuretics, steroids) potentiates toxicity Increased levels with quinidine, verapamil, amiodarone Levels may increase with spironolactone, diltiazem, triemterene, erythromycin, tetracycline, aspirin, prazosin

Diltiazem	Hypotension, sinus bradycardia, AV block, CHF, anorexia, fatigue	AV block (2nd or 3rd), hypotension, sick sinus syndrome	Increases effects of β blockers and digoxin on conduction Levels increased by cimetidine May increase digoxin levels
Dobutamine HCl	Tachyarrhythmias (high dose), vomiting, nervousness, seizures (cats)	Hypertrophic cardiomyopathy	Deceased effect with β blockers Incompatible with alkaline solutions
Dopamine HCl	Tachyarrhythmias and hypertension at high doses, vomiting	Tachyarrhythmias	Decreased effect with β blockers Incompatible with alkaline solutions
Doxapram HCl	Hyper or hypotension, seizures, bronchospasm, nausea	Seizure disorders, head trauma, severe cardiopulmonary disease, pulmonary embolism, pneumothorax	Cardiac arrhythmias: halothane, enflurane
Enalapril	Hypotension	Hyperkalemia, renal disease, COPD	Decreased vasodilation may occur with aspirin Hyperkalemia: potassium-sparing diuretics, potassium supplements Hypotension: diuretics, vasodilators, phenothiazines quinidine phenytoin, β blockers
Epinephrine	Tachydysrhythmias, tremors, restlessness, anorexia, vomiting	Cardiac disease, diabetes mellitus, hyperthyroidism	Halothane: increased potential for arrhythmias
Furosemide	Hypovolemia, electrolyte depletion, metabolic alkalosis, GI upset, weakness, lethargy, hyperglycemia	Dehydration, ascites, severe renal disease, diabetes mellitus, liver disease	Hypotension with vasodilators Increases ototoxicity and nephrotoxicity of aminoglycosides Hypokalemia potentiates digoxin toxicity Hypokalemia: steroids

(Continues)

CARDIOPULMONARY DRUGS (*Continued*)

Drug	Side Effects	Contraindications	Precautions	Drug Interactions
Glycopyrrolate	Tachycardia, constipation, dry mucous membranes	Closed angle glaucoma	Tachycardia, GI obstruction, hyperthyroid, CHF, COPD	
Heparin	Hemorrhage	Hemophilia, GI ulcers, ITP		Action decreased by digitalis, tetracyclines, antihistamines Action increased by oral anticoagulants, salicylates, dextrans, steroids, phenylbutazone
Hydralazine HCl	Hypotension, tachycardia, vomiting, anorexia		Advanced renal disease	Increased tachycardia with sympathomimetics
Hydrochlorothiazide	Hypovolemia, hypokalemia, metabolic alkalosis, hyperglycemia, vomiting, anorexia, lethargy	Renal failure	Renal or hepatic disease, diabetes mellitus, COPD, hypokalemia	Hypokalemia increases toxic potential of digoxin Hypokalemia: steroids
Hydrocodone bitartrate	Lethargy, depression, anorexia, vomiting, constipation, respiratory depression	Productive cough	Respiratory depression, increased intracranial pressure	Effects increased with other CNS depressants Cimetidine: narcotic toxicity
Isopropamide iodide	Tachycardia, constipation, dry mucous membranes, urine retention	GI or urinary obstruction Closed angle glaucoma	COPD	
Isoproterenol	Tachycardia, hypotension, vomiting, tremors	Tachyarrhythmias	Cardiac disorders, hyperthyroidism, diabetes mellitus	Effects antagonized by β blockers
Isosorbide dinitrate	Hypotension	Cerebral hemorrhage, increased intracranial pressure, severe anemia		Increased vasodilation with β blockers, diuretics, antihypertensives Decreased vasodilation with sympathomimetics
Ivermectin	Shock, listlessness, ataxia, vomiting, diarrhea, mydriasis			

Drug	Adverse effects/toxicity	Contraindications	Precautions	Drug interactions
Lidocaine	Proarrhythmia, hypotension (rapid IV), AV block, sinus bradycardia, tremors, ataxia, seizures, vomiting, drowsiness, nystagmus, respiratory arrest	Severe heart block, sick sinus syndrome	Liver disease, CHF, respiratory depression	Blood levels increased by cimetidine and β blockers Synergysm with other class 1 agents and β blockers Decreased effects with barbiturates
Marax	Tachycardia, tremors, vomiting, anorexia, diarrhea	Tachydysrhythmias	CHF	
Metoprolol	Hypotension, CHF, bradycardia, heart block, peripheral vasoconstriction, weakness, depression, bronchospasm, diarrhea	Heart block (2nd or 3rd degree), uncompensated CHF, shock	COPD, asthma, renal disease, peripheral vascular disease, compensated CHF, diabetes mellitus	Decreased bronchodilation of theophyllines Mutual inhibition: sympathomimetics Increased hypotension: vasodilators, anticholinergics Increased hypoglycemic effect of insulin Decreases lidocaine metabolism
Mexiletine	Proarrhythmia, AV block, sinus bradycardia, tremors, ataxia, vomiting, drowsiness	Severe heart block, sick sinus syndrome	Liver disease, CHF, epilepsy	Blood levels variably affected by cimetidine Synergysm with other class 1 agents and β blockers Decreased effects with barbiturates Increased theophylline levels Possible proarrhythmia with theophylline
Milbemycin	Intestinal hyperperistalsis, mild transient hypersensitivity reactions in microfilaremic animals (weakness, pale mucous membranes, dyspnea), caval syndrome		Microfilaremia	
Morphine sulfate	Respiratory and CNS depression, vomiting, constipation	Neurogenic edema, head trauma with increased intracranial pressure	Respiratory depression, Hepatic or renal disease	Excessive sedation with other CNS depressants Cimetidine: narcotic toxicity

(Continues)

CARDIOPULMONARY DRUGS (*Continued*)

Drug	Side Effects	Contraindications	Precautions	Drug Interactions
Nitroglycerin	Hypotension, rash at site of application	Cerebral hemorrhage Increased intracranial pressure, severe anemia		Increased vasodilation with β blockers, diuretics, antihypertensives Decreased vasodilation with sympathomimetics
Nitroprusside sodium	Hypotension, cyanide toxicity (dyspnea, vomiting, ataxia)		Hepatic or renal disease	Severe hypotension with inhalant anesthetics, circulatory depressants
Oxtriphylline	Tachycardia, tachypnea, restlessness, insomnia, vomiting, anorexia, seizures (rare)	Tachydysrhythmias, GI ulcers	CHF, liver disease, hyperthyroidism, diabetes mellitus	Levels increased by cimetidine, erythromycin, and propranolol
Phenytoin	IV administration: hypotension, cardiac depression, cardiac and respiratory arrest. Depression, ataxia, nystagmus, hepatopathy, seizures, nausea	Severe heart block, sick sinus syndrome	Hepatic disease, CHF	Activates hepatic microsomal enzymes Levels increased by chloramphenicol, cimetidine, phenylbutazone, sulfonamides and trimethoprim
Prazosin HCl	Hypotension, tachycardia, lethargy, nausea			Increased hypotension: β blockers, nitroglycerin
Procainamide	Hypotension (IV), CHF, proarrhythmia, prolongation of PR, QRS, QT intervals, AV block, negative inotropism, anorexia, vomiting, diarrhea, SLE (rare)	Severe heart block, sick sinus syndrome	Renal disease, CHF	Decreased effects with barbiturates Increased effects with propranolol, quinidine Increased serum levels with cimetidine, possibly trimethoprim
Propantheline bromide	Tachycardia, dry mucous membranes, constipation	Narrow angle glaucoma GI obstruction or paralytic ileus	COPD, CHF, ulcerative colitis, hepatic or renal disease	

Drug	Adverse effects	Contraindications	Cautions	Drug interactions
Propranolol	Bradycardia, AV block, hypotension, CHF, negative inotropism, depression, bronchoconstriction, peripheral vasoconstriction, GI disturbances	Asthma, advanced heart block, uncompensated CHF, sinus bradycardia, shock, peripheral claudication	Diabetes mellitus, hepatic disease, COPD, CHF	AV block: digoxin, calcium entry blockers, class 1A antiarrhythmics; Decreased effects with sympathomimetics, xanthines, NSAID, barbiturates; Increased blood levels with cimetidine; Decreased contractility with calcium entry blockers; Increases lidocaine levels
Quinidine	Hypotension, CHF, negative inotropism, proarrhythmia, AV block, sinus bradycardia, prolongation of PR, QRS, QT intervals, increase HR in atrial fibrillation, nausea, vomiting, diarrhea, depression	Advanced heart block, sick sinus syndrome	Liver disease, CHF, hyperkalemia	Increases blood levels of digoxin; Increased effects with β blockers; Decreased levels with barbiturates, phenytoin; Increased blood levels with cimetidine; Possible bleeding with aspirin
Spironolactone	Hypovolemia, hyperkalemia, diarrhea	Anuria, hyperkalemia, severe renal disease	Dehydration; Hepatic disease	Hyperkalemia with ACE inhibitors and potassium supplements; Increases digoxin levels
Taurine	None	None	None	None
Terbutaline	Tachycardia, tremors, restlessness, vomiting, nausea	Narrow angle glaucoma	Cardiac disease, diabetes mellitus, hyperthyroidism, renal disease	Mutual antagonism: β blockers; Decreases theophylline levels
Theophylline	Tachycardia, restlessness, insomnia, seizures, anorexia, vomiting, diarrhea	Tachydysrhythmias	CHF, liver disease, hyperthyroidism, diabetes mellitus	Levels increased by cimetidine erythromycin, and propranolol
Thiacetarsamide	Skin slough if perivascular injection, anorexia, vomiting, icterus, nephrotoxicity		Hepatic or renal disease	Steroids during and following administration decreases effectiveness
Tocainide	AV block, sinus bradycardia, proarrhythmia, nausea, vomiting, anorexia, ataxia	Advanced heart block, sick sinus syndrome	Hepatic disease, CHF, epilepsy	

(Continues)

CARDIOPULMONARY DRUGS (*Continued*)

Drug	Side Effects	Contraindications	Precautions	Drug Interactions
Triamterene	Hypovolemia, nausea, vomiting, anorexia, hyperkalemia	Severe hepatic or renal disease, hyperkalemia	Dehydration, hepatic or renal disease	Increases digitalis levels Hyperkalemia with ACE inhibitors and potassium supplements
Verapamil	Bradycardia, AV block, hypotension, CHF, fatigue	Advanced AV block, sick sinus syndrome, cardiogenic shock	Hypotension, β blockers, hepatic disease, CHF	Increases digoxin and theophylline levels Negative chronotropic and inotropic effects increased by β blockers Vasodilation increased by antihypertensives
Warfarin	Hemorrhage	Bleeding disorders, thrombocytopenia	CHF, hepatic and renal failure and thyrotoxicosis enhance anticoagulant effect	Increase anticoagulant effect: phenylbutazone, salicylates, sulfonamides, chloramphenicol, cimetidine, metronidazole, erythromycin, ketoconazole, propranolol, ranitidine, thyroid drugs.

Index

Page numbers followed by f indicate figures; those followed by t indicate tables.